Healthful Eating As Lifestyle (HEAL)

Integrative Prevention for Non-Communicable Diseases

Healthful Eating As Lifestyle (HEAL)

Integrative Prevention for Non-Communicable Diseases

Edited by
Shirin Anil

WITHDRAWN

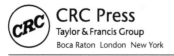

CRC Press
Taylor & Francis Group
Boca Raton London New York

CRC Press is an imprint of the
Taylor & Francis Group, an **informa** business

CRC Press
Taylor & Francis Group
6000 Broken Sound Parkway NW, Suite 300
Boca Raton, FL 33487-2742

Printed on acid-free paper
Version Date: 20161108

International Standard Book Number-13: 978-1-4987-4868-1 (paperback)

Library of Congress Cataloging-in-Publication Data

Names: Anil, Shirin, editor.
Title: Healthful eating as lifestyle (HEAL) : integrative prevention for
non-communicable diseases / edited by Shirin Anil.
Other titles: HEAL
Description: Boca Raton : CRC Press, 2016. | Includes bibliographical
references and index.
Identifiers: LCCN 2016028349| ISBN 9781498748681 (hardback : alk. paper) |
ISBN 9781315368511 (ebook)
Subjects: | MESH: Diet Therapy | Chronic Disease--prevention & control |
Attitude to Health | Life Style
Classification: LCC RM216 | NLM WB 400 | DDC 615.8/54--dc23
LC record available at https://lccn.loc.gov/2016028349

Visit the Taylor & Francis Web site at
http://www.taylorandfrancis.com

and the CRC Press Web site at
http://www.crcpress.com

Printed and bound in the United States of America
by Edwards Brothers Malloy on sustainably sourced paper

Dedicated to His Highness Prince Karim Aga Khan—the founder and chairman of the Aga Khan Development Network, my idol and inspiration to bring about a positive change and improve the quality of lives for all humans. This is my humble contribution, like a star in the galaxy of your work impacting the lives of millions.

Contents

Editor

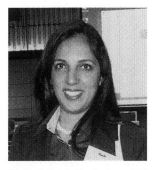

Shirin Anil, MBBS, MSc, is a medical doctor, an epidemiologist and biostatistician, and an Endeavour Executive Fellow in nutritional epidemiology, with extensive experience in the fields of global health, nutrition, non-communicable diseases (NCDs), infectious diseases, and mother and child health in developed and developing countries. She has conducted and presented more than 50 research projects in Australia, the United States, the United Kingdom, Spain, France, China, Pakistan, Malaysia, Saudi Arabia, and the United Arab Emirates, with publications in peer-reviewed journals including *Lancet*, *BMC Gastroenterology*, *BMC Pregnancy and Childbirth*, the *British Journal of Surgery*, *Frontiers of Medicine*, *Global Health Action*, and the *Journal of Human Hypertension*. Her major projects include project LIFE (Lifestyle Interventions For Eradication of NCDs), a community-led intervention for the control of diabetes, obesity, hypertension, and hypercholesterolemia, dietary patterns associated with high blood pressure, smoking in the general population, preventive medicine education for chronic diseases, complementary and alternative medicine in cancer patients, the association of artificial night light and cancer in 158 countries globally, factors associated with nonalcoholic fatty liver disease, hepatocellular cancer, nutrition in celiac disease in children, randomized control trials for the early screening and management of diabetes, hypertension, chronic respiratory diseases, and early childhood development interventions in primary health-care settings.

Dr. Anil manages the Victorian Congenital Anomalies Register, with more than 3,000 notifications of congenital anomalies in over 75,000 births per year at the Department of Health and Human Services in Victoria, Australia. She is a consulting epidemiologist and statistician at the Association for Social Development, Pakistan. In an honorary capacity, she serves on the True Health Initiative Council, a coalition of more than 250 global health experts from 30 countries, and also as the team leader for NCD prevention and control at the Aga Khan Development Network (a community health team) in Australia and the UAE. Dr. Anil is also a reviewer of many journals, including the *Journal of the American College of Nutrition*, *SAGE Open Medicine*, the *Saudi Journal of Gastroenterology*, the *Journal of Patient Safety*, and the *Journal of Royal Society of Medicine*. She is on the editorial board of *MOJ Public Health*, and was an advisor to the editorial board for the *International Journal of Medical Students* and a regional advisor for *Lancet Student*.

Contributors

Muna Ibrahim Atalla Al Baloushi
Department of Nutrition and Health
College of Food and Agriculture
United Arab Emirates University
Al Ain, UAE

Ayesha Salem Al Dhaheri
Department of Nutrition and Health
College of Food and Agriculture
United Arab Emirates University
Al Ain, UAE

Redhwan Al Naggar
Faculty of Medicine
Universiti Teknologi MARA (UiTM)
Shah Alam, Malaysia

Ranjit Mohan Anjana
Madras Diabetes Research Foundation
Chennai, India

Alvaro Avezum
Research Division
Dante Pazzanese Institute of Cardiology
São Paulo, Brazil

Ioanna Bakogianni
Department of Food Science and
   Human Nutrition
Agricultural University of Athens
Athens, Greece

David Benton
Department of Psychology
Swansea University
Swansea, Wales, United Kingdom

Karen M. Davison
School of Nursing
University of British Columbia
Vancouver, Canada

Zhizhong Dong
COFCO Nutrition and Health Research
   Institute
Beijing, China

Sara Habib
Aga Khan University
Karachi, Pakistan

Ann S. Hatcher
Center for Addiction Studies
Department of Human Services
Metropolitan State University–Denver
Denver, Colorado

Romaina Iqbal
Aga Khan University
Department of Community Health
   Sciences
Karachi, Pakistan

Leila Cheikh Ismail
Nuffield Department of Obstetrics and
   Gynaecology
University of Oxford
Oxford, United Kingdom

Zaid Kajani
Columbia University
New York, New York

Dimitra Karageorgou
Department of Food Science and
   Human Nutrition
Agricultural University of Athens
Athens, Greece

Bart Kay
School of Allied Health Sciences
de Montfort University
Leicester, United Kingdom

Claudia Stefani Marcilio
Research Division
Dante Pazzanese Institute of Cardiology
São Paulo, Brazil

Antonio Cordeiro Mattos
Research Division
Dante Pazzanese Institute of
 Cardiology
São Paulo, Brazil

Gustavo B.F. Oliveira
Research Division
Dante Pazzanese Institute of
 Cardiology
São Paulo, Brazil

Rajendra Pradeepa
Madras Diabetes Research
 Foundation
Chennai, India

Unnikrishnan Ranjit
Madras Diabetes Research
 Foundation
Chennai, India

Vaidya Ruchi
Madras Diabetes Research
 Foundation
Chennai, India

Vasudevan Sudha
Madras Diabetes Research
 Foundation
Chennai, India

Sivakumar Sudhakaran
Texas A&M University Health Science
 Center
Houston Methodist Hospital
Houston, Texas

Salim Surani
Texas A&M University
Houston, USA & University of North
 Texas
Houston, Texas

Saman Tahir
Department of Community Health
 Sciences
Aga Khan University
Karachi, Pakistan

Chunling Wang
COFCO Nutrition and Health Research
 Institute
Beijing, China

Zhe Yi
COFCO Nutrition and Health Research
 Institute
Beijing, China

Jian Ying
COFCO Nutrition and Health Research
 Institute
Beijing, China

Antonis Zampelas
Department of Food Science and
 Human Nutrition
Agricultural University of Athens
Athens, Greece
and
Department of Nutrition and Health
College of Food and Agriculture
United Arab Emirates University
Al Ain, UAE

Geng Zhang
COFCO Nutrition and Health Research
 Institute
Beijing, China

1 HEAL for Non-Communicable Diseases

Shirin Anil

CONTENTS

1.1 NON-COMMUNICABLE DISEASES: GLOBAL HEALTH CHALLENGE

Non-communicable diseases (NCDs)—diseases that are chronic in nature, slow in progression, cannot be transmitted from one person to another, yet can be inherited—are a global public health challenge. NCDs caused 38 million (68%) of 56 million deaths worldwide in 2012, of which 28 million (approximately three-quarters) occurred in lower- and middle-income countries, and 16 million (more than 40%) premature deaths—that is, the death of people less than 70 years of age (World Health Organization [WHO] 2014). Four major diseases that account for 82% of NCD deaths are (1) cardiovascular disease (CVD) (e.g., heart disease and stroke; 17.5 million deaths), (2) cancer (8.2 million deaths), (3) chronic respiratory diseases (e.g., asthma and chronic obstructive pulmonary disease [COPD]; 4 million deaths), and (4) diabetes (1.5 million deaths) (WHO 2014). If the same trend continues, CVD deaths are expected to rise to 23.3 million and cancer deaths to 11.5 million in the year 2030 (Mathers and Loncar 2006).

In addition to mortality, NCDs are responsible for worldwide morbidity. Global disability-adjusted life years (DALYs) due to NCDs increased from 43% in 1990 to 54% in 2010. Ischemic heart disease is the leading cause of DALYs, showing a 29% increase in 10 years, and stroke is the fifth leading cause, claiming 19% more DALYs in 2010 compared with that in 1990 (Murray et al. 2013).

NCDs are a threat to economic and human development. The economic growth rate is expected to decrease by half a percent for every 10% rise in NCD mortality in the working-age population (Stuckler 2008). It has been estimated that heart disease, stroke, and diabetes have led to an economic loss of USD 84 billion in the 23 lower- and middle-income countries with a high burden of NCDs from 2006 to 2015, spanning a duration of 10 years alone (Abegunde et al. 2007). If this goes unchecked without any interventions to decrease the burden of NCDs, it will not only widen the economic gap between developing and developed countries, but will also hamper the achievement of the Millennium Development Goals (MDGs) (Beaglehole et al. 2011a).

1.2 PREVENTION OF NON-COMMUNICABLE DISEASES

NCDs can be prevented by controlling their risk factors. These diseases can be attributed to four major risk factors: unhealthy diet, insufficient physical activity, smoking, and alcohol consumption, which contribute to the development of metabolic risk factors such as high blood pressure, obesity, high blood lipids, and high glucose level (Beaglehole et al. 2011b; Wagner and Brath 2012). People with ≥3 of these risk factors (abdominal obesity [>40 in. in males, >35 in. in females]; fasting glucose ≥100 mg/dl or on pharmacological treatment [Rx]; triglycerides ≥150 mg/dl or on Rx; HDL cholesterol <40 mg/dl in males or <30 mg/dl in females or on Rx; systolic blood pressure >130 mm Hg or diastolic blood pressure >85 mm Hg or on Rx) are labeled as having metabolic syndrome (MetS), according to the National Cholesterol Education Program's Adult Treatment Panel III (ATP III) (Grundy et al. 2005).

These risk factors interact with each other to impact morbidity or mortality due to NCDs. Meta-analysis of 87 studies with 951,083 participants showed that MetS increases the risk of CVD twofold (relative risk [RR] 2.35; 95% confidence interval [CI] 2.02–2.73), CVD mortality (RR 2.40; 95% CI 1.87–3.08), all-cause mortality (RR 1.58; 95% CI 1.39–1.78), stroke (RR 2.27; 95% CI 1.80–2.85), and myocardial infarction (RR 1.99; 95% CI 1.61–2.46) (Mottillo et al. 2010).

When the individual effects of the risk factors are added together, the attributable risk of a disease in the population (population attributable fraction [PAF]) may account for more than 100%, but their combined effect is less than the individual effect added together, as these risk factors overlap in disease causation (Danaei et al. 2005; WHO 2009). For example, the PAFs of smoking and unsafe sex for cervical cancer uteri are 2% and 100%, respectively, but their combined PAF is 100%, as the cancer patient may have the presence of both the risk factors, which leads to disease causation (Danaei et al. 2005). The interrelation of the risk factors also means that various interventions can be used for disease prevention depending on the resources available (Danaei et al. 2005). The intervention emphasized in this book is "healthful eating," the impact of which will be discussed on the prevention and control of NCDs as well as the risk factors mentioned previously.

1.3 HEALTHFUL EATING AS LIFESTYLE (HEAL)

Healthful eating can be described as choosing food that makes a person healthy. "Healthful" here refers to something that "creates good health," while "Healthy" refers to someone or something that "enjoys good health." The WHO defines health as a "state of complete physical, mental and social well being, and not merely the absence of disease or infirmity" (1948).

People perceive healthful eating as the consumption of fruits and vegetables and meat; less intake of sugar, salt, and fat; and a fresh, unprocessed, homemade, natural, balanced diet composed of a variety of foods in moderation (Paquette 2005). It is important to make healthful eating a lifestyle throughout the life course to enjoy good health and prevent NCDs (Figure 1.1).

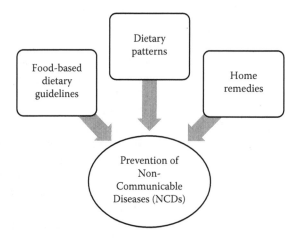

FIGURE 1.1 Healthful eating approaches for the prevention of non-communicable diseases.

1.4   DIETARY GUIDELINES

Food-based dietary guidelines (FBDGs) are defined as "simple messages on healthy eating, aimed at the general public. They give an indication of what a person should be eating in terms of foods rather than nutrients, and provide a basic framework to use when planning meals or daily menus" (European Food Information Council 2009). WHO emphasizes that FBDGs should be food based rather than nutrient based as people enjoy eating food, not nutrients. FBDGs should account for dietary patterns and the prevalence of deficiency disorders and NCDs (WHO 2003b).

WHO has given dietary recommendations for the prevention of NCDs (WHO 2015c). Many countries have developed their FBDGs specifically to their national context: for example, Dietary Guidelines for Americans (DGA) in the United States (U.S. Department of Health and Human Services 2015), Eating Well with Canada's Food Guide (Health Canada 2011a), the Eatwell Guide in the United Kingdom (NHS Choices 2016), and the Eat for Health Australian Dietary Guidelines (NHMRC 2013a). All these dietary guidelines have a primary focus of maintaining a balanced diet and healthy weight and preventing NCDs. The salient features of these guidelines are as follows.

1.4.1   WHO's Dietary Recommendations

Though FBDGs vary in different parts of the world, WHO has given the following guidelines for healthful eating to prevent and control NCDs *in adults* (WHO 2015c):

- The consumption of fruits and vegetables (at least 400 g—5 portions a day, excluding starchy roots such as potatoes, sweet potatoes, and cassava) (WHO 2003a), legumes (e.g., lentils and beans), whole grains (e.g., brown rice, millet, oats, and unprocessed maize), and nuts is recommended.
- Sugar intake should be less than 10% of total energy (approximately 50 g or 12 teaspoons for a person with healthy body weight requiring 2000 cal/day) (WHO 2003a, 2015b) and less than 5% for additional health benefits (WHO 2015b). It should be taken into consideration that sugars are naturally present in fruits, fruit juice and fruit concentrates, honey, and added by manufacturers in many packaged foods and drinks.
- Fat intake should be less than 30% of total energy (WHO 2003a; Food and Agricultural Organization 2010; Hooper et al. 2012). Saturated fats (e.g., those present in butter, coconut and palm oil, cream, cheese, ghee and lard, and fatty meat) should be avoided, and unsaturated fats (e.g., those present in avocado, nuts, canola, olive and sunflower oils, and fish) should be preferred. Trans fats (e.g., those present in processed foods, snacks, fast foods, fried food, pies, cookies, frozen pizza, margarines, and spreads) do not form a part of healthful eating.

- Salt should be restricted to 5 g/day (approximately 1 teaspoon) and iodized salt used (WHO 2012).

WHO gives a similar guideline for healthful eating *in children* to that in adults, with the following additions:

- Exclusive breast-feeding should be done in the first 6 months of life.
- Breast-feeding should continue in children up to 2 years of age and beyond.
- Breast milk should be complemented by a variety of safe and healthy foods from 6 months of age onward. Do not add salt or sugar to the complementary foods given to infants and children.

1.4.2 DIETARY GUIDELINES FOR AMERICANS

DGA is released by the secretaries of the U.S. Department of Health and Human Services (HHS) and the U.S. Department of Agriculture (USDA) every 5 years, the first edition being published in the year 1980 and the eighth in 2015. It is based on the latest/current scientific evidence and is for children and adults aged 2 years and older, including those who are at risk of developing NCDs. DGA will cover all age groups, including children less than 2 years, from the year 2020. Five major guidelines of DGA 2015–2020 (U.S. Department of Health and Human Services and U.S. Department of Agriculture 2015) are

- A healthy eating pattern consisting of appropriate calorie levels in order to maintain healthy weight supporting nutrient adequacy should be followed throughout the lifespan.
- Consume nutrient-dense foods and beverages: fruits, fruit juices, vegetables, whole grains, seafood, and fat-free and low-fat milk and milk products.
- Foods containing sodium (salt), saturated fats, trans fats, cholesterol, added sugars, and refined grains should be restricted in the diet.
- Choose healthier foods and beverages.
- Support others to have healthy eating patterns.

Table 1.1 shows the foods to decrease and increase according to DGA 2015.

1.4.3 EATING WELL WITH CANADA'S FOOD GUIDE

Eating Well with Canada's Food Guide gives recommendations for the number of servings of four groups of foods—namely, "vegetable and fruits," "grain products," "milk and alternatives," and "meat and alternatives"—to be consumed by different age groups starting from 2 years of age in males and females, separately (Health Canada 2011a). By following these recommendations, one can meet his/her requirement of vitamins, minerals, and other nutrients, reduce the risk of obesity, heart disease, type 2 diabetes, certain types of cancers, and osteoporosis, and lead a healthy

TABLE 1.1

Foods to Be Reduced and Increased in Consumption According to the Dietary Guidelines for Americans (2010)

Reduce Consumption of	Increase Consumption of
• *Salt*: Less than 2300 mg, further reduction to 1500 mg in people aged >51 years and in those of any age with hypertension, diabetes, or chronic kidney disease, or who are African Americans • *Saturated fatty acids*: Restrict to less than 10% of total calorie intake by saturated fatty acids; replace with poly- and monounsaturated fatty acids • *Cholesterol*: Less than 300 mg/day • *Trans fats* • *Sugars:* Less than 10% calories per day from added sugars • *Refined grains* • *Alcohol*: Restrict to one drink per day for women, two drinks per day for men of legal drinking age	• *Fruits* • *Vegetables*: Especially dark green, red, and orange vegetables; beans, and peas • *Whole grains*: Replace refined grains with whole grains • *Low-fat and fat-free milk and milk products* • *Proteins*: Seafood, lean meat and poultry, eggs, beans, peas, soy products, and unsalted nuts and seeds; replace protein foods containing solid fats with those containing lower solid fats and/or which are sources of oils • *Oil* to replace solid fats • Foods containing *potassium, dietary fiber, calcium, and vitamin D*

Source: USDA and U.S. HHS, *Dietary Guidelines for Americans*, Washington, DC, 2015.

life (Health Canada 2011a). Canada's Food Guide gives the following basic recommendations (Health Canada 2011b):

- At least one dark green and one orange vegetable to be consumed every day.
- Fruits and vegetables should be chosen such that they have little or no added sugar, salt, and fat.
- Fruits and vegetables should be preferred to juices.
- Half of the grain products should be whole grains.
- Consume grain products low in salt, sugar and fats.
- Consume 1% or 2% skim milk every day.
- Lower-fat alternative milk products should be preferred.
- Meat alternatives such as beans, tofu and lentils should be consumed more.
- At least 2 food guide servings of fish to be consumed every week.
- Lean meat and its alternatives should be cooked with less or no added salt and fats.
- Unsaturated fats should be restricted to 30–45 mL (2–3 tbsp) each day. Vegetable oils should be used and butter, hard margarine, shortening and lard should be avoided.
- Drink plenty of water.

1.4.4 United Kingdom: The Eatwell Guide

The Eatwell Plate was developed by the Food Standards Agency and released in 2007, to guide people toward a balanced diet and healthful eating in the United Kingdom (Food Standards Agency 2007). The Eatwell Plate has now been replaced by the Eatwell Guide (NHS Choices 2016). It is a pictorial representation of *five food groups*—namely, "fruits and vegetables," "bread, rice, potatoes, pastas and other starchy foods," "meat, fish, eggs, beans and other nondairy sources of protein," "milk and dairy foods," and "foods and drinks high in fats and/or sugar"—in the proportions they should be consumed on a plate (Food Standards Agency 2007). It emphasizes the consumption of a diet low in energy-dense food and high in fruits and vegetables (Evans 2015). As a general rule, the meal should be comprised of one-third carbohydrates, one-third fruits and vegetables, and one-third dairy, non-dairy protein food, and only a little of fatty and sugary food. It applies to most people of all ethnic groups irrespective of their weight. As children less than 2 years have different nutritional needs, the Eatwell Plate is not applicable to them (Food Standards Agency 2007). The Eatwell Guide recommends the following:

- Fruits and vegetables—at least five portions a day. Limit fruit juices and smoothies to no more than 150 ml per day.
- Meals should be based on breads, rice, pasta, potatoes, or other starchy carbohydrates. Whole grains should be chosen where possible.
- Dairy or diary alternatives (soya drinks or yogurts) should be consumed, preference should be given to lower-fat and lower-sugar options.
- Beans, pulses, fish, eggs, meat, and other protein should be added to the diet. Consume at least two portions of fish per week, one of which should be oily fish such as salmon or mackerel.
- Fats—unsaturated oils and spreads should be chosen and should be consumed in small amounts.
- Saturated fats and sugars should be reduced in the diet.
- Plenty of fluids—consume at least 6–8 cups/glasses of fluid a day.

1.4.5 Australian Dietary Guidelines—Eat for Health

The Australian Dietary Guidelines aim at promoting health and well-being, reduce the risk of NCDs, and reduce the risk of diet-related conditions (NHMRC 2013a). These guidelines apply to healthy Australians of all age groups and also to those who are overweight. It does not apply to people with medical conditions requiring dietary adjustment, nor to the frail elderly. The *five guidelines* (NHMRC 2013b) outlined are

- Maintain a healthy weight. Consume calories according to individual need and burn calories through physical activity.
- Choose nutritious foods from the *five food groups* and plenty of water.
  - Vegetables and legumes/beans

- Fruits
- Grains, mostly whole grains with high fiber content such as bread, rice, pasta, oats, quinoa, noodles, and barley
- Lean meat and poultry, eggs, fish, and nuts and seeds
- Reduced-fat dairy such as milk, cheese, and yogurt
- Limit the consumption of saturated fats, added sugar, and salt. Low-fat diets should not be considered in children less than 2 years of age.
- Breast-feed infants; breast-feed exclusively for the first 6 months of life.
- Care for food; store and prepare it safely.

The Australian Dietary Guidelines explain the servings of the food groups to be consumed according to age and gender, and give examples of daily dietary patterns for healthful eating and well-being (NHMRC 2013b).

1.5 IMPACT OF FOOD-BASED DIETARY GUIDELINES ON NON-COMMUNICABLE DISEASES

Researchers have studied the impact of FBDGs on the prevention and control of NCDs. The association of the dietary guidelines outlined previously with NCDs is highlighted as follows.

1.5.1 WHO Dietary Guidelines and NCDs

The healthy diet indicator (HDI) is a measure based on WHO's dietary guidelines for the prevention of NCDs. HDI, which is used to assess adherence to the WHO dietary guidelines of 1990 (WHO 1990), was originally developed in 1997 (Huijbregts et al. 1997). Later, when WHO revised its guidelines (WHO 2003a), HDI was adapted accordingly (Berentzen et al. 2013; Stefler et al. 2014).

The Health, Alcohol and Psychosocial Factors in Eastern Europe (HAPIEE) cohort study measured the association of HDI with all-cause mortality and CVD specific to a sample of 18,559 Central and Eastern European populations, 45–69 years of age, without major NCDs at the baseline. HDI had a statistically significant inverse association with CVD mortality (hazard ratio [HR] 0.90, 95% CI 0.81–0.99) and mortality due to chronic heart disease (CHD) (HR 0.85, 95% CI 0.74–0.97), and a marginally significant association with all-cause mortality (HR 0.95, 95% CI 0.89–1.00) (Stefler et al. 2014). An analysis of 21,142 randomly selected adults in the HAPIEE study found that HDI was significantly inversely related to metabolic syndrome, defined by the ATP III criteria (Grundy et al. 2005), in the Czech Republic (odds ratio [OR] of MetS for a 10 unit rise in HDI score 0.91, 95% CI 0.83–1.00) and Poland (OR 0.92, 95% CI 0.85–0.99) (Huangfu et al. 2014).

A meta-analysis of 11 cohort studies with 396,391 participants, 60 years or older, from Europe and the United States showed that adherence to the WHO dietary recommendations can lead to longevity in both men and women: pooled adjusted HR was 0.90 (95% CI 0.87–0.93), 0.89 (95% CI 0.85–0.92), and 0.90 (95% CI 0.85–0.95) for both genders, males, and females, respectively. According to the authors, this translates to an increase in life expectancy by 2 years at the age of 60 (Jankovic et al. 2014).

A cross-sectional study of 433 Japanese males measured the association of HDI with untreated hypertension. It found that low adherence to the WHO dietary guidelines was statistically significantly associated to the high prevalence of untreated hypertension (OR 3.33, 95% 1.39–7.94), after adjusting for age, energy consumption, physical activity, smoking, alcohol drinking, and salt intake (Kanauchi and Kanauchi 2015).

The Dutch European Prospective Investigation into Cancer and Nutrition (EPIC-NL), with 35,355 males and females with a mean follow-up of 12.7 years, explored the relation of adherence to the WHO dietary guidelines with overall cancer incidence. It found no association of HDI with overall cancer (HR 0.96, 95% CI 0.89–1.03 in males; HR 1.00, 95% CI 0.96–1.04 in females), smoking-related cancer (HR 0.94, 95% CI 0.84–1.04 in males; HR 1.00, 95% CI 0.94–1.07 in females), nor with alcohol-related cancer (HR 1.02, 95% CI 0.87–1.20 in males; HR 1.03, 95% CI 0.98–1.08 in females) (Berentzen et al. 2013).

A British cohort of 33,731 females with a mean follow-up of 9 years could not find significant association between adherence to the WHO dietary guidelines as assessed by HDI and risk of breast cancer (Cade et al. 2011).

1.5.2 DIETARY GUIDELINES FOR AMERICANS AND NCDS

Two measures have been developed by researchers to assess diet quality and adherence to DGA. These are the Healthy Eating Index (HEI) (Guenther et al. 2008) and the Dietary Guidelines Adherence Index (DGAI) (Fogli-Cawley et al. 2006). These have been revised from time to time following revision of DGA (Guenther et al. 2013; Troy and Jacques 2012).

The Health Professionals Follow-Up Study (HPFS), a cohort of 51,529 U.S. male doctors aged 40–75 years, assessed the association of HEI, calculated from a validated food frequency questionnaire (HEI-f) measuring adherence to DGA 1995, with major chronic diseases (defined as incident CVD [stroke and myocardial infarction], cancer, and nontrauma-related deaths) in 38,622 participants with a mean follow-up of 8 years (McCullough et al. 2000a). HEI-f had inverse association that was marginally significant with major chronic diseases (RR 0.89, 95% CI 0.79–1.00) and statically significant with CVD (RR 0.72, 95% CI 0.60–0.88), while no significant association with cancer (RR 1.12, 95% CI 0.95–1.31) was observed (McCullough et al. 2000a).

The Nurses' Health Study in the United States, a cohort of 121,700 female nurses aged 30–55 years, analyzed the association of HEI-f to assess adherence to DGA 1995 with major chronic diseases (fatal or nonfatal CVD including stroke and myocardial infarction, cancer and nontraumatic deaths) in 67,272 females with a mean follow-up of 12 years (McCullough et al. 2000b). It found no association of HEI-f with major chronic diseases (RR 0.97, 95% CI 0.89–1.06), neither with CVD (RR 0.86, 95% CI 0.72–1.03) nor with cancer (RR 1.02, 95% CI 0.93–1.12) (McCullough et al. 2000b).

The third phase of the Tehran Lipid and Glucose Study in Iran randomly selected 2540 adults (1384 females and 1120 males) aged 19–70 years and measured their adherence to DGA 2005 with the help of DGAI 2005. It found that the people more adherent to DGA 2005 had a low prevalence of MetS risk factors and a significantly lower prevalence of hyperglycemia, hypertension, and low high-density lipoprotein (HDL) cholesterol (Hosseini-Esfahani et al. 2010).

The Framingham Heart Study Offspring Cohort measured the association of DGAI 2005 and MetS risk factors in 3177 adults. Participants more adherent to DGA 2005 had lower waist circumference, triacylglycerol concentration, diastolic and systolic blood pressure, abdominal adiposity, hyperglycemia, and a lower prevalence of MetS. These associations of DGA and MetS were more pronounced in those younger than 55 years of age (Fogli-Cawley et al. 2007).

The Estrogen Replacement and Atherosclerosis Study in the United States studied the association of adherence to DGA 2005 with atherosclerotic progression in 224 postmenopausal females with already established coronary artery disease (Imamura et al. 2009). DGAI in which each component was weighted pertaining to its relation to atherosclerotic progression (wDGAI) was found to be inversely associated to the narrowing of the coronary arteries (0.049 mm less narrowing with 1 standard deviation [SD] difference in wDGAI, standard error [SE] 0.017, p value 0.004), adjusting for age, study site, education, smoking, frequency of walking, energy intake, systolic blood pressure, glucose concentration, self-reported intake of cholesterol-lowering drugs, and self-reported chest pain (Imamura et al. 2009).

The Southern Community Cohort Study studied the association of HEI 2010 and HEI 2005 with all-cause and case-specific mortality in low-income populations from the Southeastern United States, including 50,434 African Americans, 24,054 white individuals, and 3,084 individuals from other racial/ethnic groups, 40–79 years of age, followed up for a mean duration of 6.2 years (Yu et al. 2015). The authors reported that a higher adherence to DGA 2010 was associated with lower risk of all-cause mortality (HR 0.80, 95% CI 0.73–0.86), CVD mortality (HR 0.81, 95% CI 0.70–0.94), cancer mortality (HR 0.81, 95% CI 0.69–0.95), and other disease mortality (HR 0.77, 95% CI, 0.67–0.88), comparing the highest quintile of the HEI 2010 score with the lowest. These significant inverse associations existed even after adjustment for age, gender, and income. HEI 2005 also depicted significant inverse association with all-cause mortality in this study population (Yu et al. 2015).

1.5.3 EAT WELL WITH CANADA'S FOOD GUIDE AND NCDs

Various measures are available to measure adherence to Canada's Food Guide, including the Canadian Healthy Eating Index (HEI-C or CHEI) (Nkondjock and Ghadirian 2007; Woodruff et al. 2008), adapted from the American HEI to suit to the dietary recommendations by Canada's Food Guide, and the Canada's Food Guide (CFG) index (Hajna et al. 2012).

A cross-sectional survey conducted in school settings in the Niagara region (Ontario, Canada) studied the association of adherence to Canada's Food Guide as measured by the CFG index and anthropometric measures in 1570 children (782 girls and 788 boys) with a mean age of 12.4 years (Hajna et al. 2012). The researchers found a significant inverse association of the CFG index with waist-to-height ratio (β −0·001, 95% CI −0·002, −0·0004), waist-to-hip ratio (β −0·001, 95% CI −0·002, −0·001), and waist girth (β −0·18, 95% CI −0·30, −0·07) in girls (Hajna et al. 2012). No significant association was observed in boys.

A case control study among 80 French Canadian families—with 250 people composed of 89 BRCA gene carriers who had breast cancer (cases), 48 BRCA gene carriers without breast cancer (control 1), and 46 participants not carrying the BRCA gene and not having breast cancer (control 2)—studied the association of adherence to Canada's Food Guide measured by CHEI with the risk of developing breast cancer. It showed a significant inverse relationship between CHEI and BRCA-associated breast cancer risk (OR 0.18, 95% CI 0.05–0.68, p value .006 for trend) when comparing the highest tertile of CHEI with the lowest tertile, controlling for age, physical activity, and total energy intake (Nkondjock and Ghadirian 2007).

The data from 33,664 respondents from the Canadian Community Health Survey—Nutrition showed that CHEI was significantly higher in nonsmokers compared with smokers, lower in people consuming alcohol, and had a statistically significant positive association with the level of physical activity (Garriguet 2009).

1.5.4 THE EATWELL GUIDE AND NCDs

Data on the association of adherence with the Eatwell Guide (previously Eatwell Plate) and NCDs and its risk factors is scarce. This may be due to the fact that very few people strictly adhere to the consumption of all the five food groups in the proportions recommended by the Eatwell Guide. An analysis of 807 adults aged 19–64 years, included in the National Diet and Nutrition Survey (NDNS) rolling program, showed that only 4% of them adhered to the five dietary targets of the Eatwell Guide, and with the exception of protein intake, 51% did not follow any of the recommendations (Harland et al. 2012). Those who achieved the targets for fats, saturated fatty acids, and fruits and vegetables intake (12%) were more likely to be nonsmokers (a significant difference); no statistically significant difference was observed in terms of waist circumference or body mass index (BMI) in this group compared with people who did not achieve these three targets (Harland et al. 2012).

While working out the cost of a healthy diet, using data from the UK Women's Cohort Study, researchers from the University of Leeds in the United Kingdom developed a healthiness index, an increasing score of which shows increased adherence to the food groups of the Eatwell Guide (Morris et al. 2014). The healthiness index score was positively associated with physical activity levels. It also showed a significant association with BMI: the lowest BMI with the vegetarian dietary pattern and the highest with the traditional meat, chips, and pudding dietary pattern (Morris et al. 2014).

1.5.5 AUSTRALIAN DIETARY GUIDELINES AND NCDs

Adherence to the Australian Dietary Guidelines in adults can be measured by a dietary guideline index (DGI), a higher value of which shows greater adherence (McNaughton et al. 2008). The Dietary Guideline Index for Children and Adolescents (DGI-CA) is a tool to measure adherence to the Australian Dietary Guidelines in children aged 4–16 years (Golley et al. 2011).

Data from the Australian National Nutritional Survey (ANNS) 1995, including 10,851 adults ≥19 years of age, was utilized to explore the association between adherence to the Australian Dietary Guidelines and health status, including blood pressure, smoking status, physical activity, and BMI (McNaughton et al. 2008). It found that DGI was positively associated to physical activity levels. Higher DGI scores were inversely related to systolic and diastolic blood pressure. There were more smokers and ex-smokers among adults with lower DGI scores than those with higher DGI scores.

The Australian National Children's Nutrition and Physical Activity Survey 2007, which included 3416 children and adolescents aged 4–16 years, studied the relationship of DGI-CA with anthropometric measures (Golley et al. 2011). Researchers observed a weak positive association between DGI-CA and BMI and waist circumference z-scores in children aged 4–10 years and 12–16 years.

Analyses of 7441 males and females aged ≥25 years who participated in the Australian Diabetes, Obesity and Lifestyle (AusDiab) study showed the association between DGI and NCDs (McNaughton et al. 2009). It was found that less adherence to the Australian Dietary Guidelines (low DGI scores) was positively associated with waist circumference in males. DGI scores were inversely related to systolic and diastolic blood pressure in males, systolic blood pressure in females, and total cholesterol, triglycerides, and fasting blood sugar level in both genders.

1.6 DIETARY PATTERNS TO PREVENT NON-COMMUNICABLE DISEASES

"Dietary pattern" refers to the pattern or combination in which nutrients or food groups are consumed. It represents a broader picture of food consumption. As nutrients interact with one another to complement or inhibit each other in the foods we eat, our dietary pattern is more predictive of the risk of NCDs (Hu 2002). Dietary patterns can be predefined, such as the summation of recommendations in the dietary guidelines mentioned previously or specific food models historically linked to health (e.g., the Mediterranean diet), or can be extracted from the population's eating behaviors by statistical techniques such as factor analysis, cluster analysis, and reduced rank regression (Tucker 2010). Two famous dietary patterns and their associations with NCDs are elaborated as follows.

1.6.1 MEDITERRANEAN DIET

The Mediterranean diet is characterized by an abundance of plant foods (vegetables, fruits, breads, cereals, beans, nuts, and seeds); olive oil; fresh fruits consumed as desserts; dairy products, principally yogurt and cheese; fish and poultry in moderate amounts; red meat in low amounts; zero to four eggs weekly; and wine in low-to-moderate amounts, normally with meals (Willett et al. 1995). The Mediterranean diet has been shown to reduce overall mortality, decrease the risk of CVD incidence and mortality, reduce cancer incidence and mortality, and reduce neurodegenerative diseases (Sofi et al. 2010). It also reduces the risk of stroke, depression, and cognitive impairment (Psaltopoulou et al. 2013).

1.6.2 DIETARY APPROACHES TO STOP HYPERTENSION (DASH)

The DASH diet is rich in fruits and juices, vegetables, grains, and low-fat dairy products; small amounts of meat, poultry and fish; nuts, seeds, and legumes; and very small amounts of sugar and snacks (Appel et al. 1997). The DASH diet plays a role in the reduction of systolic and diastolic blood pressure (Appel et al. 1997) and the reduction of the risk of CVD, chronic heart disease, stroke, and heart failure (Salehi-Abargouei et al. 2013). It has also been shown to reduce the risk of type 2 diabetes in whites (Liese et al. 2009).

1.7 HOME REMEDIES TO PREVENT NON-COMMUNICABLE DISEASES

Many home remedies have been suggested to prevent individual NCDs. Precaution should be taken due to safety concerns as food ingredients, like medicines, interact with each other to inhibit or exacerbate each other's effects and disease conditions. Also, NCDs tend to occur in clusters; for example, a person with type 2 diabetes may also have hypertension, and hence may not be able to use the remedy for one disease that might adversely affect the other. Evidence regarding home remedies is scarce and needs more rigorous research, taking safety concerns into consideration. Some scientifically proven remedies are as follows.

1.7.1 REMEDIES FOR DIABETES

The following foods/food ingredients have been shown to reduce blood sugar levels:

- *Cinnamon* has been found to have a modest lowering effect on blood sugar (Pham et al. 2007).
- *Ginger*, administered at 2 g/day for at least 12 weeks, has been shown to decrease fasting blood sugar and hemoglobin A1c levels compared with placebo in type 2 diabetes patients (Khandouzi et al. 2015).
- *Green tea extract* consisting of 544 mg of polyphenols (456 mg of catechins) taken daily for a duration of at least 2 months can reduce hemoglobin A1c levels in borderline diabetics aged 32–73 years (Fukino et al. 2008).
- *Bitter gourd*, also known as bitter melon or karla, has been shown to reduce blood sugar levels in rats without causing nephrotoxicity and hepatotoxicity (Virdi et al. 2003). In a concentration of at least 2000 mg/day for 4 weeks, it can reduce the levels of fructosamine in newly diagnosed type 2 diabetes patients compared with 1000 mg/day of metformin (Fuangchan et al. 2011).

1.7.2 REMEDIES FOR HYPERTENSION

The following food/food ingredients have been reported to reduce blood pressure levels:

- *Garlic*: A meta-analysis of 11 studies has reported that garlic significantly reduces systolic blood pressure compared with placebo; its effect on the reduction of diastolic blood pressure is marginally significant (Ried et al. 2008).

- *Dark chocolate*: A meta-analysis of 13 studies showed that cocoa chocolate reduces systolic and diastolic blood pressure in prehypertensive and hypertensive patients, having no significant lowering effect on blood pressure in normotensive subjects (Ried et al. 2010).
- *Tea*: Green tea and British tea have been shown to reduce the risk of hypertension in Singaporean Chinese adults ≥40 years of age (Li et al. 2015).

1.7.3 REMEDIES FOR HYPERCHOLESTEROLEMIA

Research shows evidence of the following foods to be effective in the lowering of serum lipid levels:

- *Garlic*: A meta-analysis of 39 clinical trials indicates that if people with high total cholesterol level (>200 mg/dL) use garlic for more than 2 months, it reduces total serum cholesterol by 17 ± 6 mg/dL and low-density lipoprotein (LDL) by 9 ± 6 mg/dL (Ried et al. 2013).
- *Coriander*: The intake of two tablets of coriander seed powder per day for 6 weeks has been shown to significantly lower serum lipid levels in type 2 diabetes patients (Parsaeyan 2012).
- *Cinnamon*: Meta-analysis of 10 trials shows that the consumption of 0.12–6.0 g of cinnamon per day for 4–18 weeks can reduce total cholesterol by 15.6 mg/dL, LDL by 9.42 mg/dL, and triglycerides by 29.59 mg/dL and increases high-density lipoprotein (HDL) by 1.66 mh/dL in patients with type 2 diabetes (Allen et al. 2013).
- *Oatmeal*: 100 g of instant oatmeal per day for 6 weeks has been found to be effective in reducing total cholesterol, LDL, and triglyceride, and increasing HDL compared with those consuming 100 g of wheat flour–based noodles everyday for 6 weeks (Zhang et al. 2012).
- *Onions*: Researchers have reported a marked decrease in serum triglyceride levels after consumption of 200 mL/day of onion extract, corresponding to 500 g of onions/day for 8 weeks (Nam et al. 2007).

1.7.4 REMEDIES FOR CARDIOVASCULAR DISEASE (HEART DISEASE AND STROKE)

Studies have reported the following to be effective in the prevention of cardiovascular diseases:

- *Pomegranate*: Due to its antioxidant properties, pomegranate has been found to attenuate atherosclerosis and cardiovascular events related to it. The consumption of 240 mL of pomegranate juice per day for 1 year can increase arterial elasticity (Aviram and Rosenblat 2013).
- *Aged garlic extract*: 4 mL/day of aged garlic extract for 1 year was found to decrease the rate of progression of coronary artery calcification compared with the placebo (Budoff et al. 2004).
- *Vinegar*: In a large cohort study of women it was found that those who consumed vinegar and oil salad dressing ≥5–6 times/week had a lower risk of

fatal ischemic heart disease compared with those who rarely consumed it (RR 0.46, 95% CI 0.27–0.76) (Hu et al. 1999).

- *Fish*: The Health Professionals Follow-Up Study in men reported that eating fish once a month or more decreases the risk of ischemic stroke (He et al. 2002). A meta-analysis of cohort studies found that increased fish consumption is inversely related to the risk of stroke, especially ischemic stroke (He et al. 2004).
- *Ginger*: Pharmacologists have suggested that ginger extract can reduce the risk of stroke (Chang et al. 2011).

1.7.5 REMEDIES FOR OBESITY

Obesity, one of the risk factors for NCDs, can be prevented and controlled by the following remedies:

- *Lemons*: Lemon phenol has been shown to suppress weight gain and body fat accumulation in animal models (Fukuchi et al. 2008). The lemon detox program has been reported to reduce body fat in premenopausal Korean women (Kim et al. 2015).
- *Green tea*: 379 mg of green tea extract daily for 3 months has been shown to decrease waist circumference and BMI in male and female obese patients 30–60 years of age (Suliburska et al. 2012).
- *Kanuka honey with cinnamon, chromium, and magnesium*: In a randomized crossover trial, it was found that a kanuka honey formula with cinnamon, chromium, and magnesium at a dose of 53.5 g for 40 days decreased weight significantly by an average of 2.2 kg compared with kanuka honey alone in type 2 diabetes patients (Whitfield et al. 2015). Some types of honey contain toxic substances and hence precaution should be taken to avoid these (Islam et al. 2014).

1.7.6 REMEDIES FOR ASTHMA

Some natural remedies for asthma in scientific literature are as follows:

- *Licorice root and turmeric root*: In patients with bronchial asthma, licorice root and turmeric root combined have been found to reduce leukotriene C4, nitric oxide, and malondialdehyde significantly compared with those receiving placebo (Houssen et al. 2010).
- *Caffeine (contained in coffee and other beverages)*: A systematic Cochrane review of six randomized controlled trials reported that even low doses of caffeine (5 mg/kg body weight) can improve lung functions in asthmatic patients for up to 4 h (Welsh et al. 2010).
- *Fish oil*: Fish oil is rich in polyunsaturated fatty acids. The consumption of fish oil from the 30th week of gestation to pregnancy can reduce the risk of asthma in children by 63% and of allergic asthma by 87% compared with olive oil intake during the same period in pregnancy (Olsen et al. 2008).

1.7.7 REMEDIES FOR CANCERS

The following have been researched as a part of healthful eating for the prevention of cancers:

- *Green tea*: Green tea extract has been shown to inhibit tumor development in animal models at sites including the skin, oral cavity, esophagus, lung, stomach, intestine, colon, mammary gland, bladder, and prostate (Yang and Wang 2010). Green tea consumption has also been found to decrease overall cancer incidences in a population cohort study in Japan with 8552 participants (Nakachi et al. 2000).
- *Olive oil*: Researchers from Italy, through a large case control study, have reported that increased olive oil consumption is inversely related to the risk of breast cancer in a dose–response way (La Vecchia et al. 1995).
- *Tomatoes*: A meta-analysis of observational studies has shown that raw and cooked tomatoes can reduce the risks of prostate cancer (Etminan et al. 2004).
- *Grapes*: The resveratrol present in grapes can reduce the risk of breast cancer in women (Levi et al. 2005).

Hence, a variety of home remedies in the form of foods can be used for the prevention and control of NCDs.

1.8 NUTRITIONAL COUNSELING FOR NON-COMMUNICABLE DISEASES

Nutritional counseling starts with asking the patient/client about the symptoms, such as heaviness in the head, headache, blurred vision, increased thirst, frequent urination, vertigo, numbness in the extremities, and the like in patients with hypertension, diabetes, or CVD. Asthma presents with a cough, especially at night, during exercise, or when laughing, shortness of breath, chest tightening, and wheezing. COPD usually presents with a chronic cough that produces a lot of mucus, often referred to as a smoker's cough. Cancers present with lumps, weight loss, tiredness, blood in stools or any orifice of the body, pale skin, and localized symptoms depending on the site involved. Mental health disorders such as depression present with a lack of interest in daily activities, a sense of hopelessness, changes in eating and sleeping patterns, anger or irritability, and reckless behavior. Sometimes no symptom might be present and an NCD might be detected as an incidental finding.

Health professionals, including medical students, nurses, doctors, nutritionists, and community health workers should advise their clients and the general population to be screened for NCDs. Some routine tests that should be performed in screening for NCDs are

- *Weight and height*: BMI should be calculated by dividing weight in kg by height in m^2. Obesity should be identified by the following cutoff values, as suggested by WHO (WHO 2015a):

- <18.5 kg/m²: Underweight
- 18.5–24.9 kg/m²: Normal weight
- 25.0–29.9 kg/m²: Overweight (preobese)
- ≥30.0 kg/m²: Obese

As some ethnic groups, such as Asians, have an increased risk of type 2 diabetes and CVD at a lower BMI value, it is suggested that cutoff levels of 23 and 27.5 kg/m² for overweight and obesity, respectively, should be used for taking public health action (WHO 2015a).

- *Blood pressure*: According to the 7th Report of the Joint National Committee (JNC 7) (Chobanian et al. 2003), blood pressure is measured at two or more visits after the initial blood pressure screening and the average of these is then considered to define the following:
  - Normal blood pressure: Systolic blood pressure (SBP) <120 mm of Hg and diastolic blood pressure (DBP) <80 mm of Hg
  - Prehypertension: SBP 120–139 mm of Hg and/or DBP 80–89 mm of Hg
  - Hypertension: SBP ≥140 mm of Hg and/or DBP ≥90 mm of Hg
- *Fasting blood sugar (FBS) test*: This test measures blood glucose level and is usually done after 8 h of fasting. It is the first test of choice for the diagnosis of prediabetes and diabetes. The cutoff levels for diagnosis are (American Diabetes Association 2014):
  - Prediabetes: FBS level 100 mg/dl to 125 mg/dl, indicating impaired glucose tolerance (IGT) or impaired fasting glucose (IFG). People with prediabetes are at increased risk of developing type 2 diabetes and CVD.
  - Diabetes: FBS ≥126 mg/dl.
- *Fasting lipid profile*: Serum lipids including cholesterol, low-density lipoprotein (LDL), high-density lipoprotein (HDL), and triglycerides are usually measured in blood after 9–12 h of fasting. Lipid cutoff levels are defined as the following according to the ATP III guidelines (Grundy et al. 2004):
  - Total cholesterol: Desirable ≤200 mg/dl; borderline 200–239 mg/dl; high ≥240 mg/dl
  - LDL: Optimal <100 mg/dl; near/above optimal 100–129 mg/dl; borderline high 130–159 mg/dl; high 160–189 mg/dl; very high >190 mg/dl
  - HDL: Low <40 mg/dl; high ≥60 mg/dl
  - Triglyceride: Normal <150 mg/dl; borderline high 150–199 mg/dl; high 200–499 mg/dl; very high ≥500 mg/dl

For the prevention and control of NCDs by healthful eating, inquiries should be made about eating behaviors and the types of food consumed. Once a detailed history and investigations have been done, clients should be given recommendations based on the dietary guidelines, evidence-based dietary patterns, and evidence-based home remedies for the prevention of NCDs and their risk factors.

Table 1.2 gives a description of nutritional counseling for the Healthful Eating As Lifestyle (HEAL) program for the prevention of non-communicable diseases.

TABLE 1.2

Nutritional Counseling for Healthful Eating As Lifestyle for the Prevention and Control of Non-Communicable Diseases

Components of Counseling	Description
Symptoms that the patient tells	• *Hypertension*: Headache, dizziness, heaviness in the head, chest pain, palpitations, shortness of breath, nose bleed • *Diabetes*: Increased thirst, frequent urination, tiredness, numbness in the extremities, blurred vision, wounds that take time to heal • *Hypercholesterolemia*: Fatty skin tags (i.e., xanthelasmas) over the eyelids, xanthomas on the elbows, back, trunk, knees, buttocks, feet, or hands • *Heart disease*: Chest pain, palpitations, sweating and anxiety, epigastric pain, pain in the left side of the neck radiating to the left arm, shortness of breath • *Stroke*: Sudden weakness of any part of the body on one or both sides, confusion, slurred speech, dizziness • *Chronic lung diseases*: Cough and shortness of breath, chest tightness, wheezing • *Cancers*: Lumps, weight loss, tiredness, blood from any orifice of the body such as in stools, loss of appetite, localized symptoms depending on the site of cancer • *Mental health disorders such as depression*: Lack of interest in daily activities, feelings of helplessness, changes in eating and sleeping patterns, aggressive behavior, recklessness, anxiety, low moods
Nutritional history: Questions to be asked by health experts	Dietary assessments can be done in the form of a *diet history*, *24-hour recall*, *dietary log*, and *food frequency questionnaire*. These should inquire about • Frequency/serves of fruits and vegetables • Types and amounts of fat consumption • Salt intake • Types and amounts of meat, fish, and poultry • Grains and lentils, nuts, and seeds • Alcohol use • Sugar content in diet • Refined products consumed Some important questions to be asked are • Have you had any issues with weight? Are you underweight or overweight? • Have you been on any diets? If yes, then what diets have you followed? • Do you skip meals? How often? • Do you take breakfast regularly? • Are you a vegetarian or nonvegetarian? • Do you take snacks in between meals? What types of snacks?
Examinations and investigations	These consist of examinations from head to toe to look for anemia, signs of dehydration, checking for blurred vision, xanthomas as seen in hyperlipidemia, cyanosis indicating heart disease, weight and height for calculating BMI, blood pressure, pulse, respiratory rate, wounds on the body that have not healed, edema in the limbs, lumps anywhere in the body. Perform fasting blood sugar and lipid profiles.
Diagnosis	If you diagnose any of NCDs, refer to the concerned physician.
Nutritional management	Advise patients about Healthful Eating As Lifestyle (HEAL) based on the *food-based dietary guidelines*, *evidence-based dietary patterns*, and *home remedies* as explained in this chapter. Give precautionary guidelines about safety concerns when recommending home-based remedies.

1.9 CASE STUDIES

Based on the information given in this chapter about NCDs and Healthful Eating As Lifestyle (HEAL) for NCDs, try to analyze the following case study and respond to the questions accordingly.

1.9.1 CASE STUDY 1

A 59-year-old white male comes to you with complaints of tiredness and numbness in his extremities. He has no previous history of hypertension, diabetes, heart disease, stroke, or chronic lung diseases. His family history of hypercholesterolemia is positive. On examination, his blood pressure is normal and he has no xanthelasmas anywhere on the body. (Pointer: Numbness of the extremities may point toward diabetes.)

Give responses to the following:

1. Which investigations would you perform?
2. What information would you like to gather in nutritional history?
3. Based on your assessment, what dietary recommendations you will make if the patient is found to have a fasting blood sugar level more than 126 mg/dl?

1.9.2 CASE STUDY 2

A 30-year-old Asian female presents to you with shortness of breath while climbing stairs. She has a sedentary lifestyle and has gained weight over the previous 5 years. Her family history of heart disease is positive. She has never been diagnosed with diabetes, hyperlipidemia, or hypertension. On examination, her systolic blood pressure is 135 mm of Hg and diastolic blood pressure 85 mm of Hg. (Pointer: a sedentary lifestyle is a cause of obesity.)

Give responses to the following:

1. What more would you like to see on examination?
2. What questions would you like to ask her for nutritional assessment?
3. Given that her BMI is 32 mg/kg^2, what dietary recommendations would you give?

REFERENCES

Abegunde, D. O., C. D. Mathers, T. Adam et al. 2007. The burden and costs of chronic diseases in low-income and middle-income countries. *Lancet* 370 (9603):1929–1938.

Allen, R. W., E. Schwartzman, W. L. Baker, C. I. Coleman, and O. J. Phung. 2013. Cinnamon use in type 2 diabetes: An updated systematic review and meta-analysis. *Ann Fam Med* 11 (5):452–459.

American Diabetes Association. 2014. Diagnosing diabetes and learning about prediabetes. Accessed August 7, 2015. http://www.diabetes.org/are-you-at-risk/prediabetes.

Appel, L. J., T. J. Moore, E. Obarzanek, W. M. Vollmer, L. P. Svetkey, F. M. Sacks, G. A. Bray, T. M. Vogt, J. A. Cutler, and M. M. Windhauser. 1997. A clinical trial of the effects of dietary patterns on blood pressure. *N Engl J Med* 336 (16):1117–1124.

Aviram, M., and M. Rosenblat. 2013. Pomegranate for your cardiovascular health. *Rambam Maimonides Med J* 4 (2):e0013.

Beaglehole, R., R. Bonita, G. Alleyne et al. 2011a. UN high-level meeting on non-communicable diseases: Addressing four questions. *Lancet* 378 (9789):449–455.

Beaglehole, R., R. Bonita, R. Horton et al. 2011b. Priority actions for the non-communicable disease crisis. *Lancet* 377 (9775):1438–1447.

Berentzen, N. E., J. W. Beulens, M. P. Hoevenaar-Blom, E. Kampman, H. B. Bueno-de-Mesquita, D. Romaguera-Bosch, P. H. M. Peeters, and A. M. May. 2013. Adherence to the WHO's healthy diet indicator and overall cancer risk in the EPIC-NL cohort. *PloS One* 8 (8):e70535.

Budoff, M. J., J. Takasu, F. R. Flores, Y. Niihara, B. Lu, B. H. Lau, R. T. Rosen, and H. Amagase. 2004. Inhibiting progression of coronary calcification using aged garlic extract in patients receiving statin therapy: A preliminary study. *Prev Med* 39 (5):985–991.

Cade, J. E., E. F. Taylor, V. J. Burley, and D. C. Greenwood. 2011. Does the Mediterranean dietary pattern or the Healthy Diet Index influence the risk of breast cancer in a large British cohort of women? *Eur J Clin Nutr* 65 (8):920–928.

Chang, T.-T., K.-C. Chen, K.-W. Chang, H.-Y. Chen, F.-J. Tsai, M.-F. Sun, and C. Y.-C. Chen. 2011. *In silico* pharmacology suggests ginger extracts may reduce stroke risks. *Mol Biosyst* 7 (9):2702–2710.

Chobanian, A. V., G. L. Bakris, H. R. Black, W. C. Cushman, L. A. Green, J. L. Izzo Jr, D. W. Jones, B. J. Materson, S. Oparil, and J. T. Wright Jr. 2003. The 7th Report of the Joint National Committee on Prevention, Detection, Evaluation, and Treatment of High Blood Pressure: The JNC 7 Report. *JAMA* 289 (19):2560–2571.

Danaei, G., S. Vander Hoorn, A. D. Lopez et al.; and Comparative Risk Assessment Collaborating Group. 2005. Causes of cancer in the world: Comparative risk assessment of nine behavioural and environmental risk factors. *Lancet* 366 (9499):1784–1793.

Etminan, M., B. Takkouche, and F. Caamano-Isorna. 2004. The role of tomato products and lycopene in the prevention of prostate cancer: A meta-analysis of observational studies. *Cancer Epidemiol Biomarkers Prev* 13 (3):340–345.

European Food Information Council. 2009. Food-based dietary guidelines in Europe. Accessed June 17, 2015. http://www.eufic.org/article/en/expid/food-based-dietary-guidelines-in-europe.

Evans, C. 2015. Improving nutritional behaviour. *Food Science and Technology.* 29:16–19 Accessed July 16, 2015.

Food and Agricultural Organization (FAO). 2010. Fats and fatty acids in human nutrition: Report of an expert consultation. Rome, Italy: FAO of the United Nations.

Fogli-Cawley, J. J., J. T. Dwyer, E. Saltzman et al. 2007. The 2005 Dietary Guidelines for Americans and risk of the metabolic syndrome. *Am J Clin Nutr* 86 (4):1193–1201.

Fogli-Cawley, J. J., J. T. Dwyer, E. Saltzman, M. L. McCullough, L. M. Troy, and P. F. Jacques. 2006. The 2005 Dietary Guidelines for Americans adherence index: Development and application. *J Nutr* 136 (11):2908–2915.

Food Standards Agency. 2007. The Eatwell Plate. Accessed July 7, 2015. http://tna.europarchive.org/20100929190231/http://www.eatwell.gov.uk/healthydiet/eatwellplate.

Fuangchan, A., P. Sonthisombat, T. Seubnukarn, R. Chanouan, P. Chotchaisuwat, V. Sirigulsatien, K. Ingkaninan, P. Plianbangchang, and S. T. Haines. 2011. Hypoglycemic effect of bitter melon compared with metformin in newly diagnosed type 2 diabetes patients. *J Ethnopharmacol* 134 (2):422–428.

Fukino, Y., A. Ikeda, K. Maruyama, N. Aoki, T. Okubo, and H. Iso. 2008. Randomized controlled trial for an effect of green tea–extract powder supplementation on glucose abnormalities. *Eur J Clin Nutr* 62 (8):953–960.

Fukuchi, Y., M. Hiramitsu, M. Okada, S. Hayashi, Y. Nabeno, T. Osawa, and M. Naito. 2008. Lemon polyphenols suppress diet-induced obesity by up-regulation of mRNA Levels of the enzymes involved in betaoxidation in mouse white adipose tissue. *J Clin Biochem Nutr* 43 (3):201–209.

Garriguet, D. 2009. Diet quality in Canada. *Health Rep* 20 (3):41–52.

Golley, R. K., G. A. Hendrie, and S. A. McNaughton. 2011. Scores on the dietary guideline index for children and adolescents are associated with nutrient intake and socio-economic position but not adiposity. *J Nutr* 141 (7):1340–1347.

Grundy, S. M., J. I. Cleeman, C. N. Bairey Merz, H. B. Brewer, L. T. Clark, D. B. Hunninghake, R. C. Pasternak, S. C. Smith, and N. J. Stone. 2004. Implications of recent clinical trials for the National Cholesterol Education Program Adult Treatment Panel III guidelines. *J Am Coll Cardiol* 44 (3):720–732.

Grundy, S. M., J. I. Cleeman, S. R. Daniels, K. A. Donato, R. H. Eckel, B. A. Franklin, D. J. Gordon, R. M. Krauss, P. J. Savage, S. C. Smith, American Heart Association, and National Heart, Lung, and Blood Institute. 2005. Diagnosis and management of the metabolic syndrome: An American Heart Association/National Heart, Lung, and Blood Institute scientific statement. *Circulation* 112 (17):2735–2752.

Guenther, P. M., K. O. Casavale, J. Reedy, S. I. Kirkpatrick, H. A. B. Hiza, K. J. Kuczynski, L. L. Kahle, and S. M. Krebs-Smith. 2013. Update of the Healthy Eating Index: HEI-2010. *J Acad Nutr Diet* 113 (4):569–580.

Guenther, P. M., J. Reedy, and S. M. Krebs-Smith. 2008. Development of the Healthy Eating Index 2005. *J Am Diet Assoc* 108 (11):1896–1901.

Hajna, S., J. Liu, P. J. LeBlanc, B. E. Faught, A. T. Merchant, J. Cairney, and J. Hay. 2012. Association between body composition and conformity to the recommendations of Canada's Food Guide and the Dietary Approaches to Stop Hypertension (DASH) diet in peri-adolescence. *Public Health Nutr* 15 (10):1890–1896.

Harland, J. I., J. Buttriss, and S. Gibson. 2012. Achieving Eatwell Plate recommendations: Is this a route to improving both sustainability and healthy eating? *Nutrition Bulletin* 37 (4):324–343.

He, K., E. B. Rimm, A. Merchant, B. A. Rosner, M. J. Stampfer, W. C. Willett, and A. Ascherio. 2002. Fish consumption and risk of stroke in men. *JAMA* 288 (24):3130–3136.

He, K., Y. Song, M. L. Daviglus, K. Liu, L. Van Horn, A. R. Dyer, U. Goldbourt, and P. Greenland. 2004. Fish consumption and incidence of stroke: A meta-analysis of cohort studies. *Stroke* 35 (7):1538–1542.

Health Canada. 2011a. Canada's Food Guide. Accessed June 30, 2015. http://www.hc-sc. gc.ca/fn-an/food-guide-aliment/order-commander/index-eng.php.

Health Canada. 2011b. Eat Well with Canada's Food Guide. Accessed July 6, 2015. http://www. hc-sc.gc.ca/fn-an/food-guide-aliment/order-commander/eating_well_bien_manger-eng.php.

Hooper, L., A. Abdelhamid, H. J. Moore et al. 2012. Effect of reducing total fat intake on body weight: Systematic review and meta-analysis of randomized controlled trials and cohort studies. *BMJ* 345 (e7666).

Hosseini-Esfahani, F., M. Jessri, P. Mirmiran et al. 2010. Adherence to dietary recommendations and risk of metabolic syndrome: Tehran Lipid and Glucose Study. *Metabolism* 59 (12):1833–1842.

Houssen, M. E., A. Ragab, A. Mesbah, A. Z. El-Samanoudy, G. Othman, A. F. Moustafa, and F. A. Badria. 2010. Natural anti-inflammatory products and leukotriene inhibitors as complementary therapy for bronchial asthma. *Clin Biochem* 43 (10–11):887–890.

Hu, F. B. 2002. Dietary pattern analysis: A new direction in nutritional epidemiology. *Curr Opin Lipidol* 13 (1):3–9.

Hu, F. B., M. J. Stampfer, J. E. Manson, E. B. Rimm, A. Wolk, G. A. Colditz, C. H. Hennekens, and W. C. Willett. 1999. Dietary intake of alpha linolenic acid and risk of fatal ischemic heart disease among women. *Am J Clin Nutr* 69 (5):890–897.

Huangfu, P., H. Pikhart, and A. Peasey. 2014. PP06 Healthy diet indicator score and metabolic syndrome in the Czech Republic, Russia, and Poland: Cross-sectional findings from the HAPIEE study. *J Epidemiol Community Health* 68 (Suppl 1):A49–A50.

Huijbregts, P., E. Feskens, L. Rasanen, F. Fidanza, A. Nissinen, A. Menotti, and D. Kromhout. 1997. Dietary pattern and 20 year mortality in elderly men in Finland, Italy, and the Netherlands: Longitudinal cohort study. *BMJ* 315 (7099):13–17.

Imamura, F., P. F. Jacques, D. M. Herrington, G. E. Dallal, and A. H. Lichtenstein. 2009. Adherence to 2005 Dietary Guidelines for Americans is associated with a reduced progression of coronary artery atherosclerosis in women with established coronary artery disease. *Am J Clin Nutr* 90 (1):193–201.

Islam, M. N., M. I. Khalil, and S. H. Gan. 2014. Toxic compounds in honey. *J Appl Toxicol* 34 (7):733–742.

Jankovic, N., A. Geelen, M. T. Streppel, L. C. de Groot, P. Orfanos, E. H. van den Hooven, H. Pikhart, P. Boffetta, A. Trichopoulou, and M. Bobak. 2014. Adherence to a healthy diet according to the WHO guidelines and all-cause mortality in elderly adults from Europe and the United States. *Am J Epidemiol* 180 (10):978–988.

Kanauchi, M., and K. Kanauchi. 2015. Diet quality and adherence to a healthy diet in Japanese male workers with untreated hypertension. *BMJ Open* 5 (7):e008404.

Khandouzi, N., F. Shidfar, A. Rajab, T. Rahideh, P. Hosseini, and M. M. Taheri. 2015. The effects of ginger on fasting blood sugar, hemoglobin A1c, apolipoprotein B, apolipoprotein A-I and malondialdehyde in type 2 diabetic patients. *Iran J Pharm Res* 14 (1):131–140.

Kim, M. J., J. H. Hwang, H. J. Ko, H. B. Na, and J. H. Kim. 2015. Lemon detox diet reduced body fat, insulin resistance, and serum HS-CRP level without hematological changes in overweight Korean women. *Nutr Res* 35 (5):409–420.

La Vecchia, C., E. Negri, S. Franceschi, A. Decarli, A. Giacosa, and L. Lipworth. 1995. Olive oil, other dietary fats, and the risk of breast cancer (Italy). *Cancer Causes Control* 6 (6):545–550.

Levi, F., C. Pasche, F. Lucchini, R. Ghidoni, M. Ferraroni, and C. La Vecchia. 2005. Resveratrol and breast cancer risk. *Eur J Cancer Prev* 14 (2):139–142.

Li, W., J. Yang, X. S. Zhu, S. C. Li, and P. C. Ho. 2015. Correlation between tea consumption and prevalence of hypertension among Singaporean Chinese residents aged ≥40 years. *J Hum Hypertens*. doi: 10.1038/jhh.2015.45. Accessed July 16, 2015.

Liese, A. D., M. Nichols, X. Sun, R. B. D'Agostino, and S. M. Haffner. 2009. Adherence to the DASH diet is inversely associated with incidence of type 2 diabetes: The insulin resistance atherosclerosis study. *Diabetes Care* 32 (8):1434–1436.

Mathers, C. D., and D. Loncar. 2006. Projections of global mortality and burden of disease from 2002 to 2030. *PLoS Med* 3 (11):e442.

McCullough, M. L., D. Feskanich, E. B. Rimm, E. L. Giovannucci, A. Ascherio, J. N. Variyam, D. Spiegelman, M. J. Stampfer, and W. C. Willett. 2000a. Adherence to the Dietary Guidelines for Americans and risk of major chronic disease in men. *Am J Clin Nutr* 72 (5):1223–1231.

McCullough, M. L., D. Feskanich, M. J. Stampfer, B. A. Rosner, F. B. Hu, D. J. Hunter, J. N. Variyam, G. A. Colditz, and W. C. Willett. 2000b. Adherence to the Dietary Guidelines for Americans and risk of major chronic disease in women. *Am J Clin Nutr* 72 (5):1214–1222.

McNaughton, S. A., K. Ball, D. Crawford, and G. D. Mishra. 2008. An index of diet and eating patterns is a valid measure of diet quality in an Australian population. *J Nutr* 138 (1):86–93.

McNaughton, S. A., D. W. Dunstan, K. Ball, J. Shaw, and D. Crawford. 2009. Dietary quality is associated with diabetes and cardio-metabolic risk factors. *J Nutr* 139 (4):734–742.

Morris, M. A., C. Hulme, G. P. Clarke, K. L. Edwards, and J. E. Cade. 2014. What is the cost of a healthy diet? Using diet data from the UK Women's Cohort Study. *J Epidemiol Community Health* 68 (11):1043–1049.

Mottillo, S., K. B. Filion, J. Genest, L. Joseph, L. Pilote, P. Poirier, S. Rinfret, E. L. Schiffrin, and M. J. Eisenberg. 2010. The metabolic syndrome and cardiovascular risk: A systematic review and meta-analysis. *Journal of the American College of Cardiology* 56 (14):1113–1132.

Murray, C. J. L., T. Vos, R. Lozano et al. 2013. Disability-adjusted life years (DALYs) for 291 diseases and injuries in 21 regions, 1990–2010: A systematic analysis for the Global Burden of Disease Study 2010. *Lancet* 380 (9859):2197–2223.

Nakachi, K., S. Matsuyama, S. Miyake, M. Suganuma, and K. Imai. 2000. Preventive effects of drinking green tea on cancer and cardiovascular disease: Epidemiological evidence for multiple targeting prevention. *Biofactors* 13 (1–4):49–54.

Nam, K. H., H. W. Baik, T. Y. Choi, S. G. Yoon, S. W. Park, and H. Joung. 2007. Effects of ethanol extract of onion on the lipid profiles in patients with hypercholesterolemia. *Korean J Nutr* 40 (3):242–248.

NHMRC. 2013a. Australian Dietary Guidelines (2013). Accessed June 30, 2015. https://www. nhmrc.gov.au/guidelines-publications/n55.

NHMRC. 2013b. *Eat for Health: Australian Dietary Guidelines; Summary.* Canberra, Australia: NHMRC.

NHS choices. 2016. The Eatwell Guide. http://www.nhs.uk/Livewell/Goodfood/Pages/the-eatwell-guide.aspx. Accessed September 12, 2016.

Nkondjock, A., and P. Ghadirian. 2007. Diet quality and BRCA-associated breast cancer risk. *Breast Cancer Res Treat* 103 (3):361–369.

Olsen, S. F., M. L. Osterdal, J. D. Salvig, L. M. Mortensen, D. Rytter, N. J. Secher, and T. B. Henriksen. 2008. Fish oil intake compared with olive oil intake in late pregnancy and asthma in the offspring: 16 y of registry-based follow-up from a randomized controlled trial. *Am J Clin Nutr* 88 (1):167–175.

Paquette, M. C. 2005. Perceptions of healthy eating: State of knowledge and research gaps. *Can J Public Health/Revue Canadienne de Sante'e Publique* 96:S15–S19.

Parsaeyan, N. 2012. The effect of coriander seed powder consumption on atherosclerotic and cardioprotective indices of type 2 diabetic patients 2. *Iranian Journal of Diabetes and Obesity* 12 (2):86–90.

Pham, A. Q., H. Kourlas, and D. Q. Pham. 2007. Cinnamon supplementation in patients with type 2 diabetes mellitus. *Pharmacotherapy* 27 (4):595–599.

Psaltopoulou, T., T. N. Sergentanis, D. B. Panagiotakos, I. N. Sergentanis, R. Kosti, and N. Scarmeas. 2013. Mediterranean diet, stroke, cognitive impairment, and depression: A meta-analysis. *Ann Neurol* 74 (4):580–591.

Ried, K., O. R. Frank, N. P. Stocks, P. Fakler, and T. Sullivan. 2008. Effect of garlic on blood pressure: A systematic review and meta-analysis. *BMC Cardiovasc Disord* 8:13.

Ried, K., T. Sullivan, P. Fakler, O. R. Frank, and N. P. Stocks. 2010. Does chocolate reduce blood pressure? A meta-analysis. *BMC Med* 8:39.

Ried, K., C. Toben, and P. Fakler. 2013. Effect of garlic on serum lipids: An updated meta-analysis. *Nutr Rev* 71 (5):282–299.

Salehi-Abargouei, A., Z. Maghsoudi, F. Shirani, and L. Azadbakht. 2013. Effects of Dietary Approaches to Stop Hypertension (DASH)-style diet on fatal or nonfatal cardiovascular diseases' incidence: A systematic review and meta-analysis on observational prospective studies. *Nutrition* 29 (4):611–618.

Sofi, F., R. Abbate, G. F. Gensini, and A. Casini. 2010. Accruing evidence on benefits of adherence to the Mediterranean diet on health: An updated systematic review and meta-analysis. *Am J Clin Nutr* 92 (5):1189–1196.

Stefler, D., H. Pikhart, N. Jankovic, R. Kubinova, A. Pajak, S. Malyutina, G. Simonova, E. J. M. Feskens, A. Peasey, and M. Bobak. 2014. Healthy diet indicator and mortality in Eastern European populations: Prospective evidence from the HAPIEE cohort. *Eur J Clin Nutr* 68 (12):1346–1352.

Stuckler, D. 2008. Population causes and consequences of leading chronic diseases: A comparative analysis of prevailing explanations. *Milbank Q* 86 (2):273–326.

Suliburska, J., P. Bogdanski, M. Szulinska, M. Stepien, D. Pupek-Musialik, and A. Jablecka. 2012. Effects of green tea supplementation on elements, total antioxidants, lipids, and glucose values in the serum of obese patients. *Biol Trace Elem Res* 149 (3):315–322.

Troy, L. M., and P. F. Jacques. 2012. Diets that follow the 2010 Dietary Guidelines for Americans (DGA) are associated with higher intakes of nutrients of concern. *FASEB J* 26 (1 Suppl):267.1.

Tucker, K. L. 2010. Dietary patterns, approaches, and multicultural perspective. *Appl Physiol Nutr Metab* 35 (2):211–218.

U.S. Department of Agriculture and U.S. Department of Health and Human Services. 2010. *Dietary Guidelines for Americans, 2010*. Washington, DC: U.S. Department of Agriculture and U.S. Department of Health and Human Services.

U.S. Department of Health and Human Services and U.S. Department of Agriculture. 2015–2020 Dietary Guidelines for Americans. 8th Edition. December 2015. Accessed September 12, 2016.

Virdi, J., S. Sivakami, S. Shahani, A. C. Suthar, M. M. Banavalikar, and M. K. Biyani. 2003. Antihyperglycemic effects of three extracts from *Momordica charantia*. *J Ethnopharmacol* 88 (1):107–111.

Wagner, K. H., and H. Brath. 2012. A global view on the development of non-communicable diseases. *Prev Med* 54:S38–S41.

Welsh, E. J., A. Bara, E. Barley, and C. J. Cates. 2010. Caffeine for asthma. *Cochrane Database Syst Rev* 20 (1):CD001112.

Whitfield, P., A. Parry-Strong, E. Walsh, M. Weatherall, and J. D. Krebs. 2015. The effect of a cinnamon-, chromium- and magnesium-formulated honey on glycaemic control, weight loss and lipid parameters in type 2 diabetes: An open-label cross-over randomized controlled trial. *Eur J Nutr* (Epub ahead of print).

Willett, W. C., F. Sacks, A. Trichopoulou, G. Drescher, A. Ferro-Luzzi, E. Helsing, and D. Trichopoulos. 1995. Mediterranean diet pyramid: A cultural model for healthy eating. *Am J Clin Nutr* 61 (6):1402S–1406S.

Woodruff, S. J., R. M. Hanning, I. Lambraki, K. E. Storey, and L. McCargar. 2008. Healthy Eating Index-C is compromised among adolescents with body weight concerns, weight loss dieting, and meal skipping. *Body Image* 5 (4):404–408.

World Health Organization. 1948. Preamble to the constitution of the WHO as adopted by the International Health Conference. New York, 19–22 June, 1946.

WHO. 1990. Diet, nutrition and the prevention of chronic diseases: Report of a joint WHO/FAO Expert Consultation. Geneva: World Health Organization.

WHO. 2003a. Diet, nutrition and the prevention of chronic diseases: Report of a Joint WHO/FAO Expert Consultation. In WHO Technical Report Series, No. 916. Geneva: World Health Organization.

WHO. 2003b. Food-based dietary guidelines in the WHO European region. Copenhagen: World Health Organization, Regional Office for Europe.

WHO. 2009. Global health risks: Mortality and burden of disease attributable to selected major risks. Geneva: World Health Organization.

WHO. 2012. Guideline: Sodium intake for adults and children. Geneva: World Health Organization.

WHO. 2014. Global status report on non-communicable diseases, 2014. Geneva, Switzerland: World Health Organization.

WHO. 2015a. BMI classification. Accessed August 6, 2015. http://apps.who.int/bmi/index. jsp?introPage=intro_3.html.

WHO. 2015b. Guideline: Sugar intake for adults and children. Geneva: World Health Organization.

WHO. 2015c. Healthy diet. Accessed June 30, 2015. http://www.who.int/mediacentre/ factsheets/fs394/en/.

Yang, C. S., and X. Wang. 2010. Green tea and cancer prevention. *Nutr Cancer* 62 (7):931–937.

Yu, D., J. Sonderman, M. S. Buchowski, J. K. McLaughlin, X.-O. Shu, M. Steinwandel, L. B. Signorello, X. Zhang, M. K. Hargreaves, and W. J. Blot. 2015. Healthy eating and risks of total and cause-specific death among low-income populations of African Americans and other adults in the Southeastern United States: A prospective cohort study. *PLoS Med* 12 (5):e1001830.

Zhang, J., L. Li, P. Song, C. Wang, Q. Man, L. Meng, J. Cai, and A. Kurilich. 2012. Randomized controlled trial of oatmeal consumption versus noodle consumption on blood lipids of urban Chinese adults with hypercholesterolemia. *Nutr J* 11:54.

2 HEAL for Hypertension

Saman Tahir, Sara Habib, and Romaina Iqbal

CONTENTS

2.1 INTRODUCTION

Raised arterial blood pressure (BP) and its consequences are known as "hypertension," which is one of the most common conditions afflicting humans worldwide. Hypertension is not only a disease in itself, but also gives rise to a myriad of other illnesses, such as stroke, chronic kidney disease, myocardial infarction, and vascular diseases. In the first chapter, page 3 of Laragh and Brenner's (1994) book on hypertension, Goerge Pickering states that: "Arterial blood pressure is a quantity, and the consequences are related to it quantitatively. The higher the blood pressure the worse the prognosis." Chronically raised blood pressure lessens life expectancy. Unfortunately, despite extensive research and the unveiling of modifiable risk factors, the control of blood pressure remains suboptimal in the general population. Currently, it is estimated that about 1 billion people worldwide are diagnosed with hypertension (>140/90 mm Hg), and this is expected to increase to 1.56 billion in the next 20 years (Sarafidis et al. 2008). The rising incidence of obesity can also increase the burden of hypertension (Kaplan and Victor 2014).

2.2 DEFINING PREHYPERTENSION AND HYPERTENSION

The National High Blood Pressure Education Program (NHBPEP), coordinated by the National Heart, Lung, and Blood Institute (NHLBI) of the U.S. National Institutes of Health, was established in 1972 with the mission of spreading awareness and to prevent, control, and treat hypertension through an evidence-based approach. NHBPEP's most notable product is the Joint National Committee (JNC) report. The JNC report was the first clinical guideline for chronic disease management and has been accepted by managed care groups, the National Committee on Quality Assurance, and regional professional societies as the standard for detecting and managing high blood pressure. The following definitions were suggested in 2003 by the 7th Report of the JNC (JNC 7) and are based on the average of two or more properly measured readings at each of the two or more office visits after an initial screening (Chobanian et al. 2003).

- *Normal blood pressure*—Systolic BP <120 mm Hg and diastolic BP <80 mm Hg
- *Prehypertension*—Systolic BP 120–139 mm Hg or diastolic BP 80–89 mm Hg
- *Hypertension*—Stage 1: Systolic BP 140–159 mm Hg or diastolic BP 90–99 mm Hg; Stage 2: Systolic BP ≥160 mm Hg or diastolic BP ≥100 mm Hg

For most studies and in clinical practice, patients who are actively taking antihypertensive medications are usually defined as having hypertension regardless of their observed BP. Although the definitions of hypertension (including stage 1 and stage 2 hypertension) and prehypertension were not specifically addressed in the 2014 "Evidenced-Based Guidelines for Management of High Blood Pressure in Adults" as reported by the panel members appointed to JNC 8, thresholds were adopted for the treatment of blood pressure that are generally consistent with these definitions (James et al. 2014). Isolated systolic hypertension is considered to be present when the BP is ≥140/<90 mm Hg, and isolated diastolic hypertension is considered to be present when the BP is <140/≥90 mm Hg. Patients with BP ≥140/≥90 mm Hg are considered to have mixed systolic/diastolic hypertension. These definitions apply to adults on no antihypertensive medication and who are not acutely ill. If there is a disparity in category between systolic and diastolic pressures, the higher value determines the severity of hypertension.

Another term that has emerged through the literature is "white-coat hypertension," which refers to BP>140/90 mm Hg in a clinical setting due to the stress of visiting a doctor. Ambulatory BP monitoring that monitors BP at regular intervals is necessary for those who develop it. JNC 7 defined the upper limits of ambulatory BP as 135/85 mm Hg when patients are awake and 120/75 mmHg when they are asleep. White-coat hypertension can also be defined as high clinical BP but normal ambulatory BP. Health-care professionals need to take it into account before diagnosing a patient with essential hypertension. Whether white-coat hypertension should be considered a prehypertensive state or one which develops into established hypertension is still under debate (Chung and Lip 2003).

2.3 PRIMARY ESSENTIAL HYPERTENSION

The maintenance of arterial BP is necessary for organ perfusion. In general, arterial BP is determined by the following equation:

$$\text{Blood pressure (BP)} = \text{cardiac output (CO)} \times \text{systemic vascular resistance (SVR)}$$

BP reacts to changes in the environment to maintain organ perfusion over a wide variety of conditions. The primary factors determining BP are the sympathetic nervous system, the renin–angiotensin–aldosterone system, and the plasma volume (largely mediated by the kidneys).

The pathogenesis of primary hypertension (formerly called "essential" hypertension) is poorly understood but is most likely the result of numerous genetic and environmental factors that have multiple compounding effects on cardiovascular and renal structure and function. Although the exact etiology of primary hypertension remains unclear, a number of risk factors are strongly and independently associated with its development, including

- *Age*: Advancing age is associated with increased BP, particularly systolic BP, and an increased incidence of hypertension.
- *Obesity*: Obesity and weight gain are major risk factors for hypertension and are also determinants of the rise in BP that is commonly observed with aging (Carnethon et al. 2010; Rapsomaniki et al. 2014).
- *Family history*: Hypertension is about twice as common in subjects who have one or two hypertensive parents, and multiple epidemiologic studies suggest that genetic factors account for approximately 30% of the variation in BP in various populations (Lloyd-Jones et al. 2002; Moran et al. 2014).

- *Race*: Hypertension tends to be more common and severe, occurs earlier in life, and is associated with greater target-organ damage in blacks.
- *Reduced nephron number*: Reduced adult nephron mass may predispose subjects to hypertension, which may be related to genetic factors, intrauterine developmental disturbance (e.g., hypoxia, drugs, and nutritional deficiency), premature birth, and the postnatal environment (e.g., malnutrition, infections).
- *Diet*: Excess sodium (Na) intake (e.g., >3000 mg/day) increases the risk of hypertension, and Na restriction lowers BP.
- *Excessive alcohol consumption*: Excess alcohol intake is associated with the development of hypertension.
- *Physical inactivity*: Physical inactivity increases the risk of hypertension, and exercise is an effective means of lowering BP (Carnethon et al. 2010; Levy et al. 1996).
- *Diabetes and dyslipidemia*: The presence of other cardiovascular risk factors, including diabetes and dyslipidemia, appear to be associated with an increased risk of developing hypertension (Haider et al. 2003).
- *Personality traits and depression*: Hypertension may be more common among those with certain personality traits, such as hostile attitudes and time urgency/impatience (MacMahon et al. 1990), as well as among those with depression (Collins et al. 1990).
- *Hypovitaminosis D*: Vitamin D deficiency increasingly appears to be associated with a higher risk of hypertension, at least in some populations.

2.4   COMPLICATIONS OF HYPERTENSION

Arterial hypertension is a major cause of morbidity and mortality because of its association with cardiovascular disease (CVD), cerebrovascular disease, and renal disease. The extent of target-organ involvement (i.e., heart, brain, and kidneys) determines the outcome. The cardiac consequences of hypertension are left ventricular hypertrophy and coronary artery disease. Left ventricular hypertrophy is caused by pressure overload and is concentric. There is an increase in muscle mass and wall thickness but not ventricular volume. Left ventricular hypertrophy is an independent risk factor for cardiovascular disease, especially sudden death. The consequences of hypertension are a function of its severity. There is no threshold for complications to occur, as the elevation of BP is associated with increased morbidity throughout the whole range of BP. Hypertension is a leading risk factor for ischemic heart disease, including myocardial infarction. The lifetime risk of developing CVD is significantly higher among patients with hypertension. In a cohort of over 1.25 million patients aged 30 years or older without baseline CVD, including 20% with baseline-treated hypertension, patients with baseline hypertension had a 63.3% lifetime risk of developing CVD compared with a 46.1% risk for those with normal baseline BP (Rapsomaniki et al. 2014). Hypertension accounts for 18% of the population attributable risk of a first myocardial infarction (Moran et al. 2014) and increases the risk of heart failure at all ages. The data from the Framingham Heart Study showed that, after 40 years, the lifetime risk of developing heart failure was twice as high in subjects with BP ≥160/100 mm Hg compared with <140/90 mm Hg (Lloyd-Jones et al. 2002). Even moderate elevations contribute to risk in the long term (Levy et al. 1996). Another analysis from the Framingham study suggests that baseline systolic pressure and pulse pressure have a greater impact on the risk of subsequent heart failure than diastolic pressure. In this analysis, 2040 participants aged 50–79 years who were initially free of heart failure were followed for 17.4 years (Haider et al. 2003). Increments of one standard deviation in systolic pressure, pulse pressure, and diastolic pressure were associated with hazard ratios for heart failure of 1.56, 1.55, and 1.24, respectively, after adjustment for other risk factors.

Hypertension is the most common and most important risk factor for stroke (Collins et al. 1990; MacMahon et al. 1990), including isolated systolic hypertension (Carnethon et al. 2010; James et al. 2014). Epidemiologic studies show that there is a gradually increasing incidence of both coronary disease and stroke as BP rises above 110/75 mm Hg (Lewington et al. 2002; MacMahon et al. 1990). Both prior and current BP are important risk factors (Seshadri et al. 2001). However, these observations do not prove a causal relationship, since increasing BP could be a marker for other risk factors such as increasing body weight, which is associated with dyslipidemia, glucose intolerance, and metabolic syndrome.

Severe uncontrolled hypertension is a strong risk factor for intracerebral hemorrhage (ICH). A young person who enters a hospital with acute onset of a focal neurologic deficit and BP >220/120 mm Hg has a high likelihood of having an ICH. In a Korean cohort study, for each 20 mm Hg increase in systolic BP, the increased relative risk of hemorrhagic stroke was greater than that for ischemic stroke (3.18 vs. 2.23) (Song et al. 2004). For BP ≥180/≥110 mm Hg, the difference in relative risk was even more pronounced between hemorrhagic and ischemic stroke (28.83 vs. 9.56, respectively).

2.5 HOME REMEDIES FOR HYPERTENSION

Faced with side effects and low socioeconomic status reducing the affordability of medication, people in developing countries have sought the use of home remedies for the treatment of hypertension. Some of these are

- *Garlic*: Garlic contains the active compound allicin, which is known to increase nitric oxide production, which relaxes the muscles and results in vasodilatation. Studies have shown mixed results for garlic, with a decrease in BP for people who have increased systolic BP. Garlic preparations have also been found to be superior to placebo in reducing hypertension.
- *Annona muricata* (a species of plant from the custard apple tree family) and *celery*: A study in China where celery juice was given to patients three times a day showed a significant decrease in BP in 16 patients.
- *Ginger*: Ginger is another common ingredient used in cooking at home, specifically in Asian cooking. It improves blood circulation and promotes vasodilatation. A study showed that crude extract of ginger (0.3–3.0 mg/kg) induced a dose-dependent decrease in the arterial BP of anesthetized rats. However, there have been few human trials with low doses and inconclusive results.

- *Dark chocolate*: A growing body of clinical research also shows that daily consumption of 46–105 g dark or milk chocolate (*Theobroma cacao*), providing 213–500 mg of cocoa polyphenols, can lower systolic BP by about 5 mm Hg and diastolic BP by about 3 mm Hg (Tabassum and Ahmad 2011; Taubert et al. 2003).

Radishes, green oats, ajwain, linseed, and flaxseed have also been investigated for their hypotensive effects, but most of these studies have been done *in vitro*. More research needs to be done to investigate the effectiveness of natural foods to lower BP.

2.6 NUTRIENTS TO PREVENT AND CONTROL HYPERTENSION

Various prospective cohort studies and randomized controlled clinical trials have shown that hypertension and its associated complications are mainly caused by modifiable lifestyle risk factors and thus are highly preventable. Among these risk factors, nutrition plays a pivotal role in the pathogenesis of the disease. Due to the high prevalence of hypertension and its significance in cardiovascular disease, Healthy People 2020 includes hypertension prevention and control as one of the most critical public health goals of the coming decade (Office of Disease Prevention and Health Promotion 2015). This section of the chapter will focus on discussing the different nutrients and how they interplay with hypertension.

2.6.1 HARMFUL NUTRIENTS

2.6.1.1 Sodium

The positive relationship between Na intake and high BP has been established through various ecological, experimental, and epidemiological human studies. The INTERSALT study on men and women aged 20–59 years from 32 different countries is one such example of a standardized global epidemiological study. A positive independent linear relation between 24-hour Na excretion and systolic BP was found for both men and women, young and elderly, in 8344 normotensive people (those having normal BP) (Stamler 1997). Meta-analysis of 34 trials to determine the effect of long-term modest salt reduction on BP, plasma renin activity, aldosterone, noradrenalin (norepinephrine), adrenaline (epinephrine), total cholesterol, low-density lipoprotein, high-density lipoprotein, and triglycerides demonstrated that long-term modest salt reduction by 4.4 g/day on average caused a significant fall in BP in both hypertensive (average of 5/3 mm Hg) and normotensive (average of 2/1 mm Hg) subjects. An overall reduction of 6 g/day in salt led to a drop in systolic BP by 5.8 mm Hg after adjusting for age, ethnicity, and BP status (He et al. 2013).

Na is usually consumed in the diet in the form of sodium chloride (NaCl; i.e., salt), which is composed of 40% Na. The following are Na equivalents for different amounts of salt: 1/4 teaspoon salt=575 mg Na; 1/2 teaspoon salt=1150 mg Na; 3/4 teaspoon salt=1725 mg Na, 1 teaspoon salt=2300 mg Na (American Heart Association 2015). According to the Dietary Guidelines for Americans 2010, the recommended amount of Na intake is 2300 mg/day for ages 2 years and above. Salt at the dinner table is not the main contributor of dietary Na. Sodium adds up quickly when consumed in various amounts in the diet, including through packaged, canned, and processed foods and restaurant meals. A lower amount of 1500 mg/day is recommended for people with greater salt sensitivity, including African Americans, anyone above 51 years, or those diagnosed with hypertension, diabetes, or chronic kidney disease (Centers for Disease Control 2012).

2.6.1.2 Saturated and Trans Fats

When it comes to how fat intake affects BP, the quantity and type of fat matters. Saturated fats are the type of fats found mostly in animal food sources such as red meat, poultry, and full-fat dairy products. From a chemical standpoint these fats have no carbon–carbon double bonds in their fatty acid chains. An excess of saturated fats and trans fats in the diet can lead to an imbalance in body cholesterol levels, tipping the balance toward the more harmful low-density lipoprotein (LDL) cholesterol (Ganguly and Pierce 2015). LDL cholesterol stimulates the process of atherosclerosis, resulting in the narrowing of the arterial lumen and the hardening of the arterial wall, thus increasing BP. A study showed a significant decrease in LDL cholesterol when trans fats were isocalorically replaced with polyunsaturated and monounsaturated fatty acids (Ganguly et al. 2013). In addition, trans fats reduce the levels of high-density lipoprotein (HDL), which is also known as the "good cholesterol." Both saturated fats and trans fats can stimulate the release of proinflammatory cytokines such as interleukin-6 (IL-6), tumor necrosis factor (TNF), intracellular adhesion molecule, and vascular adhesion molecule, resulting in inflammation. A study showed that red blood cell saturated-fat levels reflecting long-term dietary intake were positively associated with IL-6 and the composite inflammation measure and marginally associated with C-reactive protein (CRP), after adjusting for age, sex, body mass index, race, smoking, statin use, aspirin use, trans and unsaturated fatty acids, and omega 3 fatty acids (Lin et al. 2014). CRP is the inflammatory marker with the strongest association with hypertension. Many clinical trials have shown that hypertensive patients have higher plasma CRP levels than normotensive patients (Stumpf et al. 2009). Excessive inflammation also promotes atherosclerosis, eventually contributing to an increase in BP (Lusis 2000).

Most trans fats are industrially produced by partially hydrogenating vegetable oils for easier cooking and longer shelf life. Sources of trans fats include all fried foods, fast foods, pastries, margarines, shortenings, cake mixes, frozen/packaged foods, and so on. When reading food labels, caution should be exercised as foods containing less that 0.5 g trans fat are labeled as 0 g trans fat as per the Food and Drug Administration regulations. This hidden trans fat can quickly add up in the diet. It is important to check the ingredients of the food product to see if there is any hydrogenated vegetable oil included in the product (Figure 2.1).

2.6.1.3 Alcohol

Alcohol contributes 7 Kcal/g, which can lead to excessive weight gain, another risk factor for hypertension. The calories coming from alcohol are empty calories due to high amounts of sugar and provide no nutritional value (Sheps 2015). Some studies show a protective effect of moderate alcohol consumption; however, this protective

---

Making Smart Choices to Reduce Consumption of Saturated and Trans Fats

- Read nutrition labels thoroughly. Check total fat in one serving. Be sure to add up the number of servings you can consume in one sitting.
- Check saturated fats and trans fats in one serving.
- When reading food labels, caution should be exercised as foods containing less that 0.5 g trans fat are labeled as 0 g trans fat as per Food and Drug Administration regulations. This labeling is not universal.
- Check for partially hydrogenated oil in ingredients to see if the product includes trans fat.
- Make sure most of your daily fats are mono- or polyunsaturated fats.
- Read nutrition information on menus if eating out.
- Eat nuts instead of cookies for a snack.
- Add assorted nuts to salads.
- Replace some meats with fish. Consume two meals per week with fish.
- Cook in vegetable oil instead of solid fats such as butter or margarine.
- Choose lean meats as much as possible.
- Watch portion sizes.
- Choose low-fat or skim dairy products.
- Limit baked goods, packaged foods, and desserts.
- Choose healthier cooking methods such as baking, grilling, boiling, poaching, stir-frying, roasting, blanching, and so on, instead of deep frying.

FIGURE 2.1 Tips for reducing the consumption of saturated and trans fats.

effect is nullified due to unmeasured confounders such as diet, lifestyle, and patterns of drinking and reverse causality. Associations between high doses of alcohol intake and blood pressure elevation have been shown in different genders, multiple racial and ethnic groups, and disparate international populations across all adult age groups (Kiatsky and Gunderson 2008). Men who regularly consume 8 or more units of alcohol per day are four times as likely to develop hypertension. Similarly, women regularly consuming more than 6 units of alcohol per day double their risk of developing hypertension (Department of Health, Home Office, Department for Education and Skills, Department for Culture, Media and Sport 2007). The risk attributed to hypertension from regular alcohol consumption is 16%, and an approximately 1 mm Hg rise in systolic BP is observed for each 10 g of alcohol consumed. Recommendations for moderate drinking include two drinks a day for men under 65 years old and one drink a day for those 65 and over. For women, one drink a day is the cutoff point regardless of age. The grade B–level recommendation is that the total number of alcoholic drinks per week should not exceed 14 standard drinks for men and 9 standard drinks for women. One standard drink is considered to be equivalent to 13.6 g or 17.2 mL of ethanol or approximately 44 mL of 80-proof (40%) spirits, 355 mL of 5% beer, or 148 mL of 12% wine (Daskalopoulou et al. 2015). Those with hypertension should be asked about alcohol consumption and if confirmed should be given appropriate screening for alcohol dependence such as the

"Cut down, Annoyed, Guilty, and Eye-opener" (CAGE) substance abuse screening tool. Advice on avoiding or moderating drinking should be given if patients are not alcohol dependent.

2.6.2 Protective Nutrients

2.6.2.1 Potassium

In the kidney, the Na/K pump in the cells regulates BP by maintaining Na (sodium) and K (potassium) concentrations across the membrane to maintain total body fluid volume (Karlish 2008). Reduced K intake results in the retention of Na in the kidneys, which increases BP. Increasing K intake stimulates natriuresis and suppresses plasma renin function (Sharma et al. 2014). Therefore, K levels in the body play a part in BP regulation. A population-based study was done on 1285 subjects aged 25–64 years who were free from any medication affecting BP. Their BP and K excretion were measured by collecting a 12 h urine sample. An inverse association was found between urinary excretion of K and BP with adjustment for age and body mass index (BMI). BP increased as the Na:K ratio became higher (Rodriguez et al. 2014). A meta-analysis of 22 randomized clinical trials and 11 cohort studies reported that an increase in K intake decreased systolic and diastolic BP (Aburto et al. 2013) Other population-based studies have found no association between hypertension and dietary K; however, this may have been due to differences in the amount of salt consumption in each study, as K intake mitigates BP in response to a high Na diet (Sharma et al. 2014). In another study, with a large, nationally representative sample from a National Health and Nutrition Examination Survey (NHANES) group with high BP had significantly lower consumption of K and a higher Na:K ratio than those with normal BP (Zhang et al. 2013). People with impaired urinary K excretion can be at risk of hyperkalemia and hence need to be careful in monitoring their K intake (Institute of Medicine 2005). High K intake has been known to negate the effect of elevated Na intake on blood pressure (Rodriguez et al. 2014).

The dietary guideline for K is an intake of 4700 mg/day in adults (WHO 2012). Rich sources of K include sweet potatoes, potatoes, bananas, spinach, tomatoes, and other green vegetables.

2.6.2.2 Calcium

Many population studies, epidemiological studies, and clinical trials have established an inverse relationship between calcium (Ca) and BP with Ca deficiency leading to a rise in BP. Ca is found in equilibrium in the serum in its three forms: ionized, protein bound, or complexed (Hazari et al. 2012). A high-dairy diet significantly reduces systolic and diastolic BP by 2 mm Hg, which correlates with a decrease in intracellular Ca (Hilpert et al. 2009). However, with respect to dairy it is important to choose the right reduced-fat, low-Na versions, as processed cheese products and spreads can be high in Na. Ca supplementation mitigates the hypertensive effect of NaCl via changes in vitamin D and parathyroid hormone (PTH) concentration (Kotchen et al., 1998). PTH increases osteolysis from the bone and the reabsorption of Ca from the kidneys, while vitamin D promotes absorption from the intestine, thereby increasing serum Ca concentration. Ca and Na then compete for reabsorption by the kidneys and high Ca intake can stimulate urinary Na excretion.

Ca is found primarily in dairy products, including milk, yogurt, and cheese. The recommended daily allowance for adults is 1000 mg/day met by 2–3 servings of dairy. One cup of milk, yogurt, or soymilk (soy beverage), 1.5 oz of natural cheese, or 2 oz of processed cheese can be considered 1 serving from the dairy group.

2.6.2.3 Magnesium

Assessing magnesium (Mg) status is difficult as most Mg is deposited in the cells and bones. Mg deficiency can only result through poor dietary intake or chronic alcoholism, as otherwise the body has its own mechanism of conserving Mg by limiting urinary excretion. Though Mg does not directly interplay with the pathophysiology of hypertension, it plays a role in the active transport of Ca and K across cell membranes. Both Ca and K affect BP. Furthermore, Mg also is involved in the production of prostaglandin E1, which is a vasodilator and thus lowers BP. Severe Mg deficiency can lead to hypocalcemia and hypokalemia, thus raising BP.

A meta-analysis of 22 studies with 1173 normotensive and hypertensive adults provided evidence that Mg supplementation for 3–24 weeks decreases systolic BP by 3–4 mm Hg and diastolic BP by 2–3 mm Hg (Kass et al. 2012). Another systematic review and meta-analysis of prospective studies showed that increased serum Mg lowered the risk of CVD (DelGobbo et al. 2013).

Mg is abundant in the body. Due to an increase in the consumption of processed foods, most people do not have enough Mg in their diets. Mg is found in varying amounts in drinking water and is also found naturally in green leafy vegetables such as spinach, legumes, nuts, seeds, and fortified cereals and whole grains.

2.6.2.4 Monounsaturated and Polyunsaturated Fats

Monounsaturated fats are usually liquids at room temperature but have the tendency to solidify if cooled. Olive oil, canola oil, sesame oil, and safflower oil are examples of sources of monounsaturated fats. The first major study investigating diet and lifestyle as risk factors for CVD including hypertension was called the Seven Countries Study as it investigated this across contrasting cultures. It was through this study that the health benefits of monounsaturated fats were discovered, as people in the Mediterranean region consumed diets rich in fat but had minimal risk of CVD. Monounsaturated fat provides 9 cal/g as with any other fat; however, unlike saturated and trans fats, it raises "good cholesterol" (i.e., HDL levels) in the blood.

Polyunsaturated fats can be further categorized into omega-3 and omega-6, depending on the distance of the first carbon–carbon double bond from the beginning of the chain. Polyunsaturated fats are "essential fats"; that is, they are required for body functions. However, the body cannot synthesize them. Rich sources of omega-3 include fatty fish such as salmon, sardines, and mackerel and rich sources of omega-6 include soybean oil, sunflower oil, and canola oil. Both omega-3 and omega-6 fats have been shown to reduce BP to varying extents. There are no dietary recommendations for mono- and polyunsaturated fats; however, out of the 25%–50% fat in the diet, it is advisable that mono- and polyunsaturated fats constitute most of the fat sources. There are studies providing evidence that linolenic acid, EPA,

DHA, and linoleic acid reduce inflammation and LDL cholesterol, and hence BP, and raise HDL cholesterol levels. However, more research is needed for this claim to be conclusive, with more focus on whether the ratio of omega-6 to omega-3 is to be maintained at 2:1 or 4:1 (University of Maryland, Medical Center 2013).

2.7 DIETARY PATTERNS TO PREVENT AND CONTROL HYPERTENSION

2.7.1 DIETARY APPROACHES TO STOP HYPERTENSION

The BP-lowering effects of individual nutrients are difficult to observe as the effects are too small to detect. The cumulative effect can become more pronounced when several nutrients with BP-lowering capabilities are consumed together. The Dietary Approaches to Stop Hypertension (DASH) trials were a milestone in lifestyle intervention strategies for the prevention and treatment of hypertension, to the point that now the DASH trial is recognized as a separate dietary pattern called the "DASH diet." The trial was a multicenter, randomized feeding study testing the effects of dietary patterns on BP. In this trial, 8813 people were screened, out of which 459 participants were chosen whose demographic characteristics most closely resembled the target population and study requirements. The sample population consisted of healthy men and women with an average age of 46 years and with systolic BP of less than 160 mm Hg and diastolic BP within 80–95 mm Hg.

The intervention was designed to last 8 weeks. Participants were also given two packets of salt, each containing 200 mg of Na, for discretionary use. Alcohol was limited to no more than two beverages per day, and caffeine intake was limited to no more than three caffeinated beverages per day. Participants were randomly assigned to the following three dietary groups:

- *Control diet*: A typical American diet with K, Mg, and Ca levels close to the 25th percentile of U.S. adults. The macronutrient profile also corresponded with the average consumption by the population.
- *Fruit/vegetable diet*: K and Mg levels matched the 75th percentile of U.S. consumption, with high amounts of fiber and fewer snacks and sweets. The diet included 8–10 servings of fruits per day, which was twice the average level of consumption at 4.3 servings per day.
- *Combination diet*: This diet was rich in fruits, vegetables, and low-fat dairy foods, and had reduced saturated fat, total fat, and cholesterol. The diet included 2.7 servings of dairy per day. K, Mg, and Ca levels were at the 75th percentile, like the fruit and vegetable diet. Fiber and protein were also a part of this diet in substantial amounts.

The intervention consisted of a 7-day cycle menu and all diets were tailored to four caloric levels (1600, 2100, 2600, and 3100 Kcal) for adjustments to ensure weight maintenance. The foods included in the menu were commonly available in markets. All three diets used the same brands of food products. The results showed a change in gradient for BP across all three diets; however, the combination diet showed the most significant reduction of 5.5 mm Hg systolic BP and 3.0 mm Hg diastolic BP. The fruit and vegetable diet had a somewhat lesser reduction of 2.8 mm Hg systolic BP and 3.0 mm Hg diastolic BP. These reductions were observed for both normotensive and hypertensive subjects, with greater reductions in those who were hypertensive. Interaction between hypertension status and diet was significant for systolic BP and was marginally significant for diastolic BP. The results showed that the use of the DASH diet on these participants significantly lowered systolic BP compared with the fruit and vegetable diet and control diet (Moore et al. 2001). The findings remained significant even after adjustment for potential confounders, including changes in weight and urinary sodium excretion. The reductions were seen after 2 weeks of adherence and the effect was sustained for 6 weeks after. Known diet-related determinants of blood pressure such as Na intake, body weight, and alcohol consumption could not have confounded the study findings as changes in these confounders were small and similar across all three diets (Appel et al. 1997).

The DASH sodium trial was also conducted on a subset of the DASH trial sample. Participants were randomly divided into six groups: DASH diet with higher (3300 mg/day) Na intake, DASH diet with intermediate (2400 mg/day) Na intake, DASH diet with low (1500 mg/day) Na intake, control diet with high (3300 mg/day) Na intake, control diet with intermediate (2400 mg/day) Na intake, and control diet with low (1500 mg/day) Na intake. The subjects' weight was monitored and systolic BP was compared across the three sodium levels within each diet and across the two diets within each Na level. Results showed that Na reduction with the DASH diet lowered BP to an extent not demonstrated by any other nonpharmacologic treatment. Reductions were greater for hypertensive subjects compared with normotensive subjects (Svetkey et al. 1999). Compared with the higher Na control diet, the DASH diet reduced systolic BP by an average of 5.9, 7.2, and 8.9 mm Hg for the higher, intermediate, and lower Na intakes, respectively. Diastolic BP was reduced by 2.9, 3.5, and 4.5 mm Hg for the higher, intermediate, and lower Na intake levels. Reducing Na intake in the control diet from higher to intermediate levels reduced systolic BP by an average of 2.1 mm Hg and by 6.7 mm Hg with the lower Na intake. Reducing Na intakes to the lower level resulted in significantly lower systolic blood pressure in all sex, race, and hypertension status subgroups with the exception of nonblack participants without hypertension.

Recommended servings for a 2000-calorie DASH diet include the following:

- *Grains*: 6–8 servings/day—Focus on whole grains as they contribute more fiber and nutrients than their refined versions.
- *Vegetables*: 4–5 servings/day—If choosing frozen or canned vegetables, low-Na options should be chosen.
- *Fruits*: 4–5 servings/day—Fruits add fiber, K, and Mg to the diet and are low in fat, with the exception of avocadoes and coconuts. Half a cup of fruit juice can count as 1 serving of fruit; however, when choosing canned fruit or juice, "no sugar added" versions should be consumed.
- *Dairy*: 2–3 servings/day—Choose low-fat or fat-free dairy products. In case of lactose intolerance, choose lactose-free dairy products. Consume regular or fat-free cheese in moderation as cheeses are also high in Na.

- *Lean meat, poultry, fish*: ≤6 servings/day—These are a good source of protein, B vitamins, iron, and zinc. It is advisable to trim away skin and fat when cooking meat and to choose heart-healthy fish such as salmon, herring, or tuna.
- *Nuts, seeds, legumes*: 4–5 servings/week—Nuts, seeds, and legumes are a rich source of phytochemicals, K, Mg, protein, fiber, and healthy monounsaturated and polyunsaturated fats.
- *Fats and oils*: 2–3 servings/day—Avoid saturated and trans fats. Saturated fats should contribute less than 6% of total calories. The DASH diet limits calories from total fat to 27% of daily calories. Monounsaturated and polyunsaturated fats should be preferred.
- *Sweets*: ≤5 servings/week—Examples of 1 serving include 1 tbsp sugar, jelly, or jam, 1/2 cup sorbet, or 1 cup (8 oz) lemonade.
- *Alcohol*: ≤2 drinks/day for men and ≤1 drink/day for women. (Mayo Clinic 2013)

The DASH diet is to complement and not supplant current recommendations. Other versions suitable for vegetarians and for weight loss have been made (Heller 2004). The DASH diet cookbook is also available to suggest recipes that fulfill recommended servings of all food groups as per the diet protocol (Heller and Rodgers 2013).

2.7.2   MEDITERRANEAN DIET

This diet is based on traditional eating patterns of countries surrounding the Mediterranean Sea, including Greece, Italy, and Spain. The diet gained recognition in the 1990s after the findings of the Seven Countries Study, which was the world's first multicountry epidemiological study investigating the relationships between diet, lifestyle, and CVD. The findings of the study showed that coronary deaths in the United States and Northern Europe exceeded those in Southern Europe even when other risk factors such as age, cholesterol, BP, smoking status, physical activity, and weight were adjusted. The main difference was in the dietary patterns across these regions, where the dietary pattern in Southern Europe came to be known as the "Mediterranean diet."

Figure 2.2 shows the components of the Mediterranean diet in the form of a pyramid.

The diet is suitable for most adults; however, children and pregnant women may require additional supplements. The main components of the diet are as follows:

- Eating primarily plant-based foods, such as fruits and vegetables, whole grains, legumes, and nuts with high levels of antioxidants. Vegetables common to the Mediterranean diet include artichokes, arugula, beets, broccoli, Brussels sprouts, cabbage, carrots, celery, celeriac, chicory, collard greens, cucumbers, dandelion greens, eggplant, fennel, kale, leeks, lemons, lettuce, mâche, mushrooms, mustard greens, nettles, okra, onions (red, sweet, white), peas, peppers, potatoes, pumpkin, parsley, radishes, rutabaga,

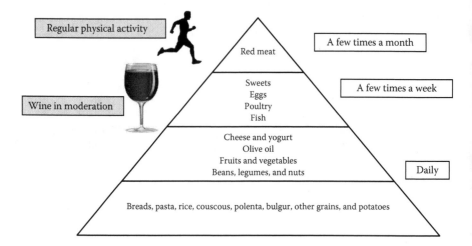

FIGURE 2.2 The Mediterranean diet pyramid. (Adapted from Oldways Preservation and Exchange Trust, Harvard School of Public Health and the European World Health Organization, The Classic Mediterranean Diet: A Cultural Model for Healthy Eating, 1994.)

scallions, shallots, spinach, sweet potatoes, turnips, and zucchini. With respect to fruits, fruit juice provides only some of the nutritional value of whole fruit. When drinking fruit juice, portion control and attention to total calories is advised. It is advisable to drink "no added sugar" versions. Fruit "drinks" do not provide the nutritional value of fruit juices. Fruits common to the traditional Mediterranean diet include apples, apricots, avocados, cherries, clementines, dates, figs, grapefruits, grapes, melons, nectarines, olives, oranges, peaches, pears, pomegranates, strawberries, tangerines, and tomatoes.

- Eating whole grains instead of refined grains—for example, oats, rice, rye, barley, corn, couscous, faro, and millet.
- Choosing low-fat or fat-free dairy products.
- Replacing butter with healthy fats such as olive oil and other healthier fats.
- Using herbs and spices instead of salt to flavor foods. Herbs and spices common to the traditional Mediterranean diet include anise, basil, bay leaf, chilies, cloves, cumin, fennel, garlic, lavender, marjoram, mint, oregano, parsley, pepper, pul biber, rosemary, sage, savory, sumac, tarragon, thyme, za'atar.
- Limiting red meat to no more than a few times a month. Choose small and lean portions. Avoid high-fat, high-sodium, and processed meats.
- Eating fish and poultry at least twice a week. Fresh or water-packed tuna, salmon, trout, mackerel, and herring are healthy choices.
- Drinking red wine in moderation (optional). No more than 148 mL of wine daily for women of all ages and men older than age 65, and no more than 296 mL of wine daily for younger men.

- Grill, boil, broil, and bake food instead of deep frying and other cooking methods using high amounts of fat.

The PREDIMED trial was a multicenter randomized parallel group study conducted in Spain to analyze the influence of the Mediterranean diet on BP. Participants were randomized into three intervention groups: Mediterranean diet plus extra virgin olive oil supplementation, Mediterranean diet plus mixed nuts, and a control diet low in fat. Results showed a greater reduction in BP in the Mediterranean diet plus extra virgin olive oil group when compared with the Mediterranean diet plus nuts group and the control group. The Mediterranean diet with extra virgin olive oil reduced diastolic BP by 1.53 mm Hg, while the Mediterranean diet with nuts reduced it by 0.65 mm Hg. But these differences were nonsignificant after multivariate adjustments. However, significant reductions were seen in diastolic BP for both Mediterranean diet groups compared with the control group, and these reductions continued to remain significant even after multivariate adjustments (Toledo et al. 2013).

Another meta-analysis looked at six randomized control trials (RCTs) investigating the effect of the Mediterranean diet on BP. Results showed a pooled estimated reduction of 1.44 mm Hg in systolic BP and 0.70 mm Hg in diastolic BP (Nissemsohn et al. 2015).

2.7.3 THERAPEUTIC LIFESTYLE CHANGES

The National Cholesterol Education Program under the U.S. National Institutes of Health developed Therapeutic Lifestyle Changes, also known as the TLC diet, which was clinically shown to lower LDL cholesterol by 20%–30%. The diet was later endorsed by the American Heart Association. The diet focuses on lowering LDL cholesterol levels. It does not target weight loss but instead promotes the maintenance of ideal body weight and recommended caloric intake to balance energy intake and expenditure. The main features of the diet are as follows:

- Intake of saturated fat should be kept below 7% of the total calorie intake: 8%–10% LDL reduction
- Daily cholesterol intake should be kept below 200 mg: 3%–5% LDL reduction
- Na intake must be limited to 2400 mg/day
- Only 25–35% of daily total calories should come from fat intake
- Calorie intake should be kept to a level needed for maintaining healthy weight: 5%–10% LDL reduction
- Physical activity must be maintained regularly along with the diet—that is, at least 30 min of exercise each day
- Healthier carbohydrate intake with a focus on whole grains instead of refined grains
- Protein: 15% within the recommended amount of 10%–35%
- Fiber: 25–30 g/day with 5–10 g soluble fibers: 3%–5% LDL reduction
- Plant stanols/sterols: 2 g/day, 5%–15% LDL reduction

- Polyunsaturated fat: Up to 10% of total calories
- Monounsaturated fat: Up to 20% of total calories

The TLC diet requires a certain literacy level, as reading nutrition facts labels, daily percentage values, and ingredients and understanding label language is a skill required to achieve the desired outcomes (U.S. Department of Health and Human Services, National Institutes of Health, National Heart Lung and Blood Institute 2005). The TLC diet has also been found to be an effective medical nutrition therapy for hypertension through an indirect reduction in cholesterol levels, which are a risk factor for hypertension.

2.7.4 Dietary Portfolio

St Michael's hospital in collaboration with the University of Toronto devised a dietary portfolio of cholesterol-lowering foods. The diet features entail what any heart-healthy diet would have, including the low consumption of saturated fat and the increased consumption of fruits, vegetables, beans, and whole grains. However, the diet has added component of consuming heart-healthy diet specific foods. On a 2000-calorie diet, apart from the heart-healthy diet, a person should add the following from the dietary portfolio:

- 2 tsp of stanol-rich margarine, such as Benecol
- A handful of nuts each day
- 2 servings/day of soy-based foods, such as soy milk or soy burgers
- 2 servings/day of foods rich in soluble fiber, such as oats, psyllium, barley, okra, and eggplant (LeWine 2011)

Though the diet is known for cholesterol reduction, secondary analysis of the data from a study conducted in 2011 showed that the dietary portfolio lowers BP by 2% in comparison with the DASH diet. This 2% reduction was in addition to the 5–10 mm Hg reduction by the DASH diet. The DASH diet had higher compliance rates than the dietary portfolio, but the BP-lowering effect of the dietary portfolio was more pronounced (Jenkins 2015).

2.8 NUTRITIONAL COUNSELING FOR HYPERTENSIVE PATIENTS

2.8.1 Nutritional History Taking

The following questions need to be asked of a hypertensive patient: age, weight and history of weight gain, height, medical history, past history of CVD—for example, stroke/heart attack/diabetes, chest pain while exercising, leg muscle tightness or fatigue when walking or climbing stairs, kidney disease/protein in urine, smoking status, cholesterol levels, BP readings, family history of CVD, psychosocial and environmental factors (employment status, family situation [married/divorced/single/children], education level)—and diet history (fat intake, servings of fruit and vegetables, fiber intake, dairy intake, intake of red meat, meal spacing, alcohol consumption, Na intake (use of salt/processed foods), fast-food consumption/eating out, reading nutrition labels).

2.8.2 PHYSICAL EXAMINATION

This should consist of a BP measurement; an examination of the heart for increased rate, size, murmurs, or arrhythmias; an examination of the abdomen for enlarged kidneys and abnormal aortic pulsation; an examination of the neck for carotid bruits, an enlarged thyroid gland, and distended veins; a peripheral pulse measurement; checking the lower extremities for edema and pulses; a neurological assessment; and an examination of optic fundi. Investigations should include urinalysis, complete blood count, blood glucose, K, Ca, creatinine, uric acid, cholesterol, HDL, LDL, triglycerides, and electrocardiograph (ECG).

2.8.3 LIFESTYLE MODIFICATIONS TO MANAGE HYPERTENSION AND PREHYPERTENSION

Key modification: DASH
Recommendations are as follows:

- Focus on heart-healthy fats: that is, polyunsaturated and monounsaturated fats (sources include olive oil, canola oil, etc.)
- Eat at least 5 servings of fruits and vegetables every day
- Consume 2–3 servings of low-fat or reduced-fat dairy per day
- Reduce Na intake to 2400 mg/day or NaCl to 6 g/day
- Maintain adequate K intake if not taking K-sparing medications (sources include bananas, kiwi, avocado, potatoes with skin, nuts, yogurt)
- Among all grains consumed, half should be whole grains
- Limit red meat: Consume moderate amounts of lean unprocessed meats, poultry, and fish (2 servings of fish per week)

Key modification: Physical activity
Recommendations are as follows:

- Avoid isometric exercises that may raise BP unless professionally super-vised—for example, weight lifting
- At least 30 min of moderate-intensity physical activity for 5 days a week—for example, brisk walking (this can be spaced into three bouts of 10 min exercise throughout the day)

Key modification: Reducing Na intake
Recommendations are as follows:

- Choose foods that say "sodium-free," "very low sodium," "reduced sodium," "light in sodium," "unsalted"
- Restrict the use of table salt

- Be spicy, not salty! Use alternative herbs and spices for flavoring—for example, bay leaves, nutmeg, basil, oregano, curry powder, ginger, garlic, and so on
- Avoid smoked, cured, frozen, canned, processed, and fast foods. When using canned foods, rinse them thoroughly with water

Key modification: Limit alcohol consumption
Recommendations are as follows:

- No more than two standard drinks per day for men and one standard drink per day for women

Key modification: Reading and understanding food labels
Recommendations are as follows:

- Reduced or less calories: At least 25% fewer calories per serving than the regular version
- Trans fat–free foods are *not* trans fat free: <0.5 g trans fat per serving can be labeled as "trans fat free." Food low in trans fat may be high in saturated fat, so be sure to check
- Only products that state "no hydrogenated oil" or "hydrogenated oil free" have 0 g trans fats
- Fat free: ≤0.5 g/serving
- Low saturated fat: ≤1 g/serving
- Low fat: ≤3 g/serving
- Reduced fat: At least 25% less fat per serving than the regular version
- Light (in fat): Half the fat of the regular version
- Low cholesterol: ≤20 mg/serving; saturated fat: ≤2 g/serving
- Low sodium: ≤140 mg/serving
- Lean: <10 g of fat, ≤4.5 g of saturated fat, <95 mg of cholesterol per serving
- Extra Lean: <5 g of fat, <2 g of saturated fat, <95 mg of cholesterol per serving
- Calorie free: <5 calories/serving
- Low calorie: ≤40 calories/serving

Key modification: Weight loss and maintenance
Recommendations are as follows:

- A 1% loss in body weight decreases systolic BP by 1 mm Hg
- Achieve and maintain BMI ≤25 kg/m^3; waist circumference <94 cm for men and <80 cm for women (Huang et al. 2008)

2.9 CASE STUDIES

2.9.1 Case Study 1

A 50-year-old male school cricket coach from Pakistan weighs 220 lbs and is 6 ft 1 in. in height. His blood pressure is 160/100 mm Hg. He has a history of stage 2 hypertension. He walks 30 min daily, four times a day. He takes 4 g of sodium in his diet per day. He was previously a chain smoker. His main complaint is that he is finding adherence to a low-salt diet difficult due to the bland taste. Give a response to the following:

- Formulate a diet plan for the patient to increase adherence and reduce sodium intake as well as meet all energy and nutrient needs.

2.9.2   CASE STUDY 2

Mr. SB is a 40-year-old male, smoker, active, with no significant medical history and who is on no medication, with confirmed elevation in blood pressure (BP) on repeated visits. He has complaints of headaches and visual disturbances. His father had hypertension and ischemic heart disease for 20 years. His brother aged 51 has hypertension too. Mr. SB was treated for mental depression for 3 years in the past. On physical examination, he weighs 96 kg, has a height of 178 cm, BP at 150/90 mm Hg, a pulse rate of 76 bpm, and a normal systematic examination. Laboratory findings are Na 140, K 3.9, Cl 102, FBS 115, OGTT 160, BUN 15, creatinine 1.1, cholesterol 270, LDL 210, HDL 45, and triglycerides 250. Give responses to the following:

1. What is the initial diagnosis for Mr. SB?
2. What lifestyle modification strategies does he need to employ?

REFERENCES

Aburto, Nancy J., Sara Hanson, Hialy Guitierrez, Lee Hopper, Paul Elliott, and Francesco P. Cappucio. 2013. Effect of increased potassium intake on cardiovascular risk factors and disease: Systematic reviews and meta-analyses. *BMJ* 346: f1374.

American Heart Association. 2015. Shaking the salt habit. Accessed April 20, 2016. http://www.heart.org/HEARTORG/Conditions/HighBloodPressure/PreventionTreatmentofHigh BloodPressure/Shaking-the-Salt-Habit_UCM_303241_Article.jsp#.VxuLXPl97IU.

Appel, Lawrence J., Thomas J. Moore, Eva Obarzanek, William M. Vollmer, Laura P. Svetkey, Frank M. Sacks, George A. Bray et al. 1997. A clinical trial of the effects of dietary patterns on blood pressure. *N Eng J Med* 336: 1117–1124.

Carnethon, Mercedes R., Natalie S. Evans, Timothy S. Church, Cora E. Lewis, Pamela J. Schreiner, David R. Jacobs, Barbara Sternfeld, and Stephen Sidney. 2010. Joint associations of physical activity and aerobic fitness on the development of incident hypertension coronary artery risk development in young adults. *Hypertension* 56 (1): 49–55.

Centers for Disease Control. 2012. Get the facts: Sodium and dietary guidelines. http://www.cdc.gov/salt/pdfs/sodium_dietary_guidelines.pdf. October 16, 2015.

Chobanian, Aram V., George L. Bakris, Henry R. Black, William C. Cushman, Lee A. Green, Joseph L. Izzo Jr, Daniel W. Jones et al. 2003. The 7th Report of the Joint National Committee on Prevention, Detection, Evaluation and Treatment of High Blood Pressure: The JNC 7 Report. *JAMA* 289 (19): 2560–2572.

Chung, Irene, and Gregory Y. H. Lip. 2003. White coat hypertension: Not so benign after all? *J Hum Hypertens* 17: 807–809.

Collins, Rory, Richard Peto, Stephen MacMahon, Jon Godwin, Nawab Qizilbash, Patricia R. Hebert, K. A. Eberlein et al. 1990. Blood pressure, stroke and coronary heart disease. Part 2: Short-term reductions in blood pressure; Overview of randomized drug trials in their epidemiological context. *Lancet* 335 (8693): 827–838.

Daskalopoulou, Stella S., Doreen M. Rabi, Kelly B. Zarnke, Kaberi Dasgupta, Kara Nerenberg, Lyne Cloutier, Mark Gelfer et al. 2015. The 2015 Canadian Hypertension Education Program recommendations for blood pressure measurement, diagnosis, assessment of risk, prevention and treatment of hypertension. *Can J Cardiol* 31 (5): 549–568.

Del Gobbo, Liana C., Fumiaki Imamura, Jason H. Y. Wu, Marcia C. de Oliveira Otto, Stephanie E. Chiuve, and Dariush Mozaffarian. 2013. Circulating and dietary magnesium and risk of cardiovascular disease: A systematic review and meta-analysis of prospective studies. *Am J Clin Nutr* 98 (1): 160–173.

Department of Health, Home Office, Department for Education and Skills, Department for Culture, Media and Sport. 2007. *Safe Sensible, Social: The Next Steps in the National Alcohol Strategy.* London: Department of Health, Home Office, Department for Education and Skills, Department for Culture, Media and Sport, Crown.

Ganguly, Riya, and Grant N. Pierce. 2015. Toxicity of dietary trans fats. *Food Chem Toxicol* 78: 170–176.

Ganguly, Riya, Matthew S. Lytwyn, and Grant N. Pierce. 2013. Differential effects of trans and polyunsaturated fatty acids in ischemia/reperfusion injury and its associated cardiovascular disease states. *Curr Pharm Des* 19 (39): 6858–6863.

Haider, Agha W., Martin G. Larson, Stanley S. Franklin, and Daniel Levy. 2003. Systolic blood pressure, diastolic blood pressure and pulse pressure as predictors of risk for congestive heart failure in the Framingham Heart Study. *Ann Intern Med* 138 (1): 10–16.

Hazari, Mohammed Abdul Hannan, Mehnaaz Sameera Arifuddin, Syed Muzzakar, and Vontela Devender Reddy. 2012. Serum calcium level in hypertension. *N Am J Med Sci* 4 (11): 569–572.

He, Feng J., Jiafu Li, and Graham A. MacGregor. 2013. Effect of long-term modest salt reduction on blood pressure: Cochrane systematic review and meta-analysis of randomized trials. *BMJ* 346: f1325.

Heller, M. 2004. What is the DASH Diet? *Dash Diet* http://dashdiet.org/what_is_the_dash_diet.asp.

Heller, M., and R. Rodgers. 2013. The everyday DASH diet cookbook. *DASH Diet.* http://dashdiet.org/everyday_dash_diet_cookbook.asp. Accessed October 20, 2015.

Hilpert, Kirsten F., Sheila G. West, Deborah M. Bagshaw, Valerie Fishell, Linda Barnhart, Michael Lefevre, Marlene M. Most et al. 2009. Effects of dairy products on intra-cellular calcium and blood pressure in adults with essential hypertension. *J Am Coll Nutr* 28 (25): 142–149.

Huang, Nancy, Karen Duggan, and Jenni Harman. 2008. Lifestyle management of hypertension. *Australian Prescriber* 31 (6): 150–153.

Institute of Medicine. 2005. *Dietary Reference Intakes for Water, Sodium, Potassium, Chloride Sulfate.* Washington, DC: National Academic Press.

James, Paul A., Suzanne Oparil, Barry L. Carter, William C. Cushman, Cheryl Dennison-Himmelfarb, Joel Handler, Daniel T. Lackland et al. 2014. Evidence based guidelines for the management of high blood pressure in adults: Report from the panel members appointed to the Eighth Joint National Committee (JNC 8). *JAMA* 311 (5): 507–520.

Jenkins, Peter, J.H. Jones, Jiri Frohlich, Benoit Lamarche, Chris Ireland, Stephanie Nishi, Korbua Srichaikul et al. 2015. Cholesterol-lowering portfolio diet also reduces blood pressure. *Nutr Metab Cardiovasc Dis* 25 (12): 1132–1139.

Kaplan, Norman M., and Ronald G. Victor. 2014. Hypertension in the population at large. In *Kaplan's Clinical Hypertension*, 11th Edition, edited by Norman M. Kaplan and Ronald G. Victor, pp. 1–18. Philadelphia, PA: Wolters Kluwer.

Karlish, Steve. 2008. The sodium potassium pump: Structure, function, regulation and pharmacology. Department of Biological Chemistry, Weizmann Institute of Science. Accessed April 20, 2016. https://www.weizmann.ac.il/Biomolecular_Sciences/scientist/Karlish/steve_karlish.pdf.

Kass, Lindsy, J. Weekes, and Lewis Carpenter. 2012. Effect of magnesium supplementation on blood pressure: A meta-analysis. *Eur J Clin Nutr* 66 (4): 411–418.

Klatsky, Arthur L., and Erica Gunderson. 2008. Alcohol and hypertension: A review. *J Am Soc Hypertens* 2 (5): 307–317.

Kotchen, Theodore A., David A. McCarron, and Nutrition Committee. 1998. Dietary electrolytes and blood pressure: A statement for healthcare professionals from AHA Nutrition Committee. *Circulation* 98 (6): 613–617.

Laragh, John H., and Barry M. Brenner, eds. 1994. *Hypertension: Pathophysiology, Diagnosis and Management*, 2nd Edition. LWW. Philadelphia, PA.

Levy, Daniel, Martin G. Larson, Ramachandran S. Vasan, William B. Kannel, and Kalon K. L. Ho. 1996. The progression from hypertension to congestive heart failure. *JAMA* 275 (20): 1557–1562.

LeWine, Howard. 2011. Portfolio beats low fat diet for lowering cholesterol. Harvard Health Blog. Accessed April 19, 2016. http://www.health.harvard.edu/blog/portfolio-beats-low-fat-diet-for-lowering-cholesterol-201108263248.

Lewington, Sarah, Robert Clarke, Nawab Qizilbash, Richard Peto, Rory Collins, and Prospective Studies Collaboration. 2002. Age-specific relevance of usual blood pressure to vascular mortality: A meta-analysis of individual data for one million adults on 61 prospective studies. *Lancet* 360 (9349): 1903–1913.

Lloyd-Jones, Donald M., Martin G. Larson, Eric P. Leip, Alexa Beiser, Ralph B. D'Agostino, William B. Kannel, Joanne M. Murabito, Ramachandran S. Vasan, Emelia J. Benjamin, and Daniel Levy. 2002. Lifetime risk for developing congestive heart failure: The Framingham Heart Study. *Circulation* 106 (24): 3068–3072.

Lusis, Aldons J. 2000. Atherosclerosis. *Nature* 407 (6801): 233–241.

MacMahon, Stephen, Richard Peto, Rory Collins, Jon Godwin, Jeffery A. Cutler, Paul Sorlie, Robert Abbott, James D. Neaton, Alan Dyer, and Jeremiah Stamler. 1990. Blood pressure, stroke and coronary heart disease, part 1: Prolonged differences in blood pressure; Prospective observational studies corrected for regression dilution bias. *Lancet* 335 (8692): 765–774.

Mayo Clinic. 2013. DASH diet: Healthy eating to lower your blood pressure. Accessed April 20, 2016. http://www.mayoclinic.org/healthy-lifestyle/nutrition-and-healthy-eating/in-depth/dash-diet/art-20048456.

Moore, Thomas J., Paul R. Conlin, Jamy Ard, Laura P. Svetkey, and DASH Collaborative Research Group. 2001. DASH (Dietary Approaches to Stop Hypertension) diet is effective treatment for stage 1 isolated systolic hypertension. *Hypertension* 38 (2): 155–158.

Moran, Andrew E., Mohammad H. Forouzanfar, Gregory Roth, George Mensah, Majid Ezzati, Christopher J. L. Murray, and Mohsen Naghavi. 2014. Temporal trends in ischemic heart disease mortality in 21 world regions: 1980–2010: The Global Burden of Disease 2010 Study. *Circulation* 129 (4): 1483–1492.

Mu, Lin, Kenneth J. Mukamal, and Asghar Z. Naqvi. 2014. Erythrocyte saturated fatty acids and systemic inflammation in adults. *Nutrition* 30 (11): 1404–1408.

Nissensohn, Mariela, Blanca Román-Viñas, Almudena Sánchez-Villegas, Suzanne Piscopo, and Lluis Serra-Majem. 2016. The effect of the Mediterranean diet on hypertension: A systematic review and meta-analysis. *J Nutr Educ Behav* 48 (1):42–53.e1.

Office of Disease Prevention and Health Promotion. 2015. *Healthy People 2020*. Washington, DC: Department of Health and Human Services.

Rapsomaniki, Eleni, Adam Timmis, Julie George, Mar Pujades-Rodriguez, Anoop D. Shah, Spiros Denaxas, Ian R. White et al. 2014. Blood pressure and incidence of twelve cardiovascular diseases: Lifetime risks, healthy life-years lost and age specific associations in 1.25 million people. *Lancet* 383 (9932): 1899–1911.

Rodrigues, Sérgio Lamêgo, Marcelo Perim Baldo, Rebeca Caldeira Machado, Ludimila Forechi, Maria del Carmem Bisi Molina, and José Geraldo Mill. 2014. High potassium intake blunts the effect of elevated sodium intake on blood pressure levels. *J Am Soc Hypertens* 8 (4): 232–238.

Sarafidis, Pantelis A., Suying Li, Shu-Cheng Chen, Allan J. Collins, Wendy W. Brown, Michael J. Klag, and George L. Bakris. 2008. Hypertension awareness, treatment and control in chronic kidney disease. *Am J Med* 121 (4): 332–340.

Seshadri, Sudha, Philip A. Wolf, Alexa Beiser, Ramachandran S. Vasan, Peter W. F. Wilson, Carlos S. Kase, Margaret Kelly-Hayes, William B. Kannel, and Ralph B. D'Agostino. 2001. Elevated midlife blood pressure increases stroke risk in elderly persons: The Framingham Study. *Arch Intern Med* 161 (19): 2343–2350.

Sharma, Shailendra, Kim McFann, Michel Chonchol, and Jessica Kendrick. Dietary sodium and potassium intake is not associated with elevated blood pressure in U.S. adults with no prior history of hypertension. 2014. *J Clin Hypertens* 16 (6): 418–423.

Sheps, Sheldon G. 2015. Does drinking alcohol affect your blood pressure? Mayo Clinic Expert Answers. Accessed April 15, 2016. http://www.mayoclinic.org/diseases-conditions/high-blood-pressure/expert-asnwers/blood-pressure/faq-20058254.

Song, Yun-Mi, Joohon Sung, Debbie A. Lawlor, George Davey Smith, Youngsoo Shin, and Shah Ebrahim. 2004. Blood pressure, haemorrhagic stroke and ischaemic stroke: The Korean national prospective occupational cohort study. BMJ 328 (7435): 324–325.

Stamler, Jeremiah. 1997. The INTERSALT study: Background, methods, findings and implications. *Am J Clin Nutr* 65 (2): 626S–642S.

Stamler, Jeremiah, Anthony R. Caggiula, Greg Grandits, Marcus O Kjelsberg, and Jeffery A. Cutler. 1996. Relationship to blood pressure of combinations of dietary macronutrients: Findings of the Multiple Risk Factor Intervention Trial (MRFIT). *Circulation* 94 (10): 2417–2423.

Stumpf, Christian, Josefine Jukic, and Atilla Yilmaz. 2009. Elevated VEGF-plasma levels in young patients with mild essential hypertension. *Eur J Clin Invest* 39 (1): 31–36.

Svetkey, Laura P., Frank M. Sacks, Eva Obarzanek, William M. Vollmer, Lawrence J. Appel, Pao-Hwa Lin, Njeri M. Karanja et al. 1999. The DASH diet sodium intake and blood pressure trial: Rationale and design. *J Am Diet Assoc* 99 (8 Suppl): S 96–104.

Tabassum, Nahida, and Feroz Ahmad. 2011. Role of natural herbs in the treatment of hypertension. *Pharmacogn Rev* 5(9):30–40.

Taubert, Dirk, Reinhard Berkels, Renate Roesen, and Wolfgang Klaus. 2003. Chocolate and blood pressure in elderly individuals with isolated systolic hypertension. *JAMA* 290 (8): 1029–1030.

Toledo, Estefania, Frank B. Hu, Ramon Estruch, Pilar Buil-Cosiales, Dolores Corella, Jordi Salas-Salvadó, M. Isabel Covas et al. 2013. Effect of the Mediterranean diet on blood pressure in the PREDIMED trial: Results from a randomized control trial. *BMC Med* 11: 207.

University of Maryland Medical Center. 2013. Omega-6 fatty acids. University of Maryland Medical Center. Accessed April 14, 2016. https://umm.edu/health/medical/altmed/supplement/omega6-fatty-acids.

U.S. Department of Health and Human Services, National Institutes of Health, National Heart Lung, and Blood Institute. 2005. *Your Guide to Lowering Your Cholesterol with TLC.* NIH. Bethesda, MD.

World Health Organization. 2012. *Guideline: Potassium Intake for Adults and Children.* Geneva: WHO Press.

Zhang, Zefeng, Mary E. Cogswell, Cathleen Gillespie, Jing Fang, Fleetwood Loustalot, Shifan Dai, Alicia L. Carriquiry et al. 2013. Association between usual sodium and potassium intake and blood pressure and hypertension among U.S. adults: NHANES 2005–2010. *PLoS One* 8 (1): e75289.

3 HEAL for Obesity

Ayesha Salem Al Dhaheri and Leila Cheikh Ismail

CONTENTS

3.1 WHAT IS OVERWEIGHT AND OBESITY?

Overweight and particularly obesity are still emerging at rapid rates and have now become epidemic throughout the world. Populations in countries with rapidly increasing wealth and changing lifestyles (especially dietary practices) are most vulnerable to obesity. Overweight and obesity are associated with increasing mortality and morbidity. The underlying process is being continuously in a positive energy balance, which in turn triggers weight gain. A positive energy balance only occurs (1) if energy intake is higher than energy expenditure, (2) if energy expenditure is lower than energy intake, or (3) a combination of the two.

Overweight and obesity are simply defined as abnormal or excessive fat accumulation to the extent that health may be adversely affected (WHO 2015). It is a chronic condition associated with an increased risk of many major diseases such as cardiovascular disease (CVD), non-insulin-dependent diabetes mellitus (NIDDM or type 2 diabetes), cancer, gallbladder disease, and hypertension. However, overweight and obese individuals are different in both the degree of excess fat they store as well as with the regional body distribution of fat. Obesity is not simply a single condition, but a group of conditions. Its etiology is complex and results from the interactions between genetics, metabolism, and the nervous system on one hand and behavior, food habits, physical activity, and sociocultural factors on the other (Demerath 2012). Factors that limit overconsumption are essential in the maintenance of a stable body weight and in the prevention of overweight and obesity (Gurnani et al. 2015). However, targeting diet and physical activity only, without considering economic, social, psychological, and cultural factors will have limited success on the prevention and treatment of obesity (Mattes and Foster 2014).

3.2 PREVALENCE OF OVERWEIGHT AND OBESITY

The prevalence of overweight and obesity is increasing worldwide at a frightening rate in both developed and developing countries. Trends in obesity are not restricted to one region, country, and racial or ethnic group. The highest levels of obesity in middle- and lower-income countries exist in the Middle East, the Western Pacific region, and Latin America (Popkin and Slining 2013). Lim et al. (2012) estimated that overweight and obesity have caused 3.4 million deaths, 4% of years of life lost, and 4% of disability-adjusted life years (DALYs) lost worldwide. In 2014, more than 1.9 billion adults were overweight, and of these over 600 million adults were clinically obese (WHO 2015). Overall, about 13% of the world's adult population (11% of men and 15% of women) are obese and 39% of adults aged 18 years and over (38% of men and 40% of women) are overweight. The overweight and obesity epidemic is not only restricted to adults, but is affecting children also. In 2013, 42 million children under the age of five were overweight or obese (WHO 2015). Most developed countries have high levels of obesity. In Europe, obesity prevalence now ranges from about 10% to 20% in men, with the lowest prevalence in Italy and the highest in the Czech Republic, while in women it ranges from 15% to 25%, with the highest prevalence in Germany and the lowest in Italy. In Canada, 15% of all adults are obese. In the United States, approximately 31.6% of men and 33.9% of women are obese.

3.3 FACTORS ASSOCIATED WITH OVERWEIGHT/OBESITY

Being overweight and/or obese are typically associated with an increased risk of mortality and a reduced quality of life. Several epidemiological studies have shown that the following factors are associated with being overweight and/or obese in the general population.

- *Age*: In men and women, overweight prevalence increases with age until 50–60 years. The often subtle nature of obesity is shown by the tendency for successive weight gain with increasing age (Hajek et al. 2015). Muscle mass usually declines with aging, so most of the increase in weight occurs in adipose tissue (Hajek et al. 2015; Thurber et al. 2015). Thus, body fat accounts for most of the weight gained with aging, because aging itself is usually accompanied by a loss of muscle mass. The BMI increase with age in women tends to continue longer than with men (Giles et al. 2015). Regardless of gender, aging is associated with a decrease in skeletal muscle.
- *Gender*: Women generally have a higher prevalence of obesity than men, especially after 50 years of age. The prevalence of obesity in Europe is 10%–20% in men and 15%–25% in women (Seidell and Halberstadt 2015). In most European countries, BMI distribution is similar for men, whereas it varies much more across countries for women (Seidell 2012). Human studies indicate that girls show a stronger preference for carbohydrates prior to puberty while boys prefer protein. After puberty, both genders display an increase in appetite for fat that occurs in response to changes in gonadal steroid levels, the onset of which is much earlier and to a greater extent in women.
- *Ethnicity*: Obesity varies across different ethnic groups (Krueger and Reither 2015). It would appear that particular ethnic groups are more susceptible to obesity when exposed to affluent lifestyles. It has been suggested that this may be due to a genetic predisposition for obesity that only becomes evident once individuals change their traditional lifestyle to a more prosperous sedentary lifestyle and its accompanying diet (WHO 2015). Research that examines the relationship between ethnicity and weight tends to produce contradictory results (Ogden and Chanana 1998). Several studies have indicated that body dissatisfaction and dieting tend to be more common in white rather than black or Asian women (Burke et al. 1992; Miller et al. 2000; Smith et al. 1999), while other studies disagree (Hill and Bhatti 1995; Striegel-Moore et al. 1995).
- *Education*: Studies have shown that education is inversely associated with BMI in women. This relation is less consistent in men, although in about half of the male population lower education is associated with higher BMI (McLaren et al. 2009; Johnson et al. 2011).

TABLE 3.1
BMI Cutoff Values in Adults for Overweight and Obesity

BMI (kg/m^2)	Classification	Health Risk
<18.5	Underweight	Increased risk
18.5–24.9	Healthy weight	Least risk
25.0–29.9	Overweight	Increased risk
30.0–34.9	Obesity I	High risk
35.0–39.9	Obesity II	Very high risk
≥40	Obesity III	Extremely high risk

Source: WHO, Obesity: Preventing and managing the global epidemic, WHO/NUT/NCD/98.1, Geneva, Switzerland, 1998.

Note: In adults, regardless of sex, a BMI between 18.5 kg/m^2 and 24.9 kg/m^2 is considered healthy, between 25.0 kg/m^2 and 29.9 kg/m^2 it is graded as overweight, and a BMI greater than 30 kg/m^2 is classified as obese.

3.4 OVERWEIGHT AND OBESITY MEASURES

3.4.1 BODY MASS INDEX

The use of body mass index (BMI) has gained scientific and mainstream acceptance as the links between BMI and disease risk (Stein et al. 2015), mortality (Winter et al. 2014), and adiposity (Krueger et al. 2014) have been shown, although the relation between body fat (generally assessed as BMI) and mortality remains a controversial topic. BMI offers a reliable and applicable measure of obesity in adults and is frequently employed in large-scale nutritional and epidemiological studies (Zong et al. 2015).

Table 3.1 shows non-gender-specific BMI criteria for overweight and obesity in adults.

3.4.2 WAIST CIRCUMFERENCE AND WAIST-TO-HIP RATIO

Circumference measurements are important tools to assess fat distribution. Research has clearly documented the link between increased abdominal fat, morbidity, and mortality (Kavak et al. 2014). The most frequently used indicators are waist circumference and waist-to-hip ratio (WHR); waist circumference is usually preferred over WHR (WHO 2008). Table 3.2 shows the cutoff values for waist circumference and WHR; and Table 3.3 shows a combination of BMI and waist circumference to assess disease risk.

3.4.3 PERCENT BODY FAT

Body fat is the most variable component of body weight and can be measured either in absolute or relative terms of total body weight (Ablove et al. 2015). On average, women have more fat than men (typically 27% vs. 15% of total body weight,

TABLE 3.2

Cutoff Values for Waist Circumference and Waist-to-Hip Ratio

Indicator	Cutoff Points	Risk of Metabolic Complications
Waist circumference	<94 cm in men <80 cm in women	"Normal"
Waist circumference	>94 cm in men >80 cm in women	Increased
Waist circumference	>102 cm in men >88 cm in women	Substantially increased
Waist-to-hip ratio	≥0.090 in men ≥0.85 in women	Substantially increased

Source: WHO, Training course on child growth assessment: WHO child growth standards, Module D; Counseling on growth and feeding, Geneva, Switzerland, 2008.

TABLE 3.3

Combination of BMI and Waist Circumference to Assess Disease Risk

BMI (kg/m²)	Classification	Disease Risk (Relative to Normal Weight and Waist Circumference)	
		Men <102 cm Women <88 cm	Men >102 cm Women >88 cm
<18.5	Underweight		
18.5–24.9	Healthy weight		
25.0–29.9	Overweight	Increased	High
30.0–34.9	Obesity I	High	Very high
35.0–39.9	Obesity II	Very high	Very high
≥40	Obesity III	Extremely high	Extremely high

Source: WHO, Training course on child growth assessment: WHO child growth standards, Module D; Counseling on growth and feeding, Geneva, Switzerland, 2008.

respectively) (Thomas et al. 2013). The various methods to measure body fat (skin-fold thickness, total body water, total body potassium, bioelectrical impedance, or dual-energy x-ray absorptiometry) greatly vary in accuracy, price, and invasiveness (Freedman et al. 2013).

3.5 HEALTH RISKS OF OBESITY

Obesity has been described as a threat to public health and its related risks should be assessed in terms of morbidity and mortality. Both the total amount and the distribution of body fat are associated with an increased risk of diseases (Eastwood et al. 2015; Redon and Lurbe 2015; Ujcic-Voortman et al. 2011).

3.5.1 CARDIOVASCULAR DISEASES

Cardiovascular diseases (CVDs) are a major cause of premature morbidity and mortality for both genders globally (Bowry et al. 2015; Stein et al. 2016). Lim (2015) states that no other factor has such a significant effect on the CVD risk profile as obesity. The risk of CVD has been correlated to

- Increasing BMI (Li et al. 2014; Manson et al. 1995; Rabkin et al. 1977)
- Regional fat distribution for both men and women (Caprio et al. 1996)—In particular, abdominal or central obesity (Donahue et al. 1987; Han et al. 1996; Okosun et al. 2004)
- Decreased high-density lipoprotein (HDL) levels and increased low-density lipoprotein (LDL) and triglyceride levels (Grundy 1998; Kannel and McGee 1979; Visscher and Seidell 2001)

3.5.2 HYPERTENSION

Obesity is significantly associated with hypertension (Hall et al. 2015; Kotsis et al. 2010) and is one of the main determinants of hypertension in the general population (DeMarco et al. 2014). Obese people have been found to have a much higher occurrence of high blood pressure (BP) (Hall et al. 2014). High BP was shown to be independently associated with high BMI (Kotsis et al. 2010) and is due to excessive fat accumulation in the heart, liver, muscle, and blood vessels (Kang 2013).

3.5.3 DIABETES MELLITUS

Type 2 diabetes has one of the strongest relationships to BMI, which also extends into childhood (Llewellyn et al. 2016). Worldwide, about 110 million patients are diabetic, and being overweight/obese with an abdominal fat distribution may well account for 80%–90% of all patients with type 2 diabetes (Esser et al. 2014). Diabetes is the most expensive public health concern of obesity (Low et al. 2014).

3.5.4 CANCER

Although other environmental and lifestyles factors (e.g., physical inactivity and diet) play significant roles in the origins of cancers (Vucenik and Stains 2012), the incidence of several major types of cancer (e.g., postmenopausal breast cancer) has been related to obesity (Davoodi et al. 2013; De Pergola and Silvestris 2013; Shanmugalingam et al. 2014).

3.6 PREVENTION AND TREATMENT OF OBESITY

The causes of obesity are diverse and multifaceted. No one solution exists; however, to fail to tackle this problem would be to condemn future generations to shorter life expectancies than their parents (House of Commons Health Committee 2004). A combination of dietary changes and physical activity, in combination with behavioral counseling, is likely to be more effective in retaining weight loss than diet or exercise alone in adults.

3.6.1 Physical Activity

An increase in physical activity is a significant part of weight loss therapy (Ladabaum et al. 2014). Most epidemiological studies have shown a reduced risk of weight gain, overweight, and obesity in people who take part on a regular basis in moderate-to-large amounts of physical activity or exercise (Brown et al. 2015).

3.6.2 Dietary Patterns for Obesity Reduction

Educating overweight and obese patients about foods and eating habits to facilitate weight control is a vital component of all weight management strategies. Education should consider the following (National Institutes of Health 1998):

- Energy values of different foods
- Food composition: fats, carbohydrates and protein
- Food labeling
- New practices of purchasing
- Food preparation
- Avoiding the overconsumption of high-calorie foods
- Adequate water intake
- Decreasing portion sizes
- Limiting alcohol consumption

Some dietary patterns for weight loss are:

- *Low-calorie diets (LCDs) and very low-calorie diets (VLCDs)*: There are essentially two forms of calorie-restricted diets that are typically used. LCDs provide 1000–1500 kcal/day and VLCDs less than 800 kcal/day. VLCDs should not be used as routine for weight loss therapy and it is not recommended generally to have a diet containing less than 1200 kcal/day (WHO 1998). Clinical trials have shown that LCDs are as effective as VLCDs in producing weight loss after 1 year (Ladabaum et al. 2014).
- *Mediterranean diet*: Research has found that high adherence to the dietary patterns of Mediterranean populations is associated with a lower prevalence of obesity in men and women (Schröder et al. 2004). Mediterranean diets are characterized by high intakes of vegetables, fruits, legumes, fish, cereals, and nuts with low-to-moderate consumption of meat and wine. This dietary pattern has been shown to significantly reduce weight, CVD, and cancer mortality rates, especially if followed for a long period (Mendez et al. 2006; Schröder et al. 2004).
- *Low-fat versus low-carbohydrate diets*: It is still rather uncertain whether one is better than the other, especially among people of African origin since the number of studies is limited (Bazzano et al. 2014). Research has shown, however, that study participants following a low-carbohydrate diet

lost more weight than those on a low-fat diet (Forster et al. 2010). Compared with a low-fat diet, a low-carbohydrate diet program tends to reduce the risk factors for CVD as well as help to maintain weight loss (Astrup et al. 2004; Bazzano et al. 2014; Yancy et al. 2004).

- *Low-glycemic index (GI) diet*: Kong et al. (2014) reported an association between a low-GI diet and decreased calorie intake with healthier dietary composition and reduced BMI in obese adolescents. In another randomized control trial where participants were randomly assigned to a high-GI diet, a low-GI diet, or a low-fat diet reported that after 6 months, there was a significant reduction in BMI in the low-GI diet group compared with the low-fat group (Juanola-Falgarona et al. 2014).

3.6.3 BEHAVIOR THERAPY

Behavior therapy is as an important component of any good obesity treatment program (Doughty et al. 2015) and aims to overcome obstacles to diet compliance and increase physical activity (WHO 1998, 2000) by teaching

- *Self-monitoring*: To observe and analyze target behaviors—for example, by using food diaries and physical activity records (Nackers et al. 2015).
- *Stimulus control*: To identify and modify environmental cues connected with a patient's overeating and their inactivity (WHO 1998)—for example, putting thought into shopping activity, ensuring problem foods are not bought, restricting the place and time of eating, as well as reducing the use of energy-saving technologies (Nackers et al. 2015).
- *Cognitive restructuring*: To improve a patient's awareness of their perceptions of themselves and their weight.
- *Social support*: People with higher levels of social support (family or friends) tend to be more successful in achieving and sustaining weight loss (Powell et al. 2015).

Behavioral treatment also includes healthy eating advice, setting eating behavior goals, mood management, and work and family management (Nackers et al. 2015).

3.6.4 DRUG TREATMENT

Drug treatment should be considered in obese adults with a BMI of 27 kg/m^2 or higher plus obesity-related medical conditions or with a BMI of 30 kg/m^2 or higher without comorbidities (Yanovski and Yanovski 2014). Weight loss medications should be used only with dietary and exercise regimes with a program of behavioral treatment and nutrition counseling (Kakkar and Dahiya 2015). The most common obesity drugs are appetite suppressants. Pharmacotherapeutic agents can be categorized as either affecting appetite or nutrient absorption or increasing thermogenesis (Smith 2014).

3.6.5 SURGICAL INTERVENTION

Surgery is generally regarded to be the best way of reducing weight and maintaining weight loss in severely obese and very severely obese patients (WHO 1998).

Although several surgical methods are available, they all either restrict energy intake or prevent nutrient absorption. The most popular surgical procedures are gastric portioning or "gastroplasty" and gastric bypass (Fruhbeck 2015). Abdominal liposuction is the most widespread aesthetic surgical practice in the U.S. but was reported to have no effects on insulin resistance and on the risk of CHD (Roslin et al. 2015). Surgical treatments for obesity generally resolve most comorbidities of severe obesity such as hypertension (Dalal and Bhattacharjee 2014), serum lipid levels (Ruiz-Tovar et al. 2014), and diabetes mellitus (Gurnani et al. 2015). However, surgery may have some serious gastric and nutritional complications (Baptista and Wassef 2013).

3.7 NUTRITIONAL INTERVENTIONS

In children and adolescents, effective intervention and prevention programs need to be in place to counter the increased prevalence of obesity. Research has shown that the lifestyle habits adopted during childhood follow through to adolescence and ultimately adulthood (Stevens et al. 2013).

3.7.1 SCHOOL-BASED PROGRAMS: LUNCH BOX AND SCHOOL LUNCH PROGRAMS

The "Lunch Box" and "School Lunch" programs target foods that are brought in or supplied by schools. It has been shown that packed lunches do not meet nutritional standards (Farris et al. 2014; Pearce et al. 2013; Stevens et al. 2013). The Lunch Box is a school-based program that provides a variety of healthy, delicious, and nutritious lunch box foods for school-aged children. It promotes the transition from processed foods in packed lunches to cooking from scratch using fresh food sources and ingredients. The program offers support to parents, food service teams, and schools by providing in-depth tools and resources to help with creating USDA-compliant menus. (For healthy school lunch box ideas, see www.thelunchbox.org.)

3.7.2 SCHOOL GARDEN

Gardening creates an opportunity for children, youth, adults, and families to gain interest in and eat fruits and vegetables. It is an excellent chance for children to engage in fun, physical activity while at the same time providing an educational tool to assist students to understand how healthy food is produced. It is important to encourage students to share their ideas and involve them every step of the way. Their engagement in the program gives them a sense of ownership and responsibility. Students will eat what they grow! Evidence demonstrates that school gardens increase the consumption of fruits and vegetables and give children a willingness to try new varieties of fruits and vegetables (Jaenke et al. 2012; Langellotto and Gupta 2012; Ratcliffe et al. 2011). School gardens can increase moderate as well as moderate-to-vigorous physical activity during the school days in elementary school children (Wells et al. 2014).

3.7.3 EAT RIGHT, GET ACTIVE

Eat Right, Get Active is a school-based program that teaches children to consume a healthy diet as well as to be physically active. The program promotes healthy foods in the school canteen and introduces regular exercise into the curriculum. It also incorporates oral health in the Schools for Health campaign. This school campaign helped eliminate junk food from the school canteens in the United Arab Emirates (HAAD-Abu Dhabi 2016). (More information on the program can be found on their website: http://schoolsforhealth.haad.ae.)

3.7.4 HEALTHY BUDDIES

The Healthy Buddies program is a school-based peer-led education program designed to promote health and wellness in youth. The curriculum-based teacher-facilitated program promotes healthy eating, physical activity, and self-esteem. The program is delivered to younger buddies with the help of older buddies. (More information on the program can be found on their website: www.healthybuddies.ca.)

Research has proved that exposure to the Healthy Buddies program resulted in a significant decrease in BMI z-score (zBMI) (1.10–1.04, p value .028) and waist circumference (77.1–75.0 cm, $p < .0001$) compared with the control group in Aboriginal children (Campbell et al. 2012; Ronsley et al. 2013).

3.7.5 MEND: MIND, EXERCISE, NUTRITION ... DO IT!

MEND is a family-based program that caters to 5–7 and 7–13-year-olds. It helps overweight children to improve their health, fitness, and self-esteem. MEND is a combination of three important aspects of safe, effective weight management and continued lifestyle change: healthy eating, regular physical activity, and behavioral change. Children and families who attend the program develop important skills and knowledge that assist them to manage their weight and feel fitter, healthier, and happier for the duration of their lives. Studies have shown that the MEND intervention was related to an improvement in BMI and psychosocial well-being (Fagg et al. 2014; Kolotourou et al. 2015). (More information about MEND can be found on the following websites: www.mendcentral.org and www.mendfoundation.org.)

3.7.6 BRIGHT BODIES

The Bright Bodies program is a comprehensive community-based 12-week weight management program that caters to obese 7–16-year-old children and their parents. The program's aims are to lose weight, build muscle, reduce stress, increase energy and self-esteem, improve family communication, and prevent future health problems. Bright Bodies uses the Smart Moves program curriculum, which employs nutrition education, behavior modification, and exercise. (More information is available from www.brightbodies.org.)

According to a recent trial in which participants were randomly assigned to either a control or Bright Bodies program for 6 months, it was demonstrated that the Bright Bodies weight management program had positive effects on body composition and insulin resistance in overweight children that were retained for up to 12 months (Santoro 2013) and even for up to 24 months after the intervention.

3.8   HOME REMEDIES FOR OVERWEIGHT AND OBESITY

Most common weight loss strategies propose lifestyle interventions customized to each individual by combining both calorie-restricted diets and exercise. Unfortunately, many have experienced disappointing results, due to diagnosis or treatments that ignored other potential causes such as "overeating" and/or the problems inherent to the therapy itself (e.g., side effects and short-lasting results). In response, people have turned toward complementary and alternative medicine (CAM). This section discusses alternative solutions such as home remedies, medicinal plant preparations, and dietary supplements, but the CAM pharmacopeia also includes other practices such as massage, acupuncture, and hypnosis. Folk and traditional (e.g., Chinese or Indian) medicines have documented since ancient times the potential of plants or plant preparations for treating obesity. Medicinal plants and plants that are used for eating purposes, as well as other natural products (e.g., honey) are typically complex and have several components comprising different chemical and pharmacological characteristics. Their usefulness is under investigation, as they may constitute excellent alternative strategies for the development of future antiobesity drugs. Some of these are

- *Lemons*: Lemon phenols have been shown to suppress weight gain and body fat accumulation in animal models (Fukuchi et al. 2008). A lemon detox program is said to reduce body fat in premenopausal Korean women (Kim et al. 2015). Other members of the citrus family are also being investigated, such as the Seville orange (*Citrus aurantium*) (Bent et al. 2004; Haaz et al. 2006; Silveira et al. 2015) and grapefruit (Dow et al. 2012; Rampersaud and Valim 2015).
- *Vinegar*: Petsiou et al. (2014) recently reviewed the evidence supporting the effects of vinegar on glucose and lipid metabolism and body weight. Included in that review was the only double-blind trial on healthy subjects. For 12 weeks, volunteers consumed 15 mL or 30 mL of apple vinegar or a daily placebo. At the end of the treatment period, subjects consuming vinegar had significantly lost a small amount of weight (1–2 kg). The effects were not sustained after the end of the treatment period and most subjects had regained the weight by the end of the 4-week post-treatment period.
- *Green tea*: Human and animal studies provide substantial evidence in support of oriental traditional customs that stem from the fact that green tea and its catechins may be helpful in the prevention or treatment of obesity. Consuming 379 mg of green tea extract daily for 3 months has been shown to decrease waist circumference and BMI in male and female obese patients 30–60 years of age (Suliburska et al. 2012).
- *Fenugreek (Trigonella foenum graecum)*: The effects of fenugreek extract on obesity and dyslipidemia induced by a high-fat diet in mice were shown by Handa et al. (2005). The authors further investigated the possible mechanisms of fenugreek and found that 4-hydroxyisoleucine was the active compound that explained the effects of lipid metabolism but not on weight.

- *Turmeric*: Turmeric (*Curcuma longa*) is possibly one of the most investigated spices. It has been shown (1) to have an *in vitro* effect on fat accumulation in adipocytes and (2) to reduce weight and inflammation on obese mice (Yun 2010).
- *Honey*: Honey is a carbohydrate-rich syrup produced by bees from floral nectars. Honey's composition is associated with its botanical origin (plant species) and geographical area (soil composition). In a crossover randomized trial, it was found that cinnamon, chromium, and magnesium-formulated kanuka honey at a dose of 53.5 g for 40 days decreased weight significantly by an average of 2.2 kg compared with kanuka honey alone in type 2 diabetic patients (Whitfield et al. 2016). Some types of honey contain toxic substances and hence precaution should be taken to avoid these (Islam et al. 2014).
- *Common beans*: Common beans (*Phaseolus vulgaris*) demonstrate a reduction of food intake in rats (Baintner et al. 2003).
- *Pine nut oil*: Korean pine nut (*Pinus koraiensis*) oil (PinnoThin) is thought to suppress appetite by acting on the release of cholecystokinin, a satiety hormone (Hughes et al. 2008; Pasman et al. 2008).
- *Caralluma fimbriata*: *C. fimbriata* is an edible cactus, traditionally known to reduce hunger and improve endurance. Caralluma extracts were tested in overweight individuals (1 g of extract per day for 60 days). At the end of the trial period there were no significant differences between the experimental and placebo groups, only a trend toward reduced body weight and composition and energy intake (Kuriyan et al. 2007).
- *Purple corn*: Purple corn (*Zea mays* L.) has shown promising effects on lipid metabolism in a mouse model. The effect was actually attributed to the color compound that makes the corn purple, cyanidin-3-glucoside. This compound belongs to the anthocyanin family which are widely distributed in human diets and used in the food industry as coloring agents (Tsuda et al. 2003).

In the future, the use of these products could be useful when associated with diet therapy. Their chief characteristics should be emphasized to reduce disappointment. Other products may be ineffective and using them must be countered to reduce negative fallout in the treatment of obesity and on the validity of phytotherapeutics.

3.9 NUTRITIONAL COUNSELING FOR OVERWEIGHT AND OBESITY

Ultimately, behavioral change should be the responsibility of the patient, but it is, however, the role of the health-care provider to bring about change with good counseling. Counseling is a talent that is not an innate but needs practice and honing. Many providers can feel that their main role is to provide help to patients in the form of advice about healthy methods of weight control. Although some education and advice may be useful, the majority of weight control patients may be aware of what they "should" eat but can be hindered by an unsupportive environment. Therefore, emphasizing questions to clarify barriers and how to overcome them can be more effective than providing advice on how to "solve" the problem. The former approach outlines for patients the manner in which a problem can be managed efficiently rather than depending on getting the right advice (Foster et al. 2005).

3.9.1 NUTRITIONAL COUNSELING IN ADULTS

Regular follow-ups of obese and overweight patients are recommended and should include BMI calculation and waist circumference measurement. Following the evaluation, appropriate treatment options can be suggested, which vary but include diet and/or dietary behavior modifications, increased physical exercise, behavioral therapy, and in some circumstances, medical treatments and surgery. Obesity counseling represents a useful and effective tool for weight loss promotion. It should be built on a longitudinal, long-lasting relationship with the health provider, enabling behavioral change management. Many well-recognized organizations, such as the U.S. Preventive Services Task Force and the Centers for Medicare and Medicaid Services, have suggested applying the "5As" model (assess advice, agree, assist, arrange) to perform effective obesity counseling (Centers for Medicare and Medicaid Services 2011). This model helps the provider to collect patient history and risk assessment, to investigate patient readiness to change, to advise specific behavioral changes, to agree on individual goals in a supportive and empathetic way, to assist the patient in identifying and overcoming barriers to change, and finally to arrange a frequent follow-up or referral to appropriate clinics/community resources. The 5As model was historically found to be effective in primary care by physicians to promote smoking cessation (Bentz et al. 2007). It has since been adapted to train primary care physicians in obesity counseling and to promote their obesity counseling competence (Goldstein et al. 2004; Jay et al. 2010a; Jay et al. 2010b; Sciamanna et al. 2002). The model is considered effective also for reminding the caregiver what has been done and what should be addressed next (Krist et al. 2008) and may therefore favorably impact a patient's long-term outcomes (Glasgow et al. 2006; Jay et al. 2010a; Whitlock et al. 2002).

Table 3.4 summarizes the 5As as adapted for obesity counseling.

3.9.2 NUTRITIONAL COUNSELING FOR CHILDREN

Various social and environmental aspects can affect a child's care, feeding, and ensuing growth. It is crucial to identify the reasons behind a child's problem before providing advice (WHO 2008). The causes of overweight and obesity are normally a result of environmental factors—for example, the family's reliance on high-energy convenience foods, a lack of safe outdoor play areas, and/or partaking in sedentary activities (watching television or playing video games). Counseling should address both environmental and dietary causes. Although the counseling should focus on the children themselves, the counselor needs to realize that parents may want to alter some of their habits to address the root causes of the child being overweight. It is essential during the counseling session to inform the parent/caregiver in a clear and sensitive way and to decide with them on actions to improve the child's nutritional status.

TABLE 3.4

THE 5As OF OBESITY COUNSELING

Components of Counseling	Description
Assess	• Calculate BMI
	• Patient history (medications, metabolic problems, family history, psychiatric illnesses)
	• Dietary habits, physical exercise
Advise	• Set the patient's weight loss target
	• Suggest changes to feeding behaviors and physical exercise
	• Inform the patient about the medical and surgical options
Agree	• Choose *with the patient* the preferred behavior change options
	• Set achievable and specific diet and exercise prescriptions
	• Follow-up on the set prescriptions during the subsequent visits
Assist	• Identify and help overcoming barriers to change
	• Be supportive and empathetic; use motivational skills
	• Describe patient support services
Arrange	• Adequately frequent follow-up
	• Refer to dedicated clinics, programs, and community resources

The action plan should contain up to three of the most important possible activities because too many of them may be forgotten or may discourage the parents/caregivers. Change may take time and the essential reasons for a growth problem are unlikely to be fixed in a one-off counseling session. Successful counseling plans should include and encourage the parents/caregivers to bring the child back for a series of follow-up sessions. In cases where many causes are applicable, try to identify the most important ones and focus on the central aspects that could be changed. Training tools have been developed by the World Health Organization (WHO) for health-care staff to support the application of the WHO growth standards. The materials teach how to measure, plot, and interpret growth indicators, and how to counsel the parents/caregivers and when to refer the child for further investigation. To counsel the parents/caregivers of children who have a problem with being overweight or obese, a health-care provider should listen to and learn from them, make sure to build confidence, and offer them support by use these counseling techniques (WHO 2008):

- Ask open questions, relevant to the child's age. Do not hesitate to ask follow-up questions as required to get the full information and to understand the causes. To identify the causes of overweight, ask questions about the child's dietary habits (type and frequency). For older children, do not forget to include questions about physical activity and how they spend their leisure time.
- Ensure that you understand what the parents/caregivers say by listening.
- Use body language and signs that show attention.
- Show that you understand how the parents/caregivers feel.
- Recognize and praise what the parents/caregivers are doing right.

- Avoid words that sound judgmental, do not place guilt on the parent/caregiver, and be sensitive to the situation.
- Accept what the parents/caregivers think and feel.
- Give related information in straightforward language.
- Offer a small number of suggestions rather than commands.
- Suggest practical help.

Educating parents/caregivers regarding their roles and responsibilities as well as the role of their children about eating can be empowering and provides a great way to preventing eating issues (Cadenhead et al. 2011).

- *Parents'/caregivers' roles*:
  - Offer three meals and two to three snacks each day, at regular times.
  - Offer healthy foods most of the time; limit less healthy foods.
  - Sit down and eat healthy foods with children.
  - Decide what foods are offered to children in the home or away from home.
  - Do not praise or punish children based on the amount of food they eat.
  - Do not use food as a reward.
  - Do not withhold food as punishment.
- *Children's roles*:
  - Decide whether to eat.
  - Decide how much to eat from the foods offered at each meal or snack.

3.10 CASE STUDIES

3.10.1 CASE STUDY 1

A 25-year-old female visits the health center with her mother. During this visit she complains about fatigue and pain in her knees, with no motivation to do exercise. Her weight is 75 kg and her height is 161 cm. Her dietary behavior is based on energy-dense, high-fat foods with unhealthy snacks between meals. Family history of diabetes and hypertension is positive. Give responses to the following:

1. Calculate the body mass index (BMI).
2. How should her weight status be classified using the WHO standard BMI cutoff points?
3. What would you recommend as a current focus for nutrition in the current case?
4. What is the relationship between diabetes, hypertension, and obesity?
5. Specify one specific physical activity recommendation for this patient.

3.10.2 CASE STUDY 2

A 10-year-old boy visits the health center with his mother for a routine well-child visit. The mother does not report any health problems for the child and there is no family history of heart disease or diabetes. During the physical examination it is noted that his weight has increased too rapidly for his height and age, with a body mass index (BMI) in the 97th percentile (above +2 z-score) for his age and sex. He is overweight and shows a positive trend toward obesity. Give responses to the following:

1. What behaviors associated with an increased risk of obesity would you look for when assessing this child and his family's diet?
2. What recommendations for changes in lifestyle would you suggest to decrease the risk of obesity?
3. Should the parents be included in the counseling session? Why or why not?
4. Will you set some goals to be achieved before the next counseling session? Mention your goal for this case.
5. Identify one school intervention program that could be recommended for policy makers to tackle obesity problems among schoolchildren.

REFERENCES

Ablove, T., N. Binkley, S. Leadley, J. Shelton, and R. Ablove. 2015. Body mass index continues to accurately predict percent body fat as women age despite changes in muscle mass and height. *Menopause* 22 (7):727–730.

Astrup, A., T. M. Larsen, and A. Harper. 2004. Atkins and other low-carbohydrate diets: Hoax or an effective tool for weight loss? *Lancet* 364 (9437):897–899.

Baintner, K., P. Kiss, U. Pfuller, S. Bardocz, and A. Pusztai. 2003. Effect of orally and intraperitoneally administered plant lectins on food consumption of rats. *Acta Physiol Hung* 90 (2):97–107.

Baptista, V., and W. Wassef. 2013. Bariatric procedures: An update on techniques, outcomes and complications. *Curr Opin Gastroenterol* 29 (6):684–693.

Bazzano, L. A., T. Hu, K. Reynolds, L. Yao, C. Bunol, Y. Liu, C.-S. Chen, M. J. Klag, P. K. Whelton, and J. He. 2014. Effects of low-carbohydrate and low-fat diets: A randomized trial. *Ann Intern Med* 161 (5):309–318.

Bent, S., A. Padula, and J. Neuhaus. 2004. Safety and efficacy of *Citrus aurantium* for weight loss. *Am J Cardiol* 94 (10):1359–1361.

Bentz, C. J., K. B. Bayley, K. E. Bonin, L. Fleming, J. F. Hollis, J. S. Hunt, B. LeBlanc, T. McAfee, N. Payne, and J. Siemienczuk. 2007. Provider feedback to improve 5A's tobacco cessation in primary care: A cluster randomized clinical trial. *Nicotine Tob Res* 9 (3):341–349.

Bowry, A. D., J. Lewey, S. B. Dugani, and N. K. Choudhry. 2015. The burden of cardiovascular disease in low- and middle-income countries: Epidemiology and management. *Can J Cardiol* 31 (9):1151–1159.

Brown, T., S. Smith, R. Bhopal, A. Kasim, and C. Summerbell. 2015. Diet and physical activity interventions to prevent or treat obesity in South Asian children and adults: A systematic review and meta-analysis. *Int J Environ Res Public Health* 12 (1):566–594.

Burke, G. L., P. J. Savage, T. A. Manolio, J. M. Sprafka, L. E. Wagenknecht, S. Sidney, L. L. Perkins, K. Liu, and D. R. Jacobs, Jr. 1992. Correlates of obesity in young black and white women: The CARDIA Study. *Am J Public Health* 82 (12):1621–1625.

Cadenhead, K., B. Leslie, B. Pawa, S. Raja, M. Yandel, and P. Yeung. 2011. Nutrition counseling strategies and resources for overweight and obese 2–5 year olds. *BC Medical Journal* 53 (1). 41–42. Accessed March 15, 2016. http://www.bcmj.org/council-health-promotion/nutrition-counseling-strategies-and-resources-overweight-and-obese-2-5-year.

Campbell, A. C., D. Barnum, V. Ryden, S. Ishkanian, S. Stock, and J. P. Chanoine. 2012. The effectiveness of the implementation of Healthy Buddies (TM), a school-based, peer-led health promotion program in elementary schools. *Can J Diabetes* 36 (4):181–186.

Caprio, S., W. V. Tamborlane, D. Silver, C. Robinson, R. Leibel, S. McCarthy, A. Grozman, A. Belous, D. Maggs, and R. S. Sherwin. 1996. Hyperleptinemia: An early sign of juvenile obesity; Relation to body fat depots and insulin concentrations. *Am J Physiol* 271(3 Pt 1):E626–E630.

Centers for Medicare and Medicaid Services. 2011. Decision memo for intensive behavioral therapy for obesity (CAG-00423N). Accessed March 3, 2016. https://www.cms.gov/medicare-coverage-database/details/nca-decision-memo.aspx?&NcaName=Intensive%20Behavioral%20Therapy%20for%20Obesity&bc=ACAAAAAAIAAA&NCAId=253&.

Dalal, P., and M. Bhattacharjee. 2014. Stroke-transient cerebral ischaemic attacks (TIAs): A medical emergency; Preventable and treatable. *J Assoc Physicians India* 62 (12):12–17.

Davoodi, S. H., T. Malek-Shahabi, A. Malekshahi-Moghadam, R. Shahbazi, and S. Esmaeili. 2013. Obesity as an important risk factor for certain types of cancer. *Iran J Cancer Prev* 6 (4):186–194.

De Pergola, G., and F. Silvestris. 2013. Obesity as a major risk factor for cancer. *J Obes* 2013, 291546.

DeMarco, V. G., A. R. Aroor, and J. R. Sowers. 2014. The pathophysiology of hypertension in patients with obesity. *Nat Rev Endocrinol* 10 (6):364–376.

Demerath, E. W. 2012. The genetics of obesity in transition. *Coll Antropol* 36 (4):1161–1168.

Donahue, R. P., E. Bloom, R. D. Abbott, D. M. Reed, and K. Yano. 1987. Central obesity and coronary heart-disease in men. *Lancet* 329 (8537):821–824.

Doughty, K. N., V. Y. Njike, and D. L. Katz. 2015. Effects of a cognitive-behavioral therapy–based immersion obesity treatment program for adolescents on weight, fitness, and cardiovascular risk factors: A pilot study. *Child Obes* 11 (2):215–218.

Dow, C. A., S. B. Going, H. H. S. Chow, B. S. Patil, and C. A. Thomson. 2012. The effects of daily consumption of grapefruit on body weight, lipids, and blood pressure in healthy, overweight adults. *Metabolism* 61 (7):1026–1035.

Eastwood, S. V., T. Tillin, H. M. Dehbi, A. Wright, N. G. Forouhi, I. Godsland, P. Whincup, N. Sattar, A. D. Hughes, and N. Chaturvedi. 2015. Ethnic differences in associations between fat deposition and incident diabetes and underlying mechanisms: The SABRE study. *Obesity (Silver Spring)* 23 (3):699–706.

Esser, N., S. Legrand-Poels, J. Piette, A. J. Scheen, and N. Paquot. 2014. Inflammation as a link between obesity, metabolic syndrome and type 2 diabetes. *Diabetes Res Clin Pract* 105 (2):141–150.

Fagg, J., P. Chadwick, T. J. Cole, S. Cummins, H. Goldstein, H. Lewis, S. Morris, D. Radley, P. Sacher, and C. Law. 2014. From trial to population: A study of a family-based community intervention for childhood overweight implemented at scale. *Int J Obes (Lond)* 38 (10):1343–1349.

Farris, A. R., S. Misyak, K. J. Duffey, G. C. Davis, K. Hosig, N. Atzaba-Poria, M. M. McFerren, and E. L. Serrano. 2014. Nutritional comparison of packed and school lunches in prekindergarten and kindergarten children following the implementation of the 2012–2013 National School Lunch Program Standards. *J Nutr Educ Behav* 46 (6):621–626.

Fitzpatrick, S. L., D. Wischenka, B. M. Appelhans, L. Pbert, M. Wang, D. K. Wilson, S. L. Pagoto, and Society of Behavioral Medicine. 2016. An evidence-based guide for obesity treatment in primary care. *Am J Med* 129 (1):115, e1–e7.

Foster, G. D, A. P. Makris, and B. A. Bailer. 2005. Behavioral treatment of obesity. *Am J Clin Nutr* 82 (1):230S–235S.

Forster G.D., Wyatt H.R., Hill J.O. et al. 2010. Weight and metabolic outcomes After 2 years on a low-carbohydrate versus low-fat diet. *Ann Intern Med.* 153(3):147–157.

Freedman, D. S., C. L. Ogden, H. M. Blanck, L. G. Borrud, and W. H. Dietz. 2013. The abilities of body mass index and skinfold thicknesses to identify children with low or elevated levels of dual-energy x-ray absorptiometry-determined body fatness. *J Pediatr* 163 (1):160–166, e1.

Fruhbeck, G. 2015. Bariatric and metabolic surgery: A shift in eligibility and success criteria. *Nat Rev Endocrinol* 11 (8):465–477.

Fukuchi, Y., M. Hiramitsu, M. Okada, S. Hayashi, Y. Nabeno, T. Osawa, and M. Naito. 2008. Lemon polyphenols suppress diet-induced obesity by up-regulation of mRNA levels of the enzymes involved in beta-oxidation in mouse white adipose tissue. *J Clin Biochem Nutr* 43 (3):201–209.

Giles, L. C., M. J. Whitrow, M. J. Davies, C. E. Davies, A. R. Rumbold, and V. M. Moore. 2015. Growth trajectories in early childhood, their relationship with antenatal and post-natal factors, and development of obesity by age 9 years: Results from an Australian birth cohort study. *Int J Obes (Lond)* 39 (7):1049–1056.

Glasgow, R. E., S. Emont, and D. C. Miller. 2006. Assessing delivery of the five "As" for patient-centered counseling. *Health Promot Int* 21 (3):245–255.

Goldstein, M. G., E. P. Whitlock, J. DePue, and Project Planning Committee of the Addressing Multiple Behavioral Risk Factors in Primary Care Project. 2004. Multiple behavioral risk factor interventions in primary care: Summary of research evidence. *Am J Prev Med* 27 (2 Suppl):61–79.

Grundy, S. M., G. J. Balady, M. H. Criqui, G. Fletcher, P. Greenland, L. F. Hiratzka, N. Houston-Miller et al. 1998. Primary prevention of coronary heart disease: Guidance from Framingham: A statement for healthcare professionals from the AHA Task Force on Risk Reduction; American Heart Association. *Circulation* 97 (18):1876–1887.

Gurnani, M., C. Birken, and J. Hamilton. 2015. Childhood obesity: Causes, consequences, and management. *Pediatr Clin North Am* 62 (4):821–840.

Han T.S., Leer E.M., Seidell J.C. et al. 1995. Waist circumference action levels in the identification of Cardiovascular risk factors: Prevalence study in a random sample. *BMJ*; 31:1401–5.

HAAD-Abu Dhabi. Eat right and get active. Accessed January 17, 2016. http://schools-forhealth.haad.ae/health-campaigns/healthy-eating.aspx.

Haaz, S., K. R. Fontaine, G. Cutter, N. Limdi, S. Perumean-Chaney, and D. B. Allison. 2006. *Citrus aurantium* and synephrine alkaloids in the treatment of overweight and obesity: An update. *Obes Rev* 7 (1):79–88.

Hajek, A., T. Lehnert, A. Ernst, C. Lange, B. Wiese, J. Prokein, S. Weyerer et al., and Group AgeCoDe Study. 2015. Prevalence and determinants of overweight and obesity in old age in Germany. *BMC Geriatr* 15:83.

Hall, J. E., J. M. do Carmo, A. A. da Silva, Z. Wang, and M. E. Hall. 2015. Obesity-induced hypertension: Interaction of neurohumoral and renal mechanisms. *Circ Res* 116 (6):991–1006.

Hall, M. E., J. M. do Carmo, A. A. da Silva, L. A. Juncos, Z. Wang, and J. E. Hall. 2014. Obesity, hypertension, and chronic kidney disease. *Int J Nephrol Renovasc Dis* 7:75–88.

Handa, T., K. Yamaguchi, Y. Sono, and K. Yazawa. 2005. Effects of fenugreek seed extract in obese mice fed a high-fat diet. *Biosci Biotechnol Biochem* 69 (6):1186–1188.

Hannon, T. S., and S. A. Arslanian. 2015. The changing face of diabetes in youth: Lessons learned from studies of type 2 diabetes. *Ann NY Acad Sci* 1353:113–137.

Hartstra, A. V., K. E. Bouter, F. Bäckhed, and M. Nieuwdorp. 2015. Insights into the role of the microbiome in obesity and type 2 diabetes. *Diabetes Care* 38 (1):159–165.

Hill, A. J., and R. Bhatti. 1995. Body shape perception and dieting in preadolescent British Asian girls: Links with eating disorders. *Int J Eat Disord* 17 (2):175–183.

House of Commons Health Committee. 2004. Obesity: Third Report of Session 2003–04, Volume 1; Report, together with formal minutes. London: The Stationery Office.

Hughes, G. M., E. J. Boyland, N. J. Williams, L. Mennen, C. Scott, T. C. Kirkham, J. A. Harrold, H. G. Keizer, and J. C. Halford. 2008. The effect of Korean pine nut oil (PinnoThin) on food intake, feeding behaviour and appetite: A double-blind placebo-controlled trial. *Lipids Health Dis* 7:6.

Islam, M. N., M. I. Khalil, and S. H. Gan. 2014. Toxic compounds in honey. *J Appl Toxicol* 34 (7):733–742.

Jaenke, R. L., C. E. Collins, P. J. Morgan, D. R. Lubans, K. L. Saunders, and J. M. Warren. 2012. The impact of a school garden and cooking program on boys' and girls' fruit and vegetable preferences, taste rating, and intake. *Health Educ Behav* 39 (2):131–141.

Jay, M., C. Gillespie, S. Schlair, S. Sherman, and A. Kalet. 2010a. Physicians' use of the 5As in counseling obese patients: Is the quality of counseling associated with patients' motivation and intention to lose weight? *BMC Health Serv Res* 10:159.

Jay, M., S. Schlair, R. Caldwell, A. Kalet, S. Sherman, and C. Gillespie. 2010b. From the patient's perspective: The impact of training on resident physician's obesity counseling. *J Gen Intern Med* 25 (5):415–422.

Johnson, W., K. O. Kyvik, A. Skytthe, I. J. Deary, and T. I. Sorensen. 2011. Education modifies genetic and environmental influences on BMI. *PLoS One* 6 (1): e16290.

Juanola-Falgarona, M., J. Salas-Salvadó, N. Ibarrola-Jurado, A. Rabassa-Soler, A. Díaz-López, M. Guasch-Ferré, P. Hernández-Alonso, R. Balanza, and M. Bulló. 2014. Effect of the glycemic index of the diet on weight loss, modulation of satiety, inflammation, and other metabolic risk factors: A randomized controlled trial. *Am J Clin Nutr* 100 (1):27–35.

Kakkar, A. K., and N. Dahiya. 2015. Drug treatment of obesity: Current status and future prospects. *Eur J Intern Med* 26 (2):89–94.

Kang, Y. S. 2013. Obesity associated hypertension: New insights into mechanism. *Electrolyte Blood Press* 11 (2):46–52.

Kannel, W. B., and D. L. McGee. 1979. Diabetes and cardiovascular disease. *JAMA* 241:2035–2038.

Kavak, V., M. Pilmane, and D. Kazoka. 2014. Body mass index, waist circumference and waist-to-hip-ratio in the prediction of obesity in Turkish teenagers. *Coll Antropol* 38 (2):445–451.

Kim, M. J., J. H. Hwang, H. J. Ko, H. B. Na, and J. H. Kim. 2015. Lemon detox diet reduced body fat, insulin resistance, and serum hs-CRP level without hematological changes in overweight Korean women. *Nutr Res* 35 (5):409–420.

Kolotourou, M., D. Radley, C. Gammon, L. Smith, P. Chadwick, and P. M. Sacher. 2015. Long-term outcomes following the MEND 7–13 child weight management program. *Child Obes* 11 (3):325–330.

Kong, A. P. S., K. C. Choi, R. S. M. Chan, K. Lok, R. Ozaki, A. M. Li, C. S. Ho et al. 2014. A randomized controlled trial to investigate the impact of a low glycemic index (GI) diet on body mass index in obese adolescents. *BMC Public Health* 14:180.

Kotsis, V., S. Stabouli, S. Papakatsika, Z. Rizos, and G. Parati. 2010. Mechanisms of obesity-induced hypertension. *Hypertens Res* 33 (5):386–393.

Krist, A. H., S. H. Woolf, C. O. Frazier, R. E. Johnson, S. F. Rothemich, D. B. Wilson, K. J. Devers, and J. W. Kerns. 2008. An electronic linkage system for health behavior counseling effect on delivery of the 5A's. *Am J Prev Med* 35 (5 Suppl):S350–S358.

Krueger, P. M., K. Coleman-Minahan, and R. N. Rooks. 2014. Race/ethnicity, nativity and trends in BMI among U.S. adults. *Obesity (Silver Spring)* 22 (7):1739–1746.

Krueger, P. M., and E. N. Reither. 2015. Mind the gap: Race/ethnic and socioeconomic disparities in obesity. *Curr Diab Rep* 15 (11):95.

Kuriyan, R., T. Raj, S. K. Srinivas, M. Vaz, R. Rajendran, and A. V. Kurpad. 2007. Effect of *Caralluma fimbriata* extract on appetite, food intake and anthropometry in adult Indian men and women. *Appetite* 48 (3):338–344.

Ladabaum, U., A. Mannalithara, P. A. Myer, and G. Singh. 2014. Obesity, abdominal obesity, physical activity, and caloric intake in U.S. adults: 1988–2010. *Am J Med* 127 (8):717–727, e12.

Langellotto, G. A., and A. Gupta. 2012. Gardening increases vegetable consumption in school-aged children: A meta-analytical synthesis. *Hort Technology* 22 (4):430–445.

Li, N., P. T. Katzmarzyk, R. Horswell, Y. Zhang, W. Li, W. Zhao, Y. Wang, J. Johnson, and G. Hu. 2014. BMI and coronary heart disease risk among low-income and underinsured diabetic patients. *Diabetes Care* 37 (12):3204–3212.

Lim, G. B. 2015. Risk factors: CVD risk and the "obesity paradox." *Nat Rev Cardiol* 12 (10):560.

Lim, S. S., T. Vos, A. D. Flaxman, G. Danaei, K. Shibuya, H. Adair-Rohani, M. A. AlMazroa et al. 2012. A comparative risk assessment of burden of disease and injury attributable to 67 risk factors and risk factor clusters in 21 regions, 1990–2010: A systematic analysis for the Global Burden of Disease Study 2010. *Lancet* 380 (9859):2224–2260.

Llewellyn, A., M. Simmonds, C. G. Owen, and N. Woolacott. 2016. Childhood obesity as a predictor of morbidity in adulthood: A systematic review and meta-analysis. *Obes Rev* 17 (1):56–67.

Low, L. L., S. F. Tong, and W. Y. Low. 2014. Mixed feelings about the diagnosis of type 2 diabetes mellitus: A consequence of adjusting to health related quality of life. *Coll Antropol* 38 (1):11–20.

Manson, J. E., M. D. Walter, C. Willet et al. 1995. Body weight and mortality among women. *N Engl J Med* 333 (11):677–685.

Masaki, K. H., J. D. Curb, D. Chiu, H. Petrovitch, and B. L. Rodriguez. 1997. Association of body mass index with blood pressure in elderly Japanese American men: The Honolulu Heart Program. *Hypertension* 29 (2):673–677.

Mattes, R., and G. D. Foster. 2014. Research issues: The food environment and obesity. *Am J Clin Nutr* 100 (6):1663–1665.

Mendez, M. A., B. M. Popkin, P. Jakszyn, A. Berenguer, M. J. Tormo, M. J. Sanchéz, J. R. Quirós et al. Adherence to a Mediterranean diet is associated with reduced 3-year incidence of obesity. *J Nutr* 136 (11):2934–2938.

McLaren, L., J. Godley, and I. A. MacNairn. 2009. Social class, gender, and time use: Implications for the social determinants of body weight? *Health Rep* 20 (4):65–73.

Miller, K. J., D. H. Gleaves, T. G. Hirsch, B. A. Green, A. C. Snow, and C. C. Corbett. 2000. Comparisons of body image dimensions by race/ethnicity and gender in a university population. *Int J Eat Disord* 27 (3):310–316.

Nackers, L. M., P. J. Dubyak, X. Lu, S. D. Anton, G. R. Dutton, and M. G. Perri. 2015. Group dynamics are associated with weight loss in the behavioral treatment of obesity. *Obesity (Silver Spring)* 23 (8):1563–1569.

National Institutes of Health. 1998. *The Practical Guide: Identification, Evaluation and Treatment of Overweight and Obesity in Adults.* Bethesda, MD: North American Association for the Study of Obesity.

Ogden, J., and A. Chanana. 1998. Explaining the effect of ethnic group on weight concern: Finding a role for family values. *Int J Obes Relat Metab Disord* 22 (7):641–647.

Okosun, I. S., K. M. Chandra, A. Boev, J. M. Boltri, S. T. Choi, D. C. Parish, and G. E. Dever. 2004. Abdominal adiposity in U.S. adults: Prevalence and trends, 1960–2000. *Prev Med* 39 (1):197–206.

Pasman, W. J., J. Heimerikx, C. M. Rubingh, R. van den Berg, M. O'Shea, L. Gambelli, H. F. Hendriks et al. 2008. The effect of Korean pine nut oil on *in vitro* CCK release, on appetite sensations and on gut hormones in post-menopausal overweight women. *Lipids Health Dis* 7:10.

Pearce, J., L. Wood, and L. Stevens. 2013. Portion weights of food served in English schools: Have they changed following the introduction of nutrient-based standard? *J Hum Nutr Diet* 26:553–562.

Petsiou, E. I., P. I. Mitrou, S. A. Raptis, and G. D. Dimitriadis. 2014. Effect and mechanisms of action of vinegar on glucose metabolism, lipid profile, and body weight. *Nutr Rev* 72 (10):651–661.

Popkin, B. M., and M. M. Slining. 2013. New dynamics in global obesity facing low- and middle-income countries. *Obes Rev* 14 (Suppl 2):11–20.

Powell, K., J. Wilcox, A. Clonan, P. Bissell, L. Preston, M. Peacock, and M. Holdsworth. 2015. The role of social networks in the development of overweight and obesity among adults: A scoping review. *BMC Public Health* 15:996.

Rabkin, S. W., F. A. L. Mathewson, and P. H. Hsu. 1977. Relation of body weight to development of ischemic heart disease in a cohort of young North American men after a 26 year observation period: The Manitoba Study. *Am J Cardiol* 39:452–458.

Rampersaud, G. C., and M. F. Valim. 2015. 100% citrus juice: Nutritional contribution, dietary benefits, and association with anthropometric measures. *Crit Rev Food Sci Nutr* 0.

Ratcliffe, M. M., K. A. Merrigan, B. L. Rogers, and J. P. Goldberg. 2011. The effects of school garden experiences on middle school–aged students' knowledge, attitudes, and behaviors associated with vegetable consumption. *Health Promot Pract* 12 (1):36–43.

Redon, J., and E. Lurbe. 2015. The kidney in obesity. *Curr Hypertens Rep* 17:43.

Ronsley, R., A. S. Lee, B. Kuzeljevic, and C. Panagiotopoulos. 2013. Healthy buddies reduces body mass index *z*-score and waist circumference in Aboriginal children living in remote coastal communities. *J Sch Health* 83 (9):605–613.

Roslin, M. S., C. Cripps, and A. Peristeri. 2015. Bariatric and metabolic surgery: Current trends and what's to follow. *Curr Opin Gastroenterol* 31 (6):513–518.

Ruiz-Tovar, J., L. Zubiaga, C. Llavero, M. Diez, A. Arroyo, and R. Calpena. 2014. Serum cholesterol by morbidly obese patients after laparoscopic sleeve gastrectomy and additional physical activity. *Obes Surg* 24 (3):385–389.

Santoro, N. 2013. Childhood obesity and type 2 diabetes: The frightening epidemic. *World J Pediatr* 9 (2):101–102.

Schröder, H., J. Marrugat, J. Vila, M. I. Covas, and R. Elosua. 2004. Adherence to the traditional Mediterranean diet is inversely associated with body mass index and obesity in a Spanish population. *J Nutr* 134 (12):3355–3361.

Sciamanna, C. N., J. D. DePue, M. G. Goldstein, E. R. Park, K. M. Gans, A. D. Monroe, and P. T. Reiss. 2002. Nutrition counseling in the promoting cancer prevention in primary care study. *Prev Med* 35 (5):437–446.

Seidell, J. C. 2012. Obesity: More nurture than nature. *Ned Tijdschr Geneeskd* 156 (31):A4679.

Seidell, J. C., and J. Halberstadt. 2015. The global burden of obesity and the challenges of prevention. *Ann Nutr Metab* 66 (Suppl 2):7–12.

Shanmugalingam, T., D. Crawley, C. Bosco, J. Melvin, S. Rohrmann, S. Chowdhury, L. Holmberg, and M. Van Hemelrijck. 2014. Obesity and cancer: The role of vitamin D. *BMC Cancer* 14:712.

Silveira, J. Q., G. K. Dourado, and T. B. Cesar. 2015. Red-fleshed sweet orange juice improves the risk factors for metabolic syndrome. *Int J Food Sci Nutr* 66 (7):830–836.

Smith, D. E., J. K. Thompson, J. M. Raczynski, and J. E. Hilner. 1999. Body image among men and women in a biracial cohort: The CARDIA Study. *Int J Eat Disord* 25 (1):71–82.

Smith, S. R. 2014. Drug treatment of obesity. *JAMA Intern Med* 174 (8):1414–1415.

Stein, A. C., C. Liao, S. Paski, T. Polonsky, C. E. Semrad, and S. S. Kupfer. 2016. Obesity and cardiovascular risk in adults with celiac disease. *J Clin Gastroenterol*. 50(7):545–550. doi: 10.1097/MCG.0000000000000422.

Stevens, L., J. Nicholas, L. Wood, and M. Nelson. 2013. School lunches v. packed lunches: A comparison of secondary schools in England following the introduction of compulsory school food standards. *Public Health Nutr* 16 (6):1037–1042.

Striegel-Moore, R. H., G. B. Schreiber, K. M. Pike, D. E. Wilfley, G. Schreiber, and J. Rodin. 1995. Drive for thinness in black and white preadolescent girls. *Int J Eat Disord* 18 (1):59–69.

Suliburska, J., P. Bogdanski, M. Szulinska, M. Stepien, D. Pupek-Musialik, and A. Jablecka. 2012. Effects of green tea supplementation on elements, total antioxidants, lipids, and glucose values in the serum of obese patients. *Biol Trace Elem Res* 149 (3):315–322.

Thomas, E. L., J. A. Fitzpatrick, S. J. Malik, S. D. Taylor-Robinson, and J. D. Bell. 2013. Whole body fat: Content and distribution. *Prog Nucl Magn Reson Spectrosc* 73:56–80.

Thurber, K. A., T. Dobbins, M. Kirk, P. Dance, and C. Banwell. 2015. Early life predictors of increased body mass index among indigenous Australian children. *PLoS One* 10 (6):e0130039.

Tsuda, T., F. Horio, K. Uchida, H. Aoki, and T. Osawa. 2003. Dietary cyanidin 3-O-beta-D-glucoside-rich purple corn color prevents obesity and ameliorates hyperglycemia in mice. *J Nutr* 133 (7):2125–2130.

Ujcic-Voortman, J. K., G. Bos, C. A. Baan, A. P. Verhoeff, and J. C. Seidell. 2011. Obesity and body fat distribution: Ethnic differences and the role of socio-economic status. *Obes Facts* 4 (1):53–60.

Visscher, T. L., and J. C. Seidell. 2001. The public health impact of obesity. *Annu Rev Public Health* 22 (1):355–375.

Vucenik, I., and J. P. Stains. 2012. Obesity and cancer risk: Evidence, mechanisms, and recommendations. *Ann NY Acad Sci* 1271:37–43.

Walker, G. E., P. Marzullo, R. Ricotti, G. Bona, and F. Prodam. 2014. The pathophysiology of abdominal adipose tissue depots in health and disease. *Horm Mol Biol Clin Investig* 19 (1):57–74.

Wells, N. M., B. M. Myers, and C. R. Henderson, Jr. 2014. School gardens and physical activity: A randomized controlled trial of low-income elementary schools. *Prev Med* 69 (Suppl 1):S27–S33.

Whitfield, P., A. Parry-Strong, E. Walsh, M. Weatherall, and J. D. Krebs. 2016. The effect of a cinnamon-, chromium- and magnesium-formulated honey on glycaemic control, weight loss and lipid parameters in type 2 diabetes: An open-label cross-over randomised controlled trial. *Eur J Nutr* 55(3):1123–1131.

Whitlock, E. P., C. T. Orleans, N. Pender, and J. Allan. 2002. Evaluating primary care behavioral counseling interventions: An evidence-based approach. *Am J Prev Med* 22 (4):267–284.

WHO. 1998. Obesity: Preventing and managing the global epidemic. WHO/NUT/NCD/98.1. Geneva, Switzerland: WHO.

WHO. 2000. Obesity: Preventing and managing the global epidemic. WHO Technical Report Series No. 894. Geneva, Switzerland: WHO.

WHO. 2008. Training course on child growth assessment: WHO child growth standards, Module D; Counseling on growth and feeding. Geneva, Switzerland: WHO.

WHO. 2015. Obesity and overweight: Fact sheet 311. Accessed March 3, 2016. http://www.who.int/mediacentre/factsheets/fs311/en.

Winter, J. E., R. J. MacInnis, N. Wattanapenpaiboon, and C. A. Nowson. 2014. BMI and all-cause mortality in older adults: A meta-analysis. *Am J Clin Nutr* 99 (4):875–890.

Yancy, W. S., M. K. Olsen, J. R. Guyton, R. P. Bakst, and E. C. Westman. A low-carbohydrate, ketogenic diet versus a low-fat diet to treat obesity and hyperlipidemia: A randomized, controlled trial. *Ann Intern Med* 140 (10):769–777.

Yanovski, S. Z., and J. A. Yanovski. 2014. Long-term drug treatment for obesity: A systematic and clinical review. *JAMA* 311 (1):74–86.

Yun, J. W. 2010. Possible anti-obesity therapeutics from nature: A review. *Phytochemistry* 71 (14–15):1625–1641.

Zong, X. N., H. Li, and Y. Q. Zhang. 2015. Family-related risk factors of obesity among preschool children: Results from a series of national epidemiological surveys in China. *BMC Public Health* 15:927.

4 HEAL for Hyperlipidemia

Bart Kay

CONTENTS

4.1 WHAT IS HYPERLIPIDEMIA?

"Hyperlipidemia" is a term that literally refers to high ("hyper-") levels of any of the lipids in the blood ("-emia"). The lipids include fats, waxes, sterols, fat-soluble vitamins (such as A, D, E, and K), monoglycerides, diglycerides, triglycerides, phospholipids, and others. Lipids are fat-soluble, hydrophobic molecules. They will not, therefore, readily dissolve into the blood plasma. For this reason a class of phospholipoproteins exist to act as carriers of the various lipids in the blood. A phospholipoprotein is a ball of phospholipids packed together to form a monolayer (hydrophilic phosphate end out, hydrophobic lipid end in). The ball structure is maintained by one or more protein structures (various proteins are synthesized that ultimately form various different phospholipoproteins), and the ball structure is also maintained by molecular cholesterol. The different phospholipoproteins exist in order to deliver the various lipid cargos to targeted cells with receptors for a specific phospholipoprotein. Phospholipoproteins are usually referred to simply as "lipoproteins." The classes of lipoproteins are chylomicrons, high-density lipoproteins (HDL), intermediate-density lipoproteins (IDL), low-density lipoproteins (LDL), and very low-density lipoproteins (VLDL). Figure 4.1 shows how various types of lipoproteins carry lipids in the blood.

Hyperlipidemia is a "medical condition" because it is defined as such by the medical profession as a fasting blood lipid level that is above a given value for that lipid. The current values are based on guidelines produced by researchers, but unfortunately without any acceptable evidentiary support (Elliott 2014), indicating that the given level is "too high" for any long-term health-related reasons, with a few exceptions. The exceptions are those indications that pancreatitis can develop at high triglyceride levels in types 1a, 2b, 4, and 5 hyperlipidemia, and that hepatosplenomegaly can be associated with type 5 hyperlipidemia.

Hyperlipidemia is typically classified as either "primary/hereditary" or "secondary/acquired." Primary or hereditary hyperlipidemia is the result of an individual's genetic makeup, when those genes interact with the environmental milieu in which that individual finds or places him/herself. Secondary or acquired hyperlipidemia is classified as that which results from sequelae of other conditions, such as type 2 diabetes mellitus. A third far less common classification for hyperlipidemia is "idiopathic," meaning of no known cause. Primary hyperlipidemia is subcategorized as one of "type 1" through "type 5" (Table 4.1).

Table 4.1 shows these classifications in terms of genetic defect, specific resultant hyperlipidemia, complications, interventions, and prevalence.

Secondary or acquired hyperlipidemias can present as the increased concentration of any of the lipoproteins affected by primary hyperlipidemias. The clinical significance of these high levels is the same as it is for primary hyperlipidemias. The most common associates to secondary hyperlipidemias have been proposed to be diabetes mellitus and the taking of thiazide diuretics, beta-blockers, or estrogens (Chait and Brunzell 1990).

4.1.1 WHAT IS DYSLIPIDEMIA?

"Dyslipidemia" is a term literally meaning "dysfunctional lipid concentrations in the blood." Dyslipidemia is often used to describe various hyperlipidemias, but it can also denote a low concentration of a given lipoprotein. An example of this is HDL, which has often been described as "good cholesterol." For a lipid level to

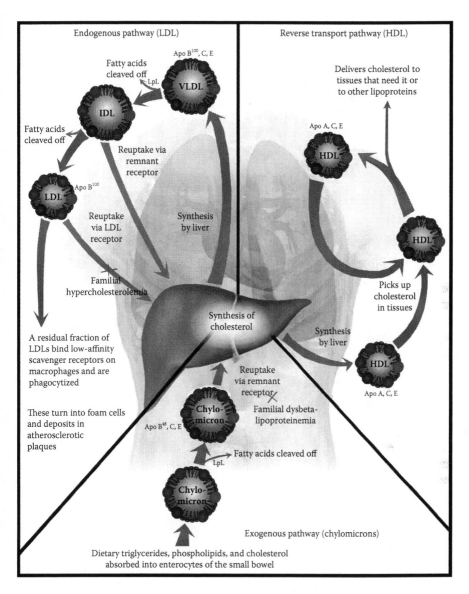

FIGURE 4.1 Lipoprotein classes. (From Npatchett, A diagram to the endogenous and exogenous pathways of lipoprotein metabolism. Own work, May 22, 2015. Licensed under CC BY-SA 3.0 via Wikimedia Commons. https://commons.wikimedia.org/wiki/File:Lipoprotein_metabolism.png#/media/File:Lipoprotein_metabol ism.png.)

be dysfunctional—that is, for the term "dyslipidemia" to be valid—the elevated (or reduced) level of that lipid in the blood must be demonstrably and causally linked to dysfunction. Failing this, it is a nonsense term. Dyslipidemia is almost invariably indicated as a "causal factor" or "risk factor" for coronary heart disease, cardiovascular disease, and cerebrovascular disease (via atherosclerosis).

TABLE 4.1
Types of Primary or Familial Hyperlipidemia

Type	Genetic Defect	Specific Resultant Hyperlipidemia	Possible Presentation	Standard Intervention(s)	Prevalence Estimate
Type 1a	Lipoprotein lipase deficiency	Chylomicrons	Can cause pancreatitis at high triglyceride levels, hepatosplenomegaly, lipemia retinalis, eruptive skin xanthomas	Dietary	1 in 1,000,000[b]
Type 1b	Altered Apo CII	Chylomicrons	"	Dietary	1 in 1,000,000[b]
Type 1c	Lipoprotein lipase inhibition	Chylomicrons	"	Dietary	1 in 1,000,000[b]
Type 2a	LDL receptor deficiency	LDL	Can cause pancreatitis at high triglyceride levels, xanthelasma, arcus senilis, tendon xanthomas	Dietary, pharmacological (bile acid sequestrants, statins, niacin)	1 in 500 heterozygotes[a]
Type 2b	LDL receptor deficiency and elevated Apo B	LDL and VLDL	"	Dietary, pharmacological (bile acid sequestrants, statins, niacin, fibrate)	1 in 100[c]
Type 3	Apo E defect	IDL	Tuboeruptive xanthomas and palmar xanthomas	Dietary, pharmacological (fibrate, statins)	1 in 10,000[c]
Type 4	Increased VLDL	VLDL	Can cause pancreatitis at high triglyceride levels	Dietary, pharmacological (fibrate, niacin, statins)	1 in 100[c]
Type 5	Increased VLDL and decreased lipoprotein lipase	VLDL and chylomicrons	Can cause pancreatitis at high triglyceride levels, hepatosplenomegaly, lipaemia retinalis, eruptive skin xanthomas	Dietary, pharmacological (fibrate, niacin)	No reference found

[a] Fung, Michelle, John Hill, Donald Cook, and Jiri Frohlich. 2011. Case series of type III hyperlipoproteinemia in children. *BMJ Case Reports 2011*; doi:10.1136/bcr.02.2011.3895.

[b] Hyperlipoproteinemia type 1, from Centre for Arab Genomic Studies. Retrieved July 2011. Citing: "About 1:1,000,000 people are affected with Hyperlipoproteinemia type I worldwide with a higher prevalence in some regions of Canada."

[c] Wikipedia. Hyperlipidemia. https://en.wikipedia.org/wiki/Hyperlipidemia. Accessed September 28, 2015.

- *In terms of raising HDL ("good cholesterol") levels using either niacin or CEPT inhibitors*, there was apparently no benefit as regards cardiovascular mortality, all-cause mortality, nonfatal heart attack incidence, or cerebrovascular accidents in a cohort of 69,515 patients followed over various numbers of person years (Verdoia et al. 2015).

- *In terms of raised LDL or triglycerides coincident with hospitalization for coronary heart disease*, the expected relationship (under the assumption that both high LDL and high blood triglycerides are valid risk factors for coronary artery disease) was absent in 136,905 admissions (Sachdeva et al. 2009, p. 117). In this study, the distributions of both blood triglyceride and LDL levels were normal in those hospitalized with atherosclerosis-related diseases. Assuming the blood lipid screening taken at hospitalization is representative of the person's chronic levels, this normal distribution of prevalence values means that one is as likely to present with coronary artery disease having maintained a low level of both triglycerides and LDL as if one had maintained a high level of both. These are not, therefore, valid risk markers. It is interesting that the authors of that study (who enjoy grants from "Big Pharma") conclude that their findings "may provide further support for recent guideline revisions with even lower LDL goals." The findings do not in fact support such a claim whatsoever. The data those authors have presented shows that the two factors are not causally related (Section 4.3.2).

- *In terms of reduced LDL and triglycerides in hospitalized patients post heart attack*, those with triglycerides less than 62.5 mg/dL and LDL less than 110 mg/dL had a 10.9-fold higher adjusted risk of mortality than patients with triglycerides greater than or equal to 62.5 mg/dL and LDL greater than or equal to 110 mg/dL (Cheng et al. 2015). This suggests that both LDL and triglyceride in the blood may actually play a vital role in survival post heart attack. Research should now investigate this possibility.

4.2 COMPLICATIONS OF HYPERLIPIDEMIA

The empirically established ramifications of the various hyperlipidemias are shown in Table 4.1. There are two ramifications of serious concern, these being (1) the indication that pancreatitis can develop in the presence of types 1a, 2b, 4, and 5 hyperlipidemias when high triglyceride levels (>11 mmol/L) are also present (Thomson 1989); and (2) hepatosplenomegaly associated with type 5 hyperlipidemia. A separate dogma often perpetuated in the literature is that elevated LDL or indeed lowered HDL are risk factors for the development of atherosclerosis over time (the "cholesterol/heart disease" hypothesis). This is an idea without acceptable empirical support (Elliott 2014). Section 4.2.1 describes what is required by way of acceptable empirical support for a notion; it also describes how the "cholesterol/heart disease" hypothesis fails to meet this burden of evidence. It should be caveated that the level of "evidence" that is "acceptable" varies between groups of professionals interested in the area. These differential standards provide for the current robust debate surrounding conclusions to the extant data. The current author is of the school requiring well-powered and well-designed meta-analyses of large subject pools over lengthy follow-up periods. Such analyses must be free from publication bias (Section 4.2.1) and should report absolute incidence rates rather than relative rates solely. Such a meta-analytical approach provides for the most robust indication of the level of coincidence between two factors, but it cannot establish causality unless the "coefficient of causality" is equal to 1.0 (Section 4.2.1.1, 1). An indication (but not "evidence") that a causal relationship is or is not possible and/or that a predictor is good enough to be of utility can be gained by applying the Bradford Hill criteria (Section 4.2.1.1).

4.2.1 EPIDEMIOLOGICAL BACKGROUND AND UNDERPINNINGS

In order for the physiological concentration of a given lipoprotein in the blood to be correctly described as "dyslipidemia" and therefore in need of intervention, there should be clear scientific support for a cause-and-effect relationship between a given risk factor and a deleterious health outcome in an adequately sized sample of individuals over adequate time. The author would like at this point to make it clear that scientific support is derived from the available valid data. "Scientific support" does not include consensus opinion. To this end, the inference that a lifestyle factor is associated with increased incidence of a given deleterious outcome is perhaps the best compromise available. This data comes in the form of meta-analyses. The meta-analytical procedure is to search for studies comparing variable "x" with outcome "y." Specific inclusion/exclusion validity criteria are determined and applied to all identified studies. Included studies are then shown on a diagram indicating the relative risk ratio or similar metric for each included study. At the bottom a single "overall result" for all included studies is shown as mathematically determined, according to result and sample size. A larger sample is weighted more than a smaller one in the overall result. Once this meta-analysis is complete, a test for "publication bias" is needed. The smaller a sample size is, the more the result for that study can be statistically expected to vary from the "overall" result. Unfortunately, small sample sizes that produce "negative" results do not tend to get published in the scientific literature. This means the "overall" result determined from a meta-analysis that includes only published literature will be biased artificially toward finding that a certain lifestyle factor is a valid associate to the deleterious health outcome at a given confidence level, when in fact it may not be at all. Once a valid (i.e., not publication-biased) meta-analysis is presented, then a number of criteria should be applied to decide whether the factor concerned should be considered a valid risk factor or not. The criteria are named for their proposer, Sir Austen Bradford Hill (1897–1991). The failure of any one of these leads to the rejection of the relationship as causal in nature and/ or of utility in the real world.

4.2.1.1 The Bradford Hill Criteria

1. *Strength (effect size)*: A small association between two factors is not of utility as a predictor. The "coefficient of causality" is equal to the correlation statistic multiplied by itself. This coefficient if multiplied by 100 renders a percentage "overlap" of variance between factors "x" and "y." To be of utility in prediction, the correlation must be very strong, and to be "causal" R^2 must equal 1.0.

2. *Consistency (reproducibility)*: Consistent findings observed by different persons in different places with different samples strengthen the likelihood of an effect.

3. *Specificity*: Causation is likely if there is a very specific population at a specific site and disease with no other likely explanation. The more specific an association between a factor and an effect is, the bigger the probability of a causal relationship.

4. *Temporality*: The effect has to occur after the cause (and if there is an expected delay between the cause and expected effect, then the effect must occur after that delay).

5. *Biological gradient*: Greater exposure should generally lead to greater incidence of the effect. However, in some cases, the mere presence of the factor can trigger the effect. In other cases, an inverse proportion is observed: greater exposure leads to lower incidence.

6. *Plausibility*: A plausible mechanism between cause and effect is helpful (but Hill noted that knowledge of the mechanism is limited by current knowledge).

7. *Coherence*: Coherence between epidemiological and laboratory findings increases the likelihood of an effect. However, Hill noted that a "lack of such [laboratory] evidence cannot nullify the epidemiological effect on associations."

8. *Experiment*: "Occasionally it is possible to appeal to experimental evidence."

9. *Analogy*: The effect of similar factors may be considered. (Hill 1965, p. 10)

4.2.2   Cholesterol as a Risk Factor for Non-Communicable Diseases

This section highlights the discussion on whether cholesterol is a risk factor for non-communicable diseases.

4.2.2.1   Cholesterol as a "Risk Factor" for Cardiovascular and Cerebrovascular Disease

Cholesterol is a sterol molecule that is hydrophobic. Cholesterol is therefore transported in the blood plasma by lipoproteins. These come in various classes, as previously described (Figure 4.1). Primarily, the classes of lipoprotein–cholesterol packages determine to which body cells the lipid payload will be delivered. Cholesterol specifically makes up 2%–3% of the body weight, 25% of which is to be found in the brain. Cholesterol is the precursor for the steroid hormones, and it is a vital structural component of all cell membranes, among other vital biological tasks. In short, too little cholesterol will lead inexorably to disease, dysfunction, decline, and ultimately increased likelihood of death (Anderson et al. 1987; Horwich et al. 2002; Steffens et al. 2003). The human body automatically synthesizes the cholesterol molecule from acetyl coenzyme A (the "first" reactant in the tricarboxylic acid cycle, also known as the TCA cycle and the "Krebs" cycle). Cholesterol is synthesized starting with two acetyl coenzyme A molecules. It makes no difference whether those particular acetyl coenzyme A molecules came originally from fat,

from carbohydrates, or from protein (or indeed alcohol). The regulation of cholesterol synthesis is managed by the activation of the genes encoding for the provision of the required enzymes. Cholesterol can also be absorbed directly from food.
Excess cholesterol is excreted in the feces. The level of cholesterol in the blood will
be determined largely by the number of each of the various lipoprotein carriers in the
blood. Chylomicrons are produced by the intestines, while the other lipoproteins are
produced by the liver, which plays a crucial role in lipoprotein–cholesterol homeostasis, signaling, and distribution. The level of the various lipoprotein subfractions
in the blood at any given point is the result of the individual genetic makeup and its
interaction with the sum of all environmental and lifestyle factors affecting the activation or suppression of the genes encoding for (1) the production of cholesterol and
(2) the production of the various lipoprotein carriers.

One hypothesis that has become popular by consensus (see the previous section
regarding consensus) for some years now is that increased concentration of cholesterol in the blood (specifically in the form of LDL) is associated with increased
risk of atherosclerosis. Atherosclerosis is a dysfunction where the immune and
inflammatory pathways are activated against a specific LDL subfraction (Phillips
and Perry 2015)—that is, the smallest and most dense of the LDL—that has
become damaged by oxidation (Chang et al. 2013), glycation (Chang et al. 2013),
or other means. In atherosclerosis the LDL must first be driven into the vascular
epithelia under pressure. This requires that the epithelial gap junctions must have
become dysfunctional or that the blood pressure has become too high (or both).
Atherosclerosis does not occur in veins whatsoever. Once driven into the gap junctions, the oxidative glycation or other derangement occurs over time. It is this
altered LDL (and actually only a subfraction of these) that have been shown to
precipitate an inflammatory/immune response. The response is the migration to
and phagocytosis of the deranged LDL by macrophages. These turn into "foam
cells," which then become encased in a fibrous tissue capsule. This capsule can
invade the lumen of the artery and occlude flow. These "plaques" can become
calcified and hence brittle, and/or the cholesterol can crystallize in the plaques,
both of which can cause rupture, bleeding, clotting, thrombosis, and infarct, and
therefore heart attack, stroke, and related emergencies. A high blood concentration
of LDL is almost universally cited as a valid risk factor in atherosclerosis. This is
despite the hypothesis being patently in breach of the Bradford Hill criteria 1, 2,
3, 5, 6, and 7 (at least).

4.2.2.2 Cholesterol/Triglycerides as "Risk Factors" for Diabetes/Hyperglycemia

Several studies have suggested an association between blood LDL level and type 2
diabetes/high fasting blood glucose (Koskinen et al. 1992; Lehto et al. 1996; Lehto
et al. 1997). Typically, such studies are small in scale. No high-quality meta-analysis
as previously described was identified by the current author. It is not inconceivable,
however, that an association between hyperglycemia/type 2 diabetes and elevated
LDL may exist. The most likely mechanism would seem to be that type 2 diabetes appears to be an inflammatory disorder at its root (Chapple and Genco 2013).

Chronic, unresolved inflammation is associated with increased LDL, with increased triglycerides, and with decreased HDL (Feingold and Grunfeld 2015). These changes are mediated by the inflammatory and immune responses, and the indicated intervention is in resolving the inflammation rather than in attempting to circumvent the symptoms either with dietary or pharmacological intervention designed to encourage opposing changes to the lipid levels. The dietary patterns associated with lowered HDL and raised triglycerides are the high-carbohydrate, low-fat approaches (see Section 4.3 for references). Conversely, the dietary patterns associated with raised HDL and with lowered triglycerides are the low-carbohydrate, high-fat approaches (see Section 4.3 for references).

4.2.2.3   Cholesterol/Triglycerides as "Risk Factors" for Hypertension

Several studies have suggested an association between blood LDL level and hypertension (Halperin et al. 2006; Laaksonen et al. 2008; Sesso et al. 2005). Similarly to other inflammatory conditions (e.g., those described in Section 4.2.2.2), it is no surprise that LDL may be elevated in hypertension via similar mechanisms. Again, the indicated course of action is ion-resolving the hypertension, not in attempting to encourage lipid profile changes.

4.2.2.4   Cholesterol/Triglycerides as "Risk Factors" for Obesity

Several studies have suggested an association between blood LDL level and obesity, the best of which in its conceptual presentation of the underlying physiology appears to be that of Klop et al. (2012). These authors correctly identify chronic unresolved inflammation as the root of lipid profile changes in obesity. The indicated intervention is in resolving the obesity, rather than attempting to modify the lipid profile. Dietary patterns associated with the amelioration of obesity and its sequelae appear to be the higher-fat (monounsaturated fatty acids [MUFAs] and saturates), moderate-protein, lower-carbohydrate (lower glycemic index/glycemic load) approaches (Nordmann et al. 2011; Schwingshackl and Hoffmann 2013).

4.2.2.5   Cholesterol/Triglycerides as "Risk Factors" for Depression

Several studies discuss the relationships between the various lipids in the brain and depression. Largely, the lipid profiles associated with adverse depression metrics are lowered HDL and raised triglycerides (Martinac et al. 2007; van Reedt Dortland et al. 2010). Müller et al. (2015) showed that diet can moderate lipid profiles in the brain. With this in mind, the dietary patterns associated with lowered HDL and raised triglycerides are the high-carbohydrate, low-fat approaches (see Section 4.3 for references). Conversely, the dietary patterns associated with raised HDL and with lowered triglycerides are the low-carbohydrate, high-fat approaches (see Section 4.3 for references). By way of caution, some persons with depression do not respond well to low-carbohydrate diets: the insulin response to glycemic loading enhances the bioavailability of tryptophan to the brain (Shabbir et al. 2013). Insufficiency of tryptophan in the brain causes low brain serotonin, a known associate to depressive symptoms. For this reason, those with depression should be under competent dietary supervision as part of their holistic treatment plan.

4.3 FOOD GROUPS AND DIETARY PATTERNS TO PREVENT HYPERLIPIDEMIA

In the case of an identified genetic or primary hyperlipidemia, the individual ought to be under competent supervision as regards their blood lipid levels. Regular checks should be undertaken, and if necessary, adjustment made to the diet. It is the increase in blood triglycerides that is associated with the accepted risks of pancreatic, liver, and spleen inflammatory dysfunctions. It appears that the maintenance of blood triglyceride levels (nominally, below 11 mmol/L) may be desirable as regards these risks (Thompson 1989). The current author suggests that the following general principles (Sections 4.3.1 through 4.3.5) apply equally to those with primary hyperlipidemias and those with secondary hyperlipidemias, as the ramifications for each population are the same. There are no apparently valid reasons to attempt to moderate phospholipoproteins directly, as described by Sections 4.1 and 4.2.

4.3.1 CARBOHYDRATES AND BLOOD TRIGLYCERIDES

It has been suggested that a diet in which carbohydrate is removed and isocalorically replaced with fat (MUFAs and saturates) nets a statistically significant improvement (reduction) in blood triglyceride levels in obese diabetic patients (Tay et al. 2015). In the case of overweight but nondiabetic persons, a low-carbohydrate diet compared with a high-carbohydrate diet (both low GI) was also associated with reduced blood triglycerides (Sacks et al. 2014). The assertion that low-carbohydrate nutrition is associated with lowered blood triglyceride levels in a more generalized population is also corroborated by Feinman et al. (2015). Those authors also suggest that the low-carbohydrate approach is coincident with better blood glucose control, with lowered levels of glycated hemoglobin, and with better fat loss. The suggestion that lowered carbohydrate intake is associated with lowered blood triglyceride is further supported by meta-analytical data of 32 published studies by Schwingshackl and Hoffmann (2013). Still other meta-analyses (Hu et al. 2012; Santos et al. 2012; Sharman et al. 2004) corroborate this also. Spreadbury and Samis (2013) have suggested that (1) CVD is still virtually absent in those rare populations with minimal Western dietary influence, and (2) the CVD risk factors for obesity and diabetes (both also risk factors for atherosclerosis in turn) are driven by increased caloric intake, with carbohydrates implicated specifically. For the reason of its association to increased blood triglyceride, the restriction of carbohydrates to as close to zero as possible/practical is indicated. There are no essential dietary carbohydrates. It should not be forgotten that there is no apparently valid reason to attempt to moderate the phospholipoprotein levels, and attempting to moderate triglycerides can be problematic also. Indeed, by way of caution described in Section 4.1.1, in terms of reduced LDL and triglycerides in hospitalized patients post heart attack, those with triglycerides less than 62.5 mg/dL and LDL less than 110 mg/dL had a 10.9-fold higher adjusted risk of mortality than patients with triglycerides greater than or equal to 62.5 mg/dL and LDL greater than or equal to 110 mg/dL (Cheng et al. 2015).

In summary, the consumption of relatively large amounts of carbohydrates is associated with reduced HDL and with increased blood triglycerides. Both are apparently symptomatic of inflammation as described in Sections 4.3.2 and 4.3.4. Although there is no direct causal evidence linking carbohydrate to inflammation indicated here, the restriction of carbohydrates is indicated as described in Sections 4.2.2.2 through 4.2.2.5.

4.3.2 SATURATED FAT AND BLOOD TRIGLYCERIDES

As described in Section 4.2, there has been a dogma in the literature for many years indicating that the consumption of saturated fat is causal in dyslipidemia—specifically hypercholesterolemia, specifically raised LDL. This hypercholesterolemia is proposed in turn to be causally related to the development of atherosclerosis. Atherosclerosis is the most common manifestation of cardiovascular/cerebrovascular disease. This dogma is perpetuated by a large (and hence powerful in terms of consensus) group of researchers. If the dogma were correct, then we should be able to identify a correlation between the intake of saturated fat in the diet and the incidence of cardiovascular and/or cerebrovascular accidents. Siri-Tarino et al. (2010) undertook just such an analysis of nearly 350,000 individuals over 6–23 years of follow-up. Their analysis showed no coincidence between increased saturated fat intake and either cerebrovascular or cardiovascular accidents. The Siri-Tarino et al. (2010) work patently suffers from publication bias (Section 4.2.1). The effect of the bias in this case is an artificially increased risk ratio, despite which their study steadfastly shows no increase in risks. The work of Siri-Tarino and colleagues has been corroborated via at least one other meta-analysis (de Souza et al. 2015). Further, there is some suggestion that lowered intake of saturated fat is associated with increased risk of death from both ischemic and hemorrhagic strokes (Yamagishi et al. 2010). A recent meta-analysis (Sachdeva et al. 2009) looks at the level of blood lipids (HDL, LDL, and triglycerides) in patients at the time of their admission to hospital for treatment of atherosclerosis-driven pathologies. The expected relationship under the lipid/CVD hypothesis is an increase in the number of patients who fall into each LDL bin range as the LDL level increases, and also an increase for each increasing triglyceride bin value, as well as a decrease for each increasing HDL bin value. Again, in short (Section 4.1.1), these relationships were absent. Finally, one of the currently accepted risk factors for cardiovascular and cerebrovascular accidents is increased adiposity (Hubert et al. 1983). With that in mind, Cohen et al. (2015) have suggested that people have been largely following the Dietary Guidelines for Americans (and presumably similar parallel Western nation documents indicating and advocating high-carbohydrate, low-fat intakes) during the period 1965–2011. This period of adherence to this apparently fallacious advice is coincidental with the onset, progression, and ever-worsening current obesity pandemic, as well as the diabetes pandemic. Both problems appear to be related to the glycemic loading concomitant with carbohydrate consumption, which was added to the diet to replace the fat erroneously removed.

In summary, there is apparently no valid reason to restrict or limit the intake of saturated fats, with the caveat that to maintain health in the long term, the restriction of carbohydrates appears critical (Section 4.3.1), as does the restriction of polyunsaturated fatty acids (PUFAs) (Section 4.3.3). Ignoring either Sections 4.3.1 or 4.3.3 may render Section 4.3.2 fruitless with respect to the long-term health of individuals.

4.3.3 Omega-6 PUFAs and Omega-3 PUFAs

Persons who follow the current Western diet will typically consume a diet that contains both omega-3 and omega-6 polyunsaturated fatty acids (PUFAs). The ratio (omega-6:omega-3) will typically exceed 20:1. A ratio in excess of 1:1 promotes inflammatory processes (Kiecolt-Glaser et al. 2007). Systemic inflammation has been implicated in processes leading to obesity, diabetes, atherosclerosis, Alzheimer's disease, mental health dysfunction, and many other complaints. Indeed, a ratio of tissue omega-6:omega-3 closer to 1:1 is associated with reduced physiological markers of atherosclerosis (Tani et al. 2015), and with reduced CVD events (Ramsden et al. 2010). Discontinuation of erroneous saturated fat avoidance in favor of PUFA, combined with using MUFA when oil is required should go a long way toward achieving a ratio closer to 1:1. In summary, the current author prefers the approach of avoiding the addition of omega-6 oil to food, and taking seafood regularly over commercially prepared supplements of omega-3.

4.3.4 Monounsaturated Fatty Acids

Degirolamo and Rudel (2010) have suggested that replacing saturated fats with MUFAs is not associated with reduced or indeed with increased atherosclerosis. The inverse is also apparently an acceptable conclusion. Therefore, it appears that neither MUFAs or saturated fats are preferable with respect to one another in terms of long-term health.

4.3.5 Trans Fats

Trans fat is found predominantly in processed foods. Usually, the manufacturers use PUFAs in "food" manufacture instead of saturated fats due to the false diet-heart hypothesis. In order to make PUFAs more like saturated fats in terms of physical properties, PUFAs are often "partially hydrogenated." As a side reaction to the catalyst used for this process, many of the remaining double bonds "twist" so that the bond loses its natural "cis" configuration and instead becomes "trans." A meta-analysis (de Souza et al. 2015) of the relationship between manufactured trans fat consumption and CHD mortality expressed as a risk ratio proved positive (1.18 [1.04–1.33]) as did the risk ratio for "CHD incidence" (1.42 [1.05–1.92]). The current author concludes that trans fats are probably absolutely contraindicated.

4.3.6 Specific Nutrients for the Adjustment of Lipid Profiles: "Home Remedies for Hyperlipidemia"

While literature exists that suggests a number of different specific foods may be associated with increased or reduced levels of the various blood lipid levels (and/ or glucose level), the previous discussion renders the description and listing of these foods redundant. It is not apparently necessary or indicated to reduce LDL, nor to increase HDL. Triglycerides can be effectively moderated using a low-carbohydrate approach to nutrition: no specific nutrient seems necessary, nor indicated. Interested readers will nonetheless find some examples of suggested "home remedies" for various conditions in Chapter 1 of this book. It is not the intention of the current author to propose that there is acceptable evidence for any of these.

4.4 OVERALL PRINCIPLES OF OPTIMAL NUTRITION TO REDUCE THE RISK OF CVD/CHD

An "ancestral" whole-food diet, however—as close as possible to grain-free, starch-free, fructose-limited, juice-free, and sugar-free—appears to represent the best lifestyle intervention for obesity, for diabetes, and for CVD/CHD (Spreadbury and Samis 2013). Those authors also suggest that such diets are typically composed of the cells of living organisms, while grains, flour, and sugar are dense, acellular powders. Bacterial inflammation of the small intestine and vagal afferents appears a crucial step in leptin resistance and obesity. Both leptin resistance and obesity are risk factors in turn for both diabetes and CVD/CHD.

4.5 AUTHOR'S CONCLUSIONS

1. There is no acceptable evidence that LDL is causal in atherosclerosis. Association does not infer causality. An LDL subfraction has been shown, rather, to play a role in the inflammatory/immune response: hence its elevation in the blood is associated with this type of dysfunction. Pharmacological or dietary intervention in this respect can be contraindicated, and competent supervision is required before attempting this.
2. None of blood LDL, HDL, or triglycerides provide valid or acceptable predictors of any adverse health outcomes according to the standards of proof imposed by the current author.
3. Dietary carbohydrate is associated with elevated triglycerides.
4. Raised triglycerides have been associated with liver, spleen, and pancreatic inflammatory dysfunction under certain circumstances. Elevated triglycerides can be ameliorated using a restricted carbohydrate nutrition plan under competent supervision.
5. Dietary carbohydrate is also associated with increased glycation of the hemoglobin (a diabetes risk factor), decreased insulin sensitivity, decreased leptin sensitivity, increased adiposity, and increased area under the insulin curve.
6. Substitution of carbohydrates for saturated fat is contraindicated, as described in conclusions 1 through 5.
7. Substitution of PUFAs (omega-6) for saturates is contraindicated with respect to inflammation (a clear risk factor for CVD/CHD).
8. Substitution of MUFAs for saturates or vice versa does not apparently meaningfully affect CVD/CHD events.
9. Trans fat is apparently absolutely contraindicated with respect to CVD/CHD outcomes, as the body recognizes this as foreign and an immune/inflammatory response occurs.
10. An "ancestral" whole-food diet, however—as close as possible to grain-free, starch-free, fructose-free, juice-free, sugar-free, and soda-free—based

on nonstarchy colorful vegetables, leafy greens, and meats, appears to represent the best lifestyle intervention for obesity, diabetes, and CVD/CHD, as well as other inflammatory-type dysfunctions, presumably.

4.6 CASE STUDIES

4.6.1 CASE STUDY 1

A 45-year-old female presents to you and says that her physician has determined that her total cholesterol, LDL cholesterol, and triglycerides are "too high" (254 mg/dL, 190 mg/dL, 500 mg/dL, respectively). The diagnosis is "secondary hyperlipidemia." The physician proposes to instigate a program of pharmacological (statins) and dietary (Dietary Guidelines for Americans 2015) intervention. Comment on this critically. See also: Bowden and Sinatra (2012).

1. Is there any valid reason to attempt to modify this person's lipid levels using dietary intervention? If so, which particular lipid(s) and using what particular intervention?
2. Is there any valid reason to attempt to modify this person's lipid levels using statin drugs?
3. If you are not a medical professional or medical prescriber (United Kingdom), should you advise anyone on pharmacological interventions?

4.6.2 CASE STUDY 2

A 60-year-old male presents to you suggesting that his recent blood lipid screen has come back with "high triglyceride levels" (15 mmol/L) and a relatively high fasting blood glucose level (6.8 mmol/L). He is confused, as he eats very little fat and follows the standard Western diet suggested by the major dietetics and diabetes associations. Explain to him how he might lower his triglyceride and fasting blood glucose levels, and why it is important to do so.

1. Discuss the association between carbohydrate consumption and each of (i) fasting blood glucose and (ii) blood triglyceride levels.
2. Describe a dietary pattern adjustment in terms of macronutrient makeup that is associated with reductions in both fasting blood glucose and blood triglycerides. Discuss at least one possible problem an individual might encounter following such a change to the diet, and how you would counsel the client through this and/or how you would moderate your approach under such circumstances.
3. Discuss the flaws in the idea that saturated fat ought to be reduced in the diet. Discuss the reasons why the use of omega-6 PUFAs is probably contraindicated for long-term health.

REFERENCES

Anderson, K. M., Castelli, W. P., Levy, D. 1987. Cholesterol and mortality: 30 years of follow-up from the Framingham Study. *JAMA* 257 (16): 2176–2180.

Bowden, J., Sinatra, S. 2012. *The Great Cholesterol Myth: Why Lowering Your Cholesterol Won't Prevent Heart Disease, and the Statin-Free Plan That Will.* Beverly, MA: Fair Winds Press.

Chait, A., and Brunzell, J. D. 1990. Acquired hyperlipidemia (secondary dyslipoproteinemias). *Endocrinol Metab Clin North Am* 19 (2): 259–278.

Chang, C., Liao, H., Chang, C., Chen, C., Chen, C., Yanga, C., Tsaih, F., Chen, C. 2013. Oxidized ApoC1 on MALDI-TOF and glycated-ApoA1 band on gradient gel as potential diagnostic tools for atherosclerotic vascular disease. *Clinica Chim Acta* 420: 69–75.

Chapple, I. L., Genco, R. 2013. Working Group of Joint EFP/AAP Workshop: Diabetes and periodontal diseases; Consensus Report of the Joint EFP/AAP Workshop on Periodontitis and Systemic Diseases. *J Clin Periodontol* 40 (Suppl 14): S106–S112.

Cheng, K., Chu, C., Lin, T., Lee, K., Sheu, S., Lai, W. 2015. Lipid paradox in acute myocardial infarction: The association with 30-day in-hospital mortality. *Crit Care Med* 43(6): 1255–1264.

Cohen, E., Cragg, M., deFonseka, J., Hite, A., Rosenberg, M., Zhou, B. 2015. Statistical review of U.S. macronutrient consumption data, 1965–2011: Americans have been following dietary guidelines, coincident with the rise in obesity. *Nutrition* 31 (5): 727–732.

Degirolamo, C., Rudel, L. L. 2010. Dietary monounsaturated fatty acids appear not to provide cardioprotection. *Curr Atheroscler Rep* 12(6): 391–396.

de Souza, R. J., Mente, A., Maroleanu, A., Cozma, A. I., Ha, V., Kishibe, T., Uleryk, E. et al. 2015. Intake of saturated and trans unsaturated fatty acids and risk of all cause mortality, cardiovascular disease, and type 2 diabetes: Systematic review and meta-analysis of observational studies. *BMJ* 351:h3978. doi:10.1136/bmj.h3978.

Elliott, J. 2014. Flaws, fallacies and facts: Reviewing the early history of the lipid and diet/heart hypotheses. *Food and Nutrition Sciences* 5: 1886–1903.

Feingold, K. R., and Grunfeld, C. 2015. In: De Groot, L. J., Beck-Peccoz, P., Chrousos, G., Dungan, K., Grossman, A., Hershman, J. M., Koch, C. et al. (eds). *The Effect of Inflammation and Infection on Lipids and Lipoproteins.* Endotext (Internet). South Dartmouth, MA: MDText.com: 2000–2015.

Feinman, R. D., Pogozelski, W. K., Astrup, A., Bernstein, R. K., Fine, E. J., Westman, E. C., Accurso, A. et al. 2015. Dietary carbohydrate restriction as the first approach in diabetes management: Critical review and evidence base. *Nutrition* 31(1): 1–13.

Fung, M., Hill, J., Cook, D., Frohlich, J. 2011. Case series of type III hyperlipoproteinemia in children. *BMJ Case Rep*: doi:10.1136/bcr.02.2011.3895.

Halperin, R. O., Sesso, H. D., Ma, J., Buring, J. E., Stampfer, M. J., Gaziano, J. M. 2006. Dyslipidemia and the risk of incident hypertension in men. *Hypertension* 47 (1): 45–50.

Hill, A. B. 1965. The environment and disease: Association or causation? *Proceedings of the Royal Society of Medicine* 58 (5): 295–300.

Horwich, T. B., Hamilton, M. A., MacLellan, W. R., Fonarow, G. C. 2002. Low serum total cholesterol is associated with marked increase in mortality in advanced heart failure. *J Card Fail* 8 (4): 216–224.

Hu, T., Mills, K. T., Yao, L., Demanelis, K., Eloustaz, M., Yancy, W. S. Jr., Kelly, T. N., He, J., Bazzano, L. A. 2012. Effects of low-carbohydrate diets versus low-fat diets on metabolic risk factors: A meta-analysis of randomized controlled clinical trials. *Am J Epidemiol* 176 (Suppl 7): S44–S54.

Hubert, H. B., Feinleib, M., McNamara, P. M., Castelli, W. P. 1983. Obesity as an independent risk factor for cardiovascular disease: A 26-year follow-up of participants in the Framingham Heart Study. *Circulation* 67(5): 968–977.

Kiecolt-Glaser, J. K., Belury, M. A., Porter, K., Beversdorf, D., Lemeshow, S., Glaser, R. 2007. Depressive symptoms, n-6: n-3 fatty acids, and inflammation in older adults. *Psychosom Med* 69 (3): 217–224.

Klop, Boudewijn, Spencer D. Proctor, John C. Mamo, Kathleen M. Botham, and Manuel Castro Cabezas. 2012. Understanding postprandial inflammation and its relationship to lifestyle behaviour and metabolic diseases. *International journal of vascular medicine* 2012:947417. doi: 10.1155/2012/947417.

Koskinen, P., Mänttäri, M., Manninen, V., Huttunen, J. K., Heinonen, O. P., Frick, M. H. 1992. Coronary heart disease incidence in NIDDM patients in the Helsinki Heart Study. *Diabetes Care* 15(7): 820–825.

Laaksonen, D. E., Niskanen, L., Nyyssönen, K., Lakka, T. A., Laukkanen, J. A., Salonen, J. T. 2008. Dyslipidemia as a predictor of hypertension in middle-aged men. *Eur Heart J* 29(20): 2561–2568.

Lehto, S., Rönnemaa, T., Pyörälä, K., Laakso, M. 1996. Predictors of stroke in middle-aged patients with non-insulin-dependent diabetes. *Stroke* 27(1): 63–68.

Lehto, S., Rönnemaa, T., Haffher, S. M., Pyörälä, K., Kallio, V., Laakso, M. 1997. Dyslipidemia and hyperglycemia predict coronary heart disease events in middle-aged patients with NIDDM. *Diabetes* 46(8): 1354–1359.

Martinac, Marko, Dalibor Karlović, Nada Vrkić, Darko Marčinko, Nada Bazina, and Dragan Babić. 2007. Serum lipids in a depressive disorder with regard to depression type. *Biochemia Medica* 17(1): 94–101.

Müller, Christian P., Martin Reichel, Christiane Muehle, Cosima Rhein, Erich Gulbins, and Johannes Kornhuber. 2015. Brain membrane lipids in major depression and anxiety disorders. *Biochimica et Biophysica Acta (BBA)-Molecular and Cell Biology of Lipids* 1851(8): 1052–1065.

Nordmann, A. J., Suter-Zimmermann, K., Bucher, H. C., Shai, I., Tuttle, K. R., Estruch, R., Briel, M. 2011. Meta-analysis comparing Mediterranean to low-fat diets for modification of cardiovascular risk factors. *Am J Med* 124(9):841–851.

Phillips, C. M., and Perry, I. J. 2015. Lipoprotein particle subclass profiles among metabolically healthy and unhealthy obese and non-obese adults: Does size matter? *Atherosclerosis* 242(2): 399–406.

Ramsden, C. E., Hibbeln, J. R., Majchrzak, S. F., Davis, J. M. 2010. N-6 fatty acid–specific and mixed polyunsaturate dietary interventions have different effects on CHD risk: A meta-analysis of randomised controlled trials. *Br J Nutr* 104(11): 1586–1600.

Sacks, F. M., Carey, V. J., Anderson, C. A. M., Miller, E. R., Copeland, T., Charleston, J., Harshfield, B. J. et al. 2014. Effects of high vs low glycemic index of dietary carbohydrate on cardiovascular disease risk factors and insulin sensitivity: The OmniCarb randomized clinical trial. *JAMA* 312(23): 2531–2541.

Sachdeva, A., Cannon, C. P., Deedwania, P. C., Labresh, K. A., Smith, S. C., Dai, D., Hernandez, A., Fonarow, G. C. 2009. Lipid levels in patients hospitalized with coronary artery disease: An analysis of 136,905 hospitalizations in Get with the Guidelines database. *Am Heart J* 157(1): 111–117.

Santos, F. L., Esteves, S. S., da Costa Pereira, A., Yancy, W. S. Jr., Nunes, J. P. 2012. Systematic review and meta-analysis of clinical trials of the effects of low carbohydrate diets on cardiovascular risk factors. *Obes Res* 13(11): 1048–1066.

Schwingshackl, L., Hoffmann, G. 2013. Comparison of effects of long-term low-fat vs high-fat diets on blood lipid levels in overweight or obese patients: A systematic review and meta-analysis. *J Acad Nutr Diet* 113(12): 1640–1661.

Sesso, H. D., Buring, J. E., Chown, M. J., Ridker, P. M., Gaziano, J. M. 2005. A prospective study of plasma lipid levels and hypertension in women. *Arch Intern Med* 165(20): 2420–2427.

Shabbir, F., Patel, A., Mattison, C., Bose, S., Krishnamohan, R., Sweeney, E., Sandhu, S. et al. 2012. Effect of diet on serotonergic neurotransmission in depression. *Neurochem Int* 62(3): 324–329.

Sharman, M. J., Gómez, A. L., Kraemer, W. J., Volek, J. S. 2004. Very low-carbohydrate and low-fat diets affect fasting lipids and postprandial lipemia differently in overweight men. *J Nutr* 134(4): 880–885.

Siri-Tarino, P. W., Sun, Q., Hu, F. B., Krauss, R. M. 2010. Meta-analysis of prospective cohort studies evaluating the association of saturated fat with cardiovascular disease. *Am J Clin Nutr* 91(3): 535–546.

Spreadbury, I., Samis, A. J. W. 2013. Evolutionary aspects of obesity, insulin resistance, and cardiovascular risk. *Curr Cardiovasc Risk Rep* 7(2): 136–146.

Steffens, D. C., McQuoid, D. R., Krishnan, K. R. 2003. Cholesterol-lowering medication and relapse of depression. *Psychopharmacol Bull* 37(4): 92–98.

Tani, S., Takahashi, A., Nagao, K., Hirayama, A. 2015. Association of fish consumption-derived ratio of serum n-3–n-6 polyunsaturated fatty acids and cardiovascular risk with the prevalence of coronary artery disease. *Int Heart J* 56(3): 260–268.

Tay, J., Luscombe-Marsh, N. D., Thompson, C. H., Noakes, M., Buckley, J. D., Wittert, G. A., Yancy, W. S. Jr, Brinkworth, G. D. 2015. Comparison of low- and high-carbohydrate diets for type 2 diabetes management: A randomized trial. *Am J Clin Nutr* 102(4): 780–790.

Thomson, G. R. 1989. *A Handbook of Hyperlipidaemia*. London: Merck Sharp & Dome.

U.S. Department of Health and Human Services and U.S. Department of Agriculture. *2015–2020 Dietary Guidelines for Americans*, 8th Edition. December 2015. Accessed September 12, 2016. http://health.gov/dietaryguidelines/2015/guidelines/

van Reedt Dortland, Arianne K. B., Erik J. Giltay, Tineke van Veen, Johannes van Pelt, Frans G. Zitman, and Brenda W. H. J. Penninx. 2010. Associations between serum lipids and major depressive disorder: Results from the Netherlands Study of Depression and Anxiety (NESDA). *J Clin Psychiatry* 71(6): 729–736.

Verdoia, M., Schaffera, A., Suryapranata, H., De Luca, G. 2015. Effects of HDL-modifiers on cardiovascular outcomes: A meta-analysis of randomized trials. *Nutr Metab Cardiovasc Dis* 25(1): 9–23.

Yamagishi, K., Iso, H., Yatsuya, H., Tanabe N., Date, C., Kikuchi, S., Yamamoto, A., Inaba, Y., Tamakoshi A. 2010. Dietary intake of saturated fatty acids and mortality from cardiovascular disease in Japanese: The Japan Collaborative Cohort Study for Evaluation of Cancer Risk (JACC) Study. *Am J Clin Nutr* 92(4): 759–765.

5 HEAL for Diabetes

Chunling Wang, Zhizhong Dong,
Zhe Yi, Jian Ying, and Geng Zhang

CONTENTS

5.1 WHAT IS DIABETES AND PREDIABETES?

5.1.1 DIABETES AND ITS CLASSIFICATION

Diabetes mellitus (DM), usually called "diabetes," is a chronic, progressive metabolic disease defined by the presence of hyperglycemia. Under this circumstance, a high level of glucose remains circulating in the blood, which leads to damage to body tissue over time. Glucose comes from the food that we eat. It is the fuel for our bodies. Diabetes occurs when the body cannot produce enough insulin or cannot respond to insulin properly (Figure 5.1). Insulin is a peptide hormone that is produced by beta cells of the pancreas. It helps glucose to be transported to skeletal muscles and fat tissue. Insulin also inhibits the liver from producing glucose. Figure 5.1 depicts the mechanism for the development of diabetes.

There are three types of diabetes. Type 1 diabetes is also called "insulin-dependent diabetes," "juvenile diabetes," or "early-onset diabetes." This type of diabetes is commonly diagnosed in teenagers and young adults. Patients with type 1 diabetes cannot produce insulin themselves: as a result, they must use external insulin. Approximately 10% of the cases of diabetes are type 1 diabetes. Type 1 diabetes is a life-long condition; patients must take insulin shots or use an insulin pump every day.

Type 2 diabetes is the most common form of diabetes. Under this condition, although the body produces insulin, it is not sensitive to the insulin. Of the total diabetes patients, 90% are diagnosed with type 2 diabetes (Centers for Disease Control and Prevention 2014). As time progresses, the insulin that is produced by type 2 diabetes patients can decrease or the body can become less sensitive to insulin. Under this circumstance, the patients must increase their medication or begin insulin therapy. Approximately 40% of type 2 diabetes patients require insulin as part of their therapy.

Gestational diabetes mellitus (GDM) occurs during pregnancy. Gestational diabetes is a circumstance in which women develop a resistance to insulin and have

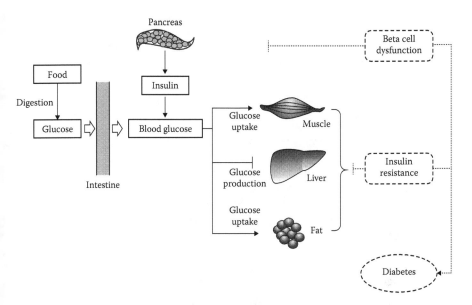

FIGURE 5.1 Mechanism for the development of diabetes.

subsequent high blood glucose during pregnancy. This circumstance is likely due to pregnancy-related factors such as the presence of human placental lactogen, which interferes with susceptible insulin receptors. This effect, in turn, elevates blood sugar levels inappropriately. Gestational diabetes usually has few symptoms and is most commonly diagnosed by screening during pregnancy. Approximately 5% of women suffer from gestational diabetes during their pregnancy without having been diagnosed with diabetes before. Most of the patients can take control of their condition with exercise and diet. However, approximately 10%–20% of patients require insulin. Gestational diabetes not only generates problems during pregnancy but also increases the risk of the baby being born with birth defects or developing childhood obesity later (Wang et al. 2015). Women with gestational diabetes usually recover after pregnancy; however, the risk of developing type 2 diabetes increases in these women compared with women without gestational diabetes.

5.1.2 PREDIABETES AND ITS CLASSIFICATION

Prediabetes is the medical stage in which an individual's blood glucose is higher than normal, but the individual does not have all of the symptoms that are required for a diagnosis of diabetes. Prediabetes is a gray zone, which implies that the individual is at a risk of getting type 2 diabetes if it is not properly controlled. Losing 7% of total body weight and engaging in moderate activities at least 150 min/week have proven to be useful in treating prediabetes. Moreover, the individual should be monitored every 1–2 years to check the situation. There are two types of prediabetes: impaired fasting glycemia/glucose (IFG), which is defined as high blood glucose after a period of fasting, and impaired glucose tolerance (IGT), which is defined as high blood glucose after eating.

5.1.3 DIAGNOSIS OF DIABETES AND PREDIABETES

The following tests are used to determine whether an individual has prediabetes or diabetes (Alberti and Zimmet 1998; Puavilai et al. 1999).

- HbA_{1C} *assay*: This is a blood test that provides information about the average blood sugar over the past 2–3 months. A result of over 5.7% indicates prediabetes, and a result of over 6.5% indicates diabetes (Gillett 2009).
- *Fasting plasma glucose test*: This test measures the blood glucose level after 12–14 h without eating or drinking. A result of over 100 mg/dL indicates prediabetes, and a result of over 126 mg/dL indicates diabetes.
- *Oral glucose tolerance test*: This test requires drinking a special sweet drink that contains a measured amount of glucose. The blood glucose level is monitored directly before drinking and 2 h after drinking. A result of over 140 mg/dL indicates prediabetes, and a result of over 200 mg/dL indicates diabetes.
- *Random plasma glucose test*: This test measures blood sugar levels at any time (2 h after a meal/postprandial) of the day and does not require fasting. A result of over 200 mg/dL indicates diabetes.

Table 5.1 shows the diagnostic criteria for diabetes according to the World Health Organization (WHO) and the International Diabetes Federation.

5.1.4 UNDERSTANDING SYMPTOMS RELATED TO HIGH BLOOD SUGAR

In addition to these tests, there are a number of symptoms that can be used to help diagnose diabetes. However, many people with untreated prediabetes or diabetes do

TABLE 5.1
Cutoff Values for Diagnosing Diabetes

Test	Prediabetes		Diabetes Mellitus
	Impaired Fasting Glycemia	Impaired Glucose Tolerance	
2 h plasma glucose	<7.8 mmol/l (<140 mg/dL)	≥7.8 mmol/l and <11.1 mmol/l (≥140 mg/dL and <200 mg/dL)	≥11.1 mmol/l (≥200 mg/dL)
Fasting glucose	6.1–6.9 mmol/l (110–125 mg/dL)	<7.0 mmol/l (<126 mg/dL)	≥7.0 mmol/l (≥126 mg/dL)

Source: WHO and IDF, *Definition and Diagnosis of Diabetes Mellitus and Intermediate Hyperglycemia: Report of a WHO/IDF Consultation*, Geneva, Switzerland, WHO, 2006.

not exhibit any of these symptoms. The tests mentioned above are the only way to obtain an accurate diagnosis.

Common symptoms of diabetes include urinating frequently; feeling very thirsty; feeling very hungry; extreme fatigue; blurry vision; cuts/bruises that are slow to heal; weight loss even when one is eating more (type 1); tingling, pain, or numbness in the hands/feet (type 2); dry, itchy skin; and more infections than usual (American Diabetes Association 2003). Typically, women with gestational diabetes exhibit no symptoms, but some women might demonstrate increased urination, fatigue, nausea and vomiting, bladder infections, yeast infections, and blurred vision.

5.1.5 Risk Factors of Diabetes

- *Type 1 diabetes*: The risk factors for type 1 diabetes are unknown. Genetic and environmental factors are possible triggers.
- *Type 2 diabetes*: Both genetic and environmental factors contribute to type 2 diabetes. An unhealthy lifestyle is the major cause. Most people who get type 2 diabetes are overweight. It is possible that obesity triggers chronic inflammation and drives the autoimmune activation of type 2 diabetes (Hemminki et al. 2015). The following risk factors are considered to be related to type 2 diabetes (Dasappa et al. 2015; Dehghani et al. 2015; Marquesim et al. 2016; Pan et al. 2015; Svensson et al. 2016): an African, Asian, Hispanic, Pacific Islander, or American Indian/Alaska Native family background; a family history of diabetes; having a baby with a birth weight of more than 9 lbs; having diabetes during pregnancy; high blood pressure; high cholesterol; inactivity (exercising less than three times a week); having other health conditions that are linked to problems with using insulin; having a history of heart disease or stroke; active or passive smoking; depression; and insomnia.
- *Gestational diabetes*: Risk factors of type 2 diabetes also contribute to gestational diabetes. Some other classical risk factors should be considered: polycystic ovary syndrome; previous diagnosis of gestational diabetes or prediabetes; maternal age over 35; a previous pregnancy that resulted in a child with a macrosomia (high birth weight: >90th centile or >4000 g [8 lbs 12.8 oz]); and/or a previous poor obstetric history.

5.1.6 Diabetes: A Global Health Challenge

Diabetes has become a serious public health problem over the past few years. Approximately, 5 million people aged between 20–79 years died from diabetes in 2015, as estimated by the International Diabetes Federation. Diabetes can induce heart disease, stroke, blindness, kidney failure, extremity amputations, and other chronic conditions. It is associated with poor performance in visuospatial skills, language, and memory (Zhao et al. 2015). The cost of diabetes treatment are very high. It was estimated by the American Diabetes Association

(ADA) that diabetes cost USD 132 billion in 2002; however, this number might underestimate the true burden of diabetes (Hogan et al. 2003). We should be aware of the following distinguishing features of type 2 diabetes:

1. The morbidity rate is increasing rapidly. The prevalence of diabetes for all age groups worldwide was estimated to be 2.8% in 2000 and 4.4% in 2030. The total number of people with diabetes is projected to rise from 171 million in 2000 to 366 million in 2030 (Wild et al. 2004). In the United States, 29.1 million people have diabetes, and 25% of them do not know that they have it (Centers for Disease Control and Prevention 2014).
2. Many people suffer from prediabetes. In 2009–2012, based on fasting glucose or HbA_{1C} levels, 37% of U.S. adults aged 20 years or older had prediabetes. Of the people with prediabetes, 9 out of 10 do not know that they have it (Centers for Disease Control and Prevention 2014).
3. Diabetes usually occurs in older people. However, increasing numbers of young people are diagnosed with diabetes today, especially in developing countries. In 2012, approximately 208,000 people who were younger than 20 years have been diagnosed as having diabetes (type 1 or type 2), which represents 0.25% of the people in this age group in the United States (Centers for Disease Control and Prevention 2014).
4. African, Asian, Hispanic, Pacific Islander, and American Indian/Alaska Natives are more prone to developing diabetes (Centers for Disease Control and Prevention 2014).
5. Men are at a higher risk of diabetes than women; however, some studies have found that the difference is diminished or even reversed in the population aged 50 and older (Bu et al. 2015).
6. People living a life of poverty are more prone to developing diabetes.

5.1.7 PREVENTION AND TREATMENT OF DIABETES: MEDICATION OR LIFESTYLE?

Most people at the prediabetes stage should focus on lifestyle changes (Gupta et al. 2014; Thomas et al. 2010). The International Diabetes Federation recommended the following to prevent the development of type 2 diabetes (International Diabetes Federation 2014):

1. Thirty minutes of exercise each day can help reduce the risk by 40%.
2. A balanced and nutritious diet is essential (Gupta et al. 2014).
3. Stop smoking if you are a smoker.
4. Live a balanced life and avoid stress and depression.
5. Have 6–9 h of good sleep each night, neither too much nor too little.

With good practices, prediabetes can be reversed, and diabetes can be prevented from progressing. Diabetes complications can also be avoided by living a healthy lifestyle (Wilson 2015). When prediabetes progresses to type 2 diabetes, then medication is needed. Medication with lifestyle modifications helps in preventing the complications of diabetes.

5.2 COMPLICATIONS OF DIABETES

5.2.1 DIABETES AND CARDIOVASCULAR DISEASE

The main cause of death in patients with diabetes is cardiovascular disease (CVD), including ischemic heart disease, stroke, and heart failure (Skyler et al. 2009). The causal relationships among hyperglycemia, insulin resistance, vascular degeneration, and atherosclerosis are well established. Hyperglycemia and insulin resistance inducing endothelial injury and dysfunction are recognized as the initial steps in the pathogenesis of atherosclerosis, followed by platelet adhesion and aggregation.

5.2.2 DIABETES AND RENAL COMPLICATIONS

Diabetic kidney disease (DKD) is defined by reduced kidney function or the presence of kidney damage for at least 3 months, regardless of kidney function. DKD has emerged as the leading cause of end-stage renal disease (Boulton et al. 2005). Diabetic patients mostly develop nephropathy after 10 years of diabetes.

5.2.3 DIABETES AND OCULAR COMPLICATIONS

Diabetic ocular complications comprise retinopathy, cataracts, lids and conjunctiva abnormalities, glaucoma, iris neovascularization, corneal diseases, ocular movement disorder, optic atrophy, and refractive error (Kyari et al. 2014).

5.2.4 DIABETES AND LOWER EXTREMITY DISEASES

People with diabetes are at a higher risk of developing lower extremity diseases, which include foot ulceration, peripheral neuropathy, and peripheral artery disease.

5.2.5 DIABETES AND NEUROPATHY

Neuropathy is one of the most common long-term complications of diabetes, which affects up to 50% of diabetic patients. Diabetic neuropathy includes distal symmetrical sensory-motor neuropathy and autonomic neuropathy (Llambes et al. 2015).

5.2.6 DIABETES AND PREGNANCY

Gestational diabetes mellitus (GDM) refers to any degree of glucose intolerance with onset or first recognition during pregnancy, which applies regardless of whether the condition persists after delivery. Usually, approximately 7% of all pregnancies are complicated with GDM (American Diabetes Association 2004a). GDM can threaten both mother and offspring, by increasing the risk of cesarean and operative vaginal delivery, macrosomia, shoulder dystocia, neonatal hypoglycemia, and hyperbilirubinemia. Women with GDM are under higher risk of type 2 diabetes after pregnancy, and the offspring is also prone to develop obesity and type 2 diabetes earlier in their life span (Kampmann et al. 2015).

5.3 FOOD GROUPS AND DIETARY PATTERNS TO PREVENT DIABETES

Although an unhealthy diet has been considered to be a predominant contributor to diabetes development, only in the past two decades has the evidence emerged from both prospective observational studies and randomized controlled trials (RCTs). Consequently, the role of diet in the prevention of diabetes is outlined as follows.

5.3.1 GLOBAL NUTRITION TRANSITION AND FOOD INTAKE TRENDS

The rapid development of economics and technologies has resulted in a worldwide revolution in food production, processing, and distribution systems and has fostered the accessibility of unhealthy foods. Characterized by high-calorie content, large portion sizes, large amounts of processed meat, highly refined carbohydrates, and sugary beverages, unhealthy diets have been popularized and have displaced fresh local food in not only developed countries but also developing countries, along with the exponential global expansion of transnational fast-food restaurants or supermarket chains (Popkin et al. 2012). Moreover, the production and consumption of animal foods, comprising beef, pork, dairy products, eggs, and poultry, have substantially increased, especially in Asian countries, where the traditional diets are plant-based (Ezzati and Riboli 2013). Another characteristic of the nutrition transition is the large shift from the intake of coarse whole grains to polished rice and refined wheat. The complete milling and processing that converts whole grains to refined grains eliminates most of the nutritional content, including fiber, essential fatty acids, micronutrients, and phytochemicals.

5.3.2 RELATED DIETARY FACTORS IN DIABETES PREVENTION

Several dietary factors in diabetes prevention will be discussed next.

5.3.2.1 Excess Energy Intake and Adiposity

In parallel with the nutrition transition discussed earlier, the prevalence of overweight and obesity has increased precipitously during the past few decades (Ezzati and Riboli 2013). Manifested by a higher body mass index (BMI), excess adiposity is the strongest risk factor for diabetes. Remarkably, a tendency toward higher rates of diabetes initiates at a much lower BMI among Asian populations compared with their Caucasian counterparts (Hu 2011). The "metabolically obese" phenotype shown by greater visceral fat depots and less muscle mass among normal-weight Asian individuals could partly explain the ethnic heterogeneity in the susceptibility to diabetes. Computed tomography has shown that East Asians present the largest abdominal and hepatic fat depots but the lowest accumulation of deep subcutaneous adipose tissue among different ethnic groups with the same waist circumference (Lear et al. 2007). Despite the discrepancy in fat mass distribution, lifestyle intervention with calorie restriction and exercise promotion to accelerate weight loss significantly reduces the risk of diabetes. For example, lifestyle modification reduced the incidence of diabetes by 58% in the Diabetes Prevention Program, which was considerably more effective than metformin (Knowler et al. 2002). Similar phenomena have been documented in various populations (Ley et al. 2014), including multiethnic American, Finnish, Chinese, and Indian.

5.3.2.2 Quantity and Quality of Dietary Fat

Although higher total fat intake was hypothesized to induce diabetes directly by triggering insulin resistance or indirectly by boosting weight gain, accumulated results from human metabolic studies do not demonstrate that high-fat diets per se have a deleterious effect on insulin sensitivity (Riserus et al. 2009). In the Women's Health Initiative, the incidence of diabetes was not decreased among generally healthy postmenopausal women assigned to a low-fat dietary pattern compared with the usual diet group (Tinker et al. 2008). Emerging evidence supports that the quality rather than the quantity of fat is more important, and diets that consist of plant-based fats instead of animal fats are more beneficial (Hu et al. 2001). The data from the Nurses' Health Study showed that a higher intake of omega-6 polyunsaturated fatty acids (PUFAs) was associated with a lower diabetes risk (Salmeron et al. 2001). Substituting saturated fat with omega-6 PUFAs could ameliorate glucose metabolism and insulin resistance (Hu et al. 2001). Nevertheless, the association between omega-3 PUFAs and diabetes risk remains controversial (Wu et al. 2012).

5.3.2.3 Quantity and Quality of Carbohydrates

Cohort studies suggest that the energy intake from carbohydrates does not appreciably influence diabetes risk (Hauner et al. 2012). However, the increased consumption of fiber, specifically cereal fiber, was associated with a reduced risk of type 2 diabetes. A meta-analysis of prospective studies revealed that higher cereal fiber intake was inversely associated with diabetes risk (relative risk [RR] for extreme quintiles 0.72; 95% confidence interval [CI] 0.56–0.93), while fruit fiber (RR 0.89; 95% CI 0.70–1.13) and vegetable fiber (RR 0.93, 95% CI 0.74–1.17) were not significantly associated (Schulze et al. 2007). Carbohydrate quality can be evaluated according to the blood glucose raising potential of carbohydrate foods, such as the glycemic index (GI) and glycemic load (GL, a product of GI and the amount of carbohydrates in a food). In a recent meta-analysis of follow-up studies, low-GI and -GL diets were associated with a decreased risk of diabetes compared with diets that have a higher GI and GL, independent of the dietary cereal fiber intake (Bhupathiraju et al. 2014).

5.3.2.4 Vitamins and Minerals

Significant associations between specific trace elements and type 2 diabetes have been reported using nutritional status assessments of either dietary intake or biomarkers or both. In a meta-analysis of 13 prospective cohort studies that involved 536,318 participants, every 100 mg/day increment in magnesium intake was associated with a 14% lower risk of incident type 2 diabetes (RR 0.86, 95% CI 0.82–0.89) (Dong et al. 2011). Notably, the observed inverse association was more pronounced in overweight than normal-weight participants (Dong et al. 2011). In contrast, higher heme-iron intake was associated with an elevated risk of diabetes (Zhao et al. 2012). Analogously, higher body iron stores displayed by increased ferritin concentrations were associated with a higher risk of diabetes (Zhao et al. 2012). An inverse association was found between circulating 25-hydroxyvitamin D concentrations and risk of diabetes in a meta-analysis of 21 prospective studies that comprised 76,220 participants (Song et al. 2013). However, the causal relationship between plasma vitamin D and diabetes has not been confirmed yet, because this biomarker might be a surrogate of an overall healthy lifestyle, including habitual outdoor physical activities and exposure to sunlight. Furthermore, small RCTs have not supported that vitamin D supplementation could improve glycated hemoglobin (HbA$_{1C}$), fasting plasma glucose, or insulin sensitivity (Mitri et al. 2011). Ongoing large RCTs might provide more informative insight with regard to the role of vitamin D in the prevention of type 2 diabetes.

5.3.3 FOOD GROUPS AND DIABETES PREVENTION

Evidence from prospective and RCT studies has indicated that the intake of several individual food items or food groups might partly contribute to diabetes prevention.

- *Whole grains*: Higher whole-grain intake has been consistently associated with a lower risk of diabetes even after adjustment for BMI (Aune et al. 2013). Otherwise, a greater consumption of white rice, a refined grain, could be a dietary trigger for type 2 diabetes, especially in Asian populations, among whom white rice is served as a staple food and is a main source of calories (Hu et al. 2012). Substituting white rice with brown rice for 5 consecutive days in Asian Indians reduced the 5-day change in the plasma glucose by 19.8% and the 5-day percentage change in the fasting insulin by 57% (Mohan et al. 2014). In a 16-week randomized trial, the participants with a high risk of diabetes in the brown-rice group had lower diastolic blood pressure and a marginally higher reversion rate of low serum HDL cholesterol than their counterparts in the white-rice group, but there was no difference between the two groups in the fasting glucose or insulin concentrations (Zhang et al. 2011).
- *Fish and seafood*: Although a high consumption of fish, fish oil, or eicosapentaenoic acid in addition to docosahexaenoic acid has been proven to be advantageous to cardiovascular health, their effects on type 2 diabetes prevention remain controversial. According to a systematic review and meta-analysis, neither fish nor seafood consumption were associated with the incidence of type 2 diabetes. A contradiction in the direction of the association between fish or seafood consumption and risk of diabetes was reported between geographical regions. Higher fish or seafood consumption was associated with a higher risk of diabetes in North America and Europe but associated with a lower risk in Asia (Wu et al. 2012). The reason for this regional variation is unclear, but the conceivable differences in the types of fish consumed, cooking methods used, and levels of exposure to pollutants in diverse locations deserve further investigation.

- *Fruits and vegetables*: Previous epidemiologic studies have generated somewhat mixed results regarding the link of fruit and vegetable intake with the risk of type 2 diabetes. Specifically, no correlation between the total intake of fruits and vegetables and risk of diabetes was found. However, a greater intake of green leafy vegetables was associated with a lower risk (Cooper et al. 2012). In addition, the consumption of specific whole fruits, especially blueberries, grapes, and apples, was significantly associated with a lower risk of type 2 diabetes, whereas greater consumption of fruit juice was associated with a higher risk, according to the results of three large-scale prospective longitudinal cohort studies (Muraki et al. 2013).
- *Dairy products*: An updated meta-analysis of 14 cohort studies elucidated that a daily intake of dairy products was associated with a moderately lower risk of diabetes, with a pooled RR of 0.94 (95% CI 0.91–0.97) and 0.88 (95% CI 0.84–0.93) for 200 g/day total and low-fat dairy consumption, respectively (Gao et al. 2013).
- *Beverages*: Greater intake of sugar-sweetened beverages has been associated with a higher risk of type 2 diabetes in a meta-analysis (Malik et al. 2010) and a pooled analysis of European cohorts (Romaguera et al. 2013). This association remains significant even after adjustment for BMI, which suggests that the deleterious effects of sugar-sweetened beverages on diabetes are not entirely mediated by bodyweight. The substitution of water, coffee, or tea for sugar-sweetened beverages was associated with a lower risk of diabetes (Pan et al. 2012). Alcohol consumption is associated with diabetes in a U-shaped manner (Baliunas et al. 2009). On the basis of findings from a meta-analysis, the amounts of alcohol consumption that were the most protective of diabetes were 24 g/day in women and 22 g/day in men, but alcohol became harmful at a consumption level above 50 g/day in women and 60 g/day in men (Baliunas et al. 2009). In a randomized trial, moderate alcohol consumption improved insulin sensitivity (Joosten et al. 2008). Coffee consumption has been consistently associated with a lower risk of diabetes. In a meta-analysis of 28 prospective cohort studies, coffee consumption was inversely associated with the risk of diabetes in a dose-responsive manner (Ding et al. 2014). Furthermore, both caffeinated and decaffeinated coffee intake were associated with a lower risk of diabetes, which suggests that bioactive compounds other than caffeine might contribute to the benefits (Ding et al. 2014). A 5-year follow-up study with a total of more than 17,000 persons found that the consumption of green tea and coffee was inversely associated with the risk of diabetes after adjustment for age, sex, body mass index, and other risk factors (Iso et al. 2006). Multivariable odds ratios (ORs) for diabetes among participants who frequently drank green tea and coffee (≥6 cups of green tea/day and ≥3 cups of coffee/day) were 0.67 (95% CI 0.47–0.94) and 0.58 (95% CI 0.37–0.90), respectively, compared with those who drank less than 1 cup/week. Null association was documented between the consumption of black or Oolong teas and the risk of diabetes. Those inverse associations were more pronounced in females and in overweight males (Iso et al. 2006).

- *Nuts*: The consumption of nuts, which are high in PUFAs and monoun-saturated fatty acids (MUFAs), could have favorable effects on diabetes prevention. Appropriately, greater nut consumption, especially walnuts, was associated with a lower risk of diabetes (Rios et al. 2015). In the PREDIMED trial, supplementation with mixed nuts (30 g/day) signifi-cantly reduced incident diabetes in a preliminary analysis from one center (multivariable adjusted hazard ratios 0.48, 95% CI 0.24–0.96) (Salas-Salvado et al. 2011) and by a nonsignificant 18% in the entire cohort (Salas-Salvado et al. 2014). However, the nuts were supplemented in the context of a Mediterranean diet in this trial and, therefore, the beneficial results might not be simply attributed to nut consumption. Despite their high fat and energy density, regular moderate consumption of nuts was not associated with increased obesity, but instead conferred benefits in weight control.

5.3.4 Dietary Patterns and Overall Diet Quality

Instead of considering individual food items in isolation, the application of food pat-tern techniques has led to a variety of different food patterns that are related to the risk of diabetes.

5.3.4.1 Mediterranean Diet

This food pattern features a good source of MUFAs, namely, olive oil, accompanied with the intake of vegetables, nuts, seeds, fruits, whole grains, low-to-moderate consumption of wine with meals, and a reduction in the consumption of red meat and unhealthy fats. A high content of fiber, magnesium, polyphenol, and antioxi-dants facilitates this diet as a useful approach to control hyperglycemia and weight maintenance (Schroder 2007). An inverse association between the Mediterranean dietary pattern and the prevalence of diabetes was observed in various multiethnic studies. A higher adherence to the Mediterranean dietary pattern was related to favorable changes in the glucose, HbA_{1C}, insulin, HOMA-IR (as one of the basic features of metabolic syndrome and diabetes), and lipid profiles (Khemayanto and Shi 2014).

5.3.4.2 Dietary Approaches to Stop Hypertension

Along with the initial known effect on blood pressure control, the Dietary Approaches to Stop Hypertension (DASH) diet (rich in fruits, vegetables, whole grains, and low-fat dairy foods, and limited in sodium, saturated fat, red meat, and sugar-sweetened foods and beverages) was also associated with beneficial effects on blood glucose and the incidence of type 2 diabetes. In the Insulin Resistance Atherosclerosis Study of 862 subjects from three different ethnicities (Hispanic, non-Hispanic white, and black), the DASH diet lowered the risk of diabetes incidence by as much as 36% in whites compared with black and Hispanic participants (Liese et al. 2009). In a 6-month RCT among 116 men and women with metabolic syndrome, the DASH diet resulted in a reduction in the fasting blood glucose by 15 and 8 mg/dL for men and women, respectively (Azadbakht et al. 2005).

5.3.4.3 Moderately Low-Carbohydrate Diet

A moderately low-carbohydrate diet is a pattern that restricts the consumption of carbohydrates by increasing the intake of fats and protein from animal or plant food sources. Prospective studies have indicated that a diet that is moderately low in total carbohydrate but high in plant-based protein and fat is associated with a lower diabetes risk (Halton et al. 2008), whereas a diet that is low in carbohydrates but high in animal fat and protein is associated with a higher risk (de Koning et al. 2011).

5.3.4.4 Vegetarian and Vegan

There are subtle differences between vegetarian and vegan. Vegetarian diets, including the lacto-ovo- (consuming dairy or eggs), pesco- (consuming fish, eggs, or dairy), and semivegetarian diets (consuming all but meat products), are devoid of some animal products, while vegan diets abstain from all animal-derived products. Vegetarian diets were associated with a lower risk of diabetes in the Adventist Health Study, which recruited 15,200 men and 26,187 women across the United States and Canada who were free of diabetes at baseline (Tonstad et al. 2013). Compared with the nonvegetarian group, the corresponding odds ratio of 2-year diabetes incidence was 0.38 (95% CI 0.23–0.61) for vegans, 0.61 (95% CI 0.50–0.76) for lacto-ovo-vegetarians, and 0.48 (95% CI 0.31–0.75) for semivegetarians, after adjustment for multiple confounding factors that include age, gender, education, income, television watching, physical activity, sleep, alcohol use, smoking, and BMI (Tonstad et al. 2013). Findings from prospective studies that use exploratory methods to identify dietary patterns further supported that those dietary patterns that favor fruits, vegetables, whole grains, and legumes at the expense of red meats, refined grains, and sugar-sweetened beverages are beneficial for diabetes prevention (Ley et al. 2014).

5.3.4.5 Prudent Pattern

The "prudent pattern" is another dietary pattern that is characterized by a higher consumption of whole grains, vegetables, fruits, poultry or seafood, legumes, and coffee. In an American prospective cohort study among 42,504 men, a higher adherence to the prudent pattern was associated with a reduced risk of diabetes by 16% after 12 years of follow-up (van Dam et al. 2002). Similar results were obtained in both the Nurses' Health Study (Fung et al. 2004) and the Atherosclerosis Risk in Communities study (Lutsey et al. 2008).

5.4 FOOD GROUPS AND DIETARY PATTERNS TO TREAT DIABETES

An individual's diet is considered to contribute to the development of type 2 diabetes, and the evidence is increasing to support the benefits of lifestyle and nutritional interventions to prevent or delay type 2 and gestational diabetes. However, there is no standard meal plan or eating pattern that works universally for all people with diabetes. Therefore, it is recommended that each person with diabetes be actively engaged in self-management, education, and treatment planning with his or her health-care provider (HCP).

5.4.1 Nutrition Therapy Recommendations for Diabetes in Adults

Medical recommendations, including those for nutrition therapy, are now being developed using an evidence-based approach (Franz et al. 2014). The Academy of Nutrition and Dietetics published evidence-based nutrition recommendations for type 1 and type 2 diabetes in 2010, and in 2013 the American Diabetes Association (ADA) published nutrition therapy recommendations for the management of adults with diabetes using a similar process (Evert et al. 2013). The ADA has long recognized the integral role of nutrition therapy in overall diabetes management and recommends that each person with diabetes receive an individualized eating plan that has been developed in collaboration with his or her health-care provider. A grading system developed by the ADA and modeled on existing methods was used to clarify and codify the evidence that forms the basis for the recommendations. Depending on the quality of evidence, recommendations were assigned ratings of A, B, C, or expert opinion or expert consensus (E) based on no evidence from clinical trials (Evert and Boucher 2014). For evidence rating at the A level, the description is clear evidence from well-conducted, generalizable RCTs that are adequately powered. The recommendations with evidence level A are summarized in Table 5.2, as adapted from the ADA recommendations (Evert and Boucher 2014). It is necessary to compare the term "nutrition therapy" with "medical nutrition therapy" (MNT). MNT is an evidence-based application of the nutrition care process provided by a registered dietitian/nutritionist (RD/N) and is the legal definition of nutrition counseling by an RD/N in the United States; nutrition therapy is the treatment of a disease or condition through the modification of nutrient or whole-food intake. Therefore, nutrition therapy has a broader definition than MNT (Evert and Boucher 2014).

Table 5.2 shows the nutrition therapy recommendations for the management of adults with diabetes, as adapted from the ADA recommendations (Evert and Boucher 2014).

5.4.2 Dietary Intake and Diabetes in Multiethnic Populations

Medical nutritional therapy is an essential component of diabetes prevention and management, and it is necessary to determine and assess dietary patterns in diabetes patients. It is necessary to consider a patient's ethnic background when addressing the prevention and treatment of diabetes. Ethnic differences play an important role in diabetes onset. For example, in a recent systematic review, the evidence suggests that the genetic background of Africans and East Asians makes them more and differentially susceptible to diabetes than Caucasians (Kodama et al. 2013). In another study, a large difference was shown between dietary intake by Japanese and Western patients (Horikawa et al. 2014). Japanese with type 2 diabetic patients had a "high-carbohydrate, low-fat" diet in comparison with Western diabetic patients but had an energy intake that was similar to Western patients with diabetes. More studies are needed to establish ethnic-specific nutritional therapies for diabetes.

TABLE 5.2

Nutrition Therapy Recommendations for the Management of Adults with Diabetes

Topic	Recommendation
Effectiveness of nutrition therapy	Nutrition therapy is recommended for all people with type 1 and type 2 diabetes as an effective component of the overall treatment plan.
	Individuals who have diabetes should receive individualized MNT as needed to achieve treatment goals, preferably provided by an RD familiar with the components of diabetes MNT.
	For individuals with type 1 diabetes, participation in an intensive flexible insulin therapy education program using the carbohydrate-counting, meal-planning approach can result in improved glycemic control.
Energy balance	For overweight or obese adults with type 2 diabetes, reducing energy intake while maintaining a healthful eating pattern is recommended to promote weight loss.
	Modest weight loss may provide clinical benefits (improved glycemia, blood pressure, and/or lipids) in some individuals with diabetes, especially those early in the disease process. To achieve modest weight loss, intensive lifestyle interventions (counseling about nutrition therapy, physical activity, and behavior change) with ongoing support are recommended.
Carbohydrates	The amount of carbohydrates and available insulin may be the most important factor influencing glycemic response after eating and should be considered when developing the eating plan.
Substitution of sucrose for starch	While substituting sucrose-containing foods for isocaloric amounts of other carbohydrates may have similar blood glucose effects, consumption should be minimized to avoid displacing nutrient-dense food choices.
Protein	For people with diabetes and diabetic kidney disease (either micro- or macro-albuminuria), reducing the amount of dietary protein below usual intake is not recommended because it does not alter glycemic measures, cardiovascular risk measures, or the course of glomerular filtration rate (GFR) decline.
Omega-3 fatty acids	Evidence does not support recommending omega-3 (EPA and DHA) supplements for people with diabetes for the prevention or treatment of cardiovascular events.
Micronutrients and herbal supplements	Routine supplementation with antioxidants, such as vitamins E and C and carotene, is not advised because of a lack of evidence of efficacy and concern related to long-term safety.

Source: Adapted from the ADA Recommendations (Evert, A. B., and J. L. Boucher, *Diabetes Spectr*, 27, 2, 2014.)

MNT: Medical nutrition therapy; RD: registered dietitian.

5.4.3 Dietary Patterns and Approaches for the Management of Adults with Diabetes

There is good evidence that lifestyle modifications, including dietary interventions, can prevent the progression of impaired glucose tolerance to diabetes (Gong et al. 2015). However, there is limited evidence on the optimal dietary approach to control hyperglycemia in type 2 diabetes.

5.4.3.1 Low-Carbohydrate, Low-GI Diet

From ADA nutrition therapy recommendations for diabetes patients, substituting low-glycemic-load foods for higher-glycemic-load foods could modestly improve glycemic control (Evert et al. 2013). In a systematic review and meta-analysis of different dietary approaches to the management of type 2 diabetes, a low-carbohydrate or low-GI diet appeared to decrease the percentage of HbA_{1C} and increase HDL, with no significant effect on weight loss and reducing LDL and triglycerides (Ajala et al. 2013). In a recent systematic review, a low-GI diet was associated with less frequent insulin use and lower birth weight than control diets, which suggests that it is the most appropriate dietary intervention to be prescribed to patients with GDM (Viana et al. 2014).

5.4.3.2 Mediterranean Diet

The Mediterranean diet is rich in olive oil, legumes, unrefined cereals, fruit, and vegetables, low in meat and meat products, and has moderate amounts of dairy products (mostly cheese and yogurt), fish, and red wine. A substantial amount of evidence supports the role of the Mediterranean diet in the improvement of various markers of cardiovascular risk in people with diabetes, showing better glycemic control, greater weight loss, and a more favorable lipid profile (Ajala et al. 2013; Khemayanto and Shi 2014). In a prospective study performed in 10 Mediterranean countries, the adherence to the Mediterranean diet was associated with a lower incidence of GDM and a better degree of glucose balance (Karamanos et al. 2014). From ADA nutrition therapy recommendations for diabetes patients, in people with type 2 diabetes, a Mediterranean-style, MUFA-rich eating pattern can benefit glycemic control and CVD risk factors and can therefore be recommended as an effective alternative to a lower-fat, higher-carbohydrate eating pattern (Evert et al. 2013).

5.4.3.3 The Benefits of Breakfast Cereal Consumption

The evidence that relates to the consumption of breakfast cereal and diabetes is summarized in a systematic review (Williams 2014). There has been one meta-analysis of the evidence of the effect of whole-grain breakfast cereal consumption on diabetes (Aune et al. 2013). The RR of incident type 2 diabetes comparing the highest versus the lowest consumption of whole-grain breakfast cereal was 0.72 (95% CI 0.55–0.93). For each additional serving of whole-grain breakfast cereal, the RR was 0.73 (95% CI 0.59–0.91; P). There was evidence for a stronger protective effect of whole-grain breakfast cereals compared with refined-grain cereals at 7 servings/week: an HR (pooled hazard ratio) of 0.60 (95% CI 0.50–0.71) for whole-grain cereals versus an HR of 0.95 (95% CI 0.73–1.3) for refined-grain cereals. The conclusion was the following: "These results suggest that intake of breakfast cereals might confer a lower risk of type 2 diabetes" (Aune et al. 2013). In summary, there is some evidence that supports the role of breakfast cereals, especially those that are higher in fiber, in the management of diabetes, but more studies in different populations will be required to confirm these effects.

5.5   FOOD GROUPS, NUTRACEUTICALS, AND REMEDIES FOR DIABETES

5.5.1   Nutraceuticals and Remedies for Diabetes Prevention

The following foods and food ingredients have been shown to reduce blood sugar levels (Rios et al. 2015):

- *Ginseng*: One clinical trial showed that taking 200 mg of *Panax ginseng* daily lowered blood glucose and HbA$_{1C}$ (Sotaniemi et al. 1995). Another trial indicated that taking 3 g of American ginseng attenuated the postprandial blood glucose response (Vuksan et al. 2000). Ginsenosides contained in both *P. ginseng* and American ginseng are considered to be bioactive compounds that are responsible for decreasing insulin resistance and improving insulin sensitivity (Rios et al. 2015).
- *Beta-glucan*: As a soluble fiber, beta-glucan is abundant in oat and barley food products. Human studies demonstrated that intact grains as well as a variety of processed oat and barley foods that contain at least 4 g of beta-glucan could significantly reduce postprandial blood glucose (Tosh 2013).
- *Phytoestrogens*: Phytoestrogens are known as polyphenols that are structurally similar to endogenous estrogen and have weak estrogenic properties. Two major types of phytoestrogens, isoflavones and lignans, have shown potentially beneficial effects on glycemic parameters among postmenopausal women in long-term intervention studies, while the results of short-term, small-size clinical trials are conflicting. Habitual consumption of phytoestrogens, especially their intact food sources such as soy and whole flaxseed, could be considered to be a component of an overall healthy dietary pattern for the prevention of diabetes (Talaei and Pan 2015).

5.5.2   Nutraceuticals and Remedies for Diabetes Treatment

The following nutraceuticals and remedies have been found to be effective in the treatment of diabetes:

- *Oat and barley foods*: Oat and barley foods have been shown to reduce the human glycemic response compared with similar wheat foods or a glucose control (Tosh 2013). One of the main active components in these foods is the soluble-fiber, mixed-linkage beta-glucan. These fibers appear to form a barrier in the small intestine that delays glucose absorption, consequently reducing the glycemia. The European Food Safety Authority (EFSA) has recognized that a cause-and-effect relationship between the consumption of oat and barley beta-glucans and a reduction in the postprandial glycemic responses has been established; the panel concludes that "in order to obtain the claimed effect, 4 g of beta-glucans from oat or barley for each 30 g of available carbohydrates should be consumed per meal." In a review of 76 human studies, intact grains as well as a variety of processed oat and barley foods that contain at least 4 g of beta-glucan and 30–80 g of available carbohydrate can significantly reduce postprandial blood glucose (Tosh 2013). The glycemic response was related to the doses of beta-glucans, and the consumption of greater doses or smaller doses for longer periods of time produced better results (Francelino Andrade et al. 2014).

- *Cinnamon*: Cinnamon has become a natural product of interest because it has been hypothesized to provide health benefits such as the ability to lower serum lipids and blood glucose. In a recent meta-analysis of 10 RCTs ($n = 543$ patients), cinnamon doses of 120–6000 mg/day for 4–18 weeks reduced the levels of fasting plasma glucose (−24.59 mg/dL; 95% CI −40.52–8.67 mg/dL), total cholesterol (−15.60 mg/dL; 95% CI −29.76–1.44 mg/dL), LDL (−9.42 mg/dL; 95% CI −17.21–1.63 mg/dL), and triglycerides (−29.59 mg/dL; 95% CI −48.27–10.91 mg/dL). Cinnamon also increased the levels of HDL (1.66 mg/dL; 95% CI 1.09–2.24 mg/dL). No significant effect on the HbA_{1C} levels (−0.16%; 95% CI −0.39%–0.02%) was seen (Allen et al. 2013).
- *Glucomannan*: Glucomannan is a soluble fiber that is derived from *Amorphophallus konjac* and is available in many over-the-counter products, such as Lipozene. Glucomannan is thought to prolong the gastric emptying time, which increases satiety, reduces body weight, decreases the ingestion of foods that increase cholesterol and glucose concentrations and reduces the postprandial rise in plasma glucose (Sood et al. 2008). A systematic review concluded that the consumption of 3–15 g of glucomannan per day appears to beneficially affect the total cholesterol, LDL cholesterol, triglycerides, body weight, and FBG, but not HDL cholesterol or blood pressure (Sood et al. 2008).
- *Legumes*: Legumes (peas, beans, lentils, peanuts) are valuable sources of dietary protein, nondigestible carbohydrates including dietary fiber, resistance starches, oligosaccharides, and bioactive compounds such as functional fatty acids (linoleic acid, alpha-linolenic acid), isoflavones (daidzein, genistein, glycitein), and alpha-amylase inhibitory peptides. Legumes are considered to be a component of a healthy diet, and there is much evidence that shows that the regular consumption of legumes has protective effects against obesity, type 2 diabetes, and cardiovascular disease (Mirmiran et al. 2014).

5.6 NUTRITIONAL COUNSELING FOR DIABETES

Nutritional counseling plays an important role in the prevention and treatment of prediabetes and diabetes. Table 5.3 shows the details of nutritional counseling for diabetes.

5.7 CASE STUDIES

Based on the information given in this chapter, try to analyze the following case studies and respond to the questions accordingly.

TABLE 5.3
Nutritional Counseling for Prevention and Treatment of Diabetes

Components of Counseling	Description
Symptoms that the patient reports	*Diabetes*: Increased thirst, frequent urination, tiredness, numbness in the extremities, blurred vision, wounds that take time to heal, feeling hungry even during eating, weight loss even when eating more (type 1), extreme fatigue, dry and itchy skin, more infections than usual.
Nutritional history: Questions to be asked by health expert	Dietary assessment can be done in the form of *diet history, 24-hour recall, dietary log,* and *food frequency questionnaire.* These should inquire about

- Types and amount of fat consumption
- Frequency/servings of fruits and vegetables
- Salt intake
- Type and amount of meat, fish, and poultry
- Grains and lentils, nuts, and seeds
- Alcohol use
- Sugar content in diet
- Refined products consumed

Some important questions to be asked are

- Do you have a previous history of hypertension, diabetes, or heart disease?
- Do you have a family history of diabetes, heart disease, hypertension, or hypercholesterolemia?
- Have you had any issues with weight? Underweight or overweight?
- Have you been on any diets? If yes, then what diets have you followed?
- Do you skip meals? How often?
- Do you eat breakfast regularly?
- Are you a vegetarian or nonvegetarian?
- Do you eat snacks in between meals? What types of snacks?

Examination and investigations	These consist of examinations from head to toe to look for anemia, signs of dehydration, checking for blurred vision, xanthomas as seen in hyperlipidemia, cyanosis indicating heart disease, weight and height for calculating BMI, blood pressure, pulse, respiratory rate, wounds on the body that are not healed, edema in the limbs, lumps anywhere in the body. Perform fasting blood sugar and lipid profiles.
Diagnosis	If you make a diagnosis of diabetes, refer to the concerned physician.
Nutritional management	Advise patients about Healthful Eating As Lifestyle (HEAL) based on the *food-based dietary guidelines, evidence-based dietary patterns,* and *home remedies* as explained in this chapter. Provide precautionary guidelines about safety concerns when recommending home-based remedies.

5.7.1 CASE STUDY 1

A 55-year-old Chinese male network engineer consults you with his health check report.

Height: 175 cm	Weight: 74 kg
Waist circumference: 90 cm	Parental history of diabetes: Yes
Blood pressure: 130/80 mm Hg	Fasting glucose: 5.6 mmol/L
Triglycerides: 1.5 mmol/L	HDL cholesterol: 1.1 mmol/L
...	...

Give responses to the following:

1. Will you suggest that he submit to further examination? Why?
2. What information on his dietary intake would you like to collect?
3. If he expresses a willingness to lose weight, what nutritional recommendations will you provide?

5.7.2 CASE STUDY 2

A 46-year-old Native American male comes to you with a complaint of numbness in the hands, urinating frequently, and feeling thirsty. He has no previous history of hypertension, diabetes, heart disease, or disease of the urinary system. His family history of diabetes is positive. On examination, his blood pressure is normal, his height is 170 cm, and his weight is 86 kg.

Give responses to the following:

1. Which further investigations would you suggest to him?
2. What information would you like to gather on his dietary intake?
3. Based on your assessment, what dietary recommendations will you make if the patient is found to have a fasting blood sugar level of more than 126 mg/dL?

REFERENCES

Ahmad, J. 2015. The diabetic foot. *Diabetes Metab Syndr* 10 (1):48–60.
Ajala, O., English, P., and Pinkney, J. 2013. Systematic review and meta-analysis of different dietary approaches to the management of type 2 diabetes. *Am J Clin Nutr* 97 (3):505–516.
Alberti, K. G., and P. Z. Zimmet. 1998. Definition, diagnosis and classification of diabetes mellitus and its complications, Part 1: Diagnosis and classification of diabetes mellitus provisional report of a WHO consultation. *Diabet Med* 15 (7):539–553.
Allen, R. W., E. Schwartzman, W. L. Baker, C. I. Coleman, and O. J. Phung. 2013. Cinnamon use in type 2 diabetes: An updated systematic review and meta-analysis. *Ann Fam Med* 11 (5):452–459.
American Diabetes Association. 2003. Standards of medical care for patients with diabetes mellitus. *Diabetes Care* 26 (Suppl 1):S33–S50.
American Diabetes Association. 2004a. Gestational diabetes mellitus. *Diabetes Care* 27 (Suppl 1):3.

Aune, D., T. Norat, P. Romundstad, and L. J. Vatten. 2013. Whole grain and refined grain consumption and the risk of type 2 diabetes: A systematic review and dose-response meta-analysis of cohort studies. *Eur J Epidemiol* 28 (11):845–58.

Azadbakht, L., P. Mirmiran, A. Esmaillzadeh, T. Azizi, and F. Azizi. 2005. Beneficial effects of a dietary approaches to stop hypertension eating plan on features of the metabolic syndrome. *Diabetes Care* 28 (12):2823–2831.

Baliunas, D. O., B. J. Taylor, H. Irving, M. Roerecke, J. Patra, S. Mohapatra, and J. Rehm. 2009. Alcohol as a risk factor for type 2 diabetes: A systematic review and meta-analysis. *Diabetes Care* 32 (11):2123–2132.

Bhupathiraju, S. N., Tobias, D. K., Malik, V. S., Pan, A., Hruby, A., Manson, J. E., Willett, W. C., and Hu, F. B. 2014. Glycemic index, glycemic load, and risk of type 2 diabetes: Results from 3 large U.S. cohorts and an updated meta-analysis. *Am J Clin Nutr* 100 (1):218–232.

Boulton, A. J., A. I. Vinik, J. C. Arezzo, V. Bril, E. L. Feldman, R. Freeman, R. A. Malik, R. E. Maser, J. M. Sosenko, and D. Ziegler. 2005. Diabetic neuropathies: A statement by the American Diabetes Association. *Diabetes Care* 28 (4):956–962.

Bu, S., Ruan, D., Yang, Z., Xing, X., Zhao, W., Wang, N., Xie, L., and Yang, W. 2015. Sex-specific prevalence of diabetes and cardiovascular risk factors in the middle-aged population of China: A subgroup analysis of the 2007–2008 China National Diabetes and Metabolic Disorders Study. *PLoS One* 10 (9):e0139039.

Centers for Disease Control and Prevention. 2014. National diabetes statistics report. Accessed June 15, 2015. http://www.cdc.gov/diabetes/data/statistics/2014statisticsreport.html.

Cooper, A. J., Forouhi, N. G., Ye, Z., Buijsse, B., Arriola, L., Balkau, B., Barricarte, A. et al. 2012. Fruit and vegetable intake and type 2 diabetes: EPIC-InterAct prospective study and meta-analysis. *Eur J Clin Nutr* 66 (10):1082–1092.

Dasappa, H., Fathima, F. N., Prabhakar, R., and Sarin, S. 2015. Prevalence of diabetes and pre-diabetes and assessments of their risk factors in urban slums of Bangalore. *J Family Med Prim Care* 4 (3):399–404.

de Koning, L., Fung, T. T., Liao, X., Chiuve, S. E., Rimm, E. B., Willett, W. C., Spiegelman, D., and Hu, F. B. 2011. Low-carbohydrate diet scores and risk of type 2 diabetes in men. *Am J Clin Nutr* 93 (4):844–850.

Dehghani, A., Kumar Bhasin, S., Dwivedi, S., and Kumar Malhotra, R. 2015. Influence of comprehensive lifestyle intervention in patients of CHD. *Glob J Health Sci* 7 (7):46852.

Ding, M., S. N. Bhupathiraju, M. Chen, R. M. van Dam, and F. B. Hu. 2014. Caffeinated and decaffeinated coffee consumption and risk of type 2 diabetes: A systematic review and a dose-response meta-analysis. *Diabetes Care* 37 (2):569–586.

Dong, J. Y., P. Xun, K. He, and L. Q. Qin. 2011. Magnesium intake and risk of type 2 diabetes: Meta-analysis of prospective cohort studies. *Diabetes Care* 34 (9):2116–2122.

Evert, A. B., and J. L. Boucher. 2014. New diabetes nutrition therapy recommendations: What you need to know. *Diabetes Spectr* 27 (2):121–310.

Evert, A. B., J. L. Boucher, M. Cypress, S. A. Dunbar, M. J. Franz, E. J. Mayer-Davis, J. J. Neumiller et al. 2013. Nutrition therapy recommendations for the management of adults with diabetes. *Diabetes Care* 36 (11):3821–42.

Ezzati, M., and E. Riboli. 2013. Behavioral and dietary risk factors for noncommunicable diseases. *N Engl J Med* 369 (10):954–964.

Francelino Andrade, E., Vieira Lobato, R., Vasques Araújo, T., Gilberto Zangerônimo, M., Vicente Sousa, R., and José Pereira, L. 2014. Effect of beta-glucans in the control of blood glucose levels of diabetic patients: A systematic review. *Nutr Hosp* 31 (1):170–177.

Franz, M. J., J. L. Boucher, and A. B. Evert. 2014. Evidence-based diabetes nutrition therapy recommendations are effective: The key is individualization. *Diabetes Metab Syndr Obes* 7:65–72.

Fung, T. T., M. Schulze, J. E. Manson, W. C. Willett, and F. B. Hu. 2004. Dietary patterns, meat intake, and the risk of type 2 diabetes in women. *Arch Intern Med* 164 (20): 2235–2240.

Gao, D., N. Ning, C. Wang, Y. Wang, Q. Li, Z. Meng, and Y. Liu. 2013. Dairy products consumption and risk of type 2 diabetes: Systematic review and dose-response meta-analysis. *PLoS One* 8 (9):e73965.

Gillett, M. J. 2009. International Expert Committee report on the role of the A_{1C} assay in the diagnosis of diabetes: Diabetes care 32 (7):1327–1334. *Clin Biochem Rev* 30 (4): 197–200.

Gong, Q. H., J. F. Kang, Y. Y. Ying, H. Li, X. H. Zhang, Y. H. Wu, and G. Z. Xu. 2015. Lifestyle interventions for adults with impaired glucose tolerance: A systematic review and meta-analysis of the effects on glycemic control. *Intern Med* 54 (3):303–310.

Gupta, A., N. K. Agarwal, and P. S. Byadgi. 2014. Clinical assessment of dietary interventions and lifestyle modifications in Madhumeha (type 2 diabetes mellitus). *Ayu* 35 (4):391–397.

Halton, T. L., Liu, S., Manson, J. E., and Hu, F. B. 2008. Low-carbohydrate-diet score and risk of type 2 diabetes in women. *Am J Clin Nutr* 87 (2):339–346.

Hemminki, K., X. Liu, A. Forsti, J. Sundquist, K. Sundquist, and J. Ji. 2015. Subsequent type 2 diabetes in patients with autoimmune disease. *Sci Rep* 5:13871.

Hogan, P., Dall, T., and Nikolov, P. 2003. Economic costs of diabetes in the U.S. in 2002. *Diabetes Care* 26 (3):917–932.

Horikawa, C., Yoshimura, Y., Kamada, C., Tanaka, S., Tanaka, S., Takahashi, A., Hanyu, O. et al. 2014. Dietary intake in Japanese patients with type 2 diabetes: Analysis from Japan Diabetes Complications Study. *J Diabetes Investig* 5 (2):176–187.

Hu, E. A., A. Pan, V. Malik, and Q. Sun. 2012. White rice consumption and risk of type 2 diabetes: Meta-analysis and systematic review. *BMJ* 344:e1454.

Hu, F. B. 2011. Globalization of diabetes: The role of diet, lifestyle, and genes. *Diabetes Care* 34 (6):1249–1257.

Hu, F. B., R. M. van Dam, and S. Liu. 2001. Diet and risk of type II diabetes: The role of types of fat and carbohydrate. *Diabetologia* 44 (7):805–817.

International Diabetes Federation. 2014. *IDF Diabetes Atlas*, 6th Edition, update poster. Brussels, Belgium: International Diabetes Federation.

Iso, H., C. Date, K. Wakai, M. Fukui, and A. Tamakoshi. 2006. The relationship between green tea and total caffeine intake and risk for self-reported type 2 diabetes among Japanese adults. *Ann Intern Med* 144 (8):554–562.

Joosten, M. M., J. W. Beulens, S. Kersten, and H. F. Hendriks. 2008. Moderate alcohol consumption increases insulin sensitivity and ADIPOQ expression in postmenopausal women: A randomised, crossover trial. *Diabetologia* 51 (8):1375–1381.

Kampmann, U., L. R. Madsen, G. O. Skajaa, D. S. Iversen, N. Moeller, and P. Ovesen. 2015. Gestational diabetes: A clinical update. *World J Diabetes* 6 (8):1065–1072.

Khemayanto, H., and B. Shi. 2014. Role of Mediterranean diet in prevention and management of type 2 diabetes. *Chin Med J* 127 (20):3651–3656.

Knowler, W. C., Barrett-Connor, E., Fowler, S. E., Hamman, R. F., Lachin, J. M., Walker, E. A., and Nathan, D. M. 2002. Reduction in the incidence of type 2 diabetes with lifestyle intervention or metformin. *N Engl J Med* 346 (6):393–403.

Kodama, K., D. Tojjar, S. Yamada, K. Toda, C. J. Patel, and A. J. Butte. 2013. Ethnic differences in the relationship between insulin sensitivity and insulin response: A systematic review and meta-analysis. *Diabetes Care* 36 (6):1789–1796.

Kyari, F., A. Tafida, S. Sivasubramaniam, G. V. Murthy, T. Peto, and C. E. Gilbert. 2014. Prevalence and risk factors for diabetes and diabetic retinopathy: Results from the Nigeria national blindness and visual impairment survey. *BMC Public Health* 14:1299.

Lear, S. A., K. H. Humphries, S. Kohli, A. Chockalingam, J. J. Frohlich, and C. L. Birmingham. 2007. Visceral adipose tissue accumulation differs according to ethnic background:

Results of the Multicultural Community Health Assessment Trial (M-CHAT). *Am J Clin Nutr* 86 (2):353–359.

Ley, S. H., Hamdy, O., Mohan, V., and Hu, F. B. 2014. Prevention and management of type 2 diabetes: Dietary components and nutritional strategies. *Lancet* 383 (9933):1999–2007.

Liese, A. D., M. Nichols, X. Sun, R. B. D'Agostino, Jr, and S. M. Haffner. 2009. Adherence to the DASH diet is inversely associated with incidence of type 2 diabetes: The insulin resistance atherosclerosis study. *Diabetes Care* 32 (8):1434–1436.

Llambes, F., S. Arias-Herrera, and R. Caffesse. 2015. Relationship between diabetes and periodontal infection. *World J Diabetes* 6 (7):927–935.

Lutsey, P. L., L. M. Steffen, and J. Stevens. 2008. Dietary intake and the development of the metabolic syndrome: The Atherosclerosis Risk in Communities study. *Circulation* 117 (6):754–761.

Malik, V. S., B. M. Popkin, G. A. Bray, J. P. Despres, W. C. Willett, and F. B. Hu. 2010. Sugar-sweetened beverages and risk of metabolic syndrome and type 2 diabetes: A meta-analysis. *Diabetes Care* 33 (11):2477–2483.

Marquesim, N. A., Cavassini, A. C., Morceli, G., Magalhaes, C. G., Rudge, M. V., Calderon, I. M., Kron, M. R., and Lima, S. A. 2016. Depression and anxiety in pregnant women with diabetes or mild hyperglycemia. *Arch Gynecol Obstet* 293 (4):833–837.

Mirmiran, P., Z. Bahadoran, and F. Azizi. 2014. Functional foods-based diet as a novel dietary approach for management of type 2 diabetes and its complications: A review. *World J Diabetes* 5 (3):267–281.

Mitri, J., M. D. Muraru, and A. G. Pittas. 2011. Vitamin D and type 2 diabetes: A systematic review. *Eur J Clin Nutr* 65 (9):1005–1015.

Mohan, V., Spiegelman, D., Sudha, V., Gayathri, R., Hong, B., Praseena, K., Anjana, R. M. et al. 2014. Effect of brown rice, white rice, and brown rice with legumes on blood glucose and insulin responses in overweight Asian Indians: A randomized controlled trial. *Diabetes Technol Ther* 16 (5):317–325.

Muraki, I., F. Imamura, J. E. Manson, F. B. Hu, W. C. Willett, R. M. van Dam, and Q. Sun. 2013. Fruit consumption and risk of type 2 diabetes: Results from three prospective longitudinal cohort studies. BMJ 347:f5001.

Pan, A., V. S. Malik, M. B. Schulze, J. E. Manson, W. C. Willett, and F. B. Hu. 2012. Plain-water intake and risk of type 2 diabetes in young and middle-aged women. *Am J Clin Nutr* 95 (6):1454–1460.

Popkin, B. M., L. S. Adair, and S. W. Ng. 2012. Global nutrition transition and the pandemic of obesity in developing countries. *Nutr Rev* 70 (1):3–21.

Puavilai, G., S. Chanprasertyotin, and A. Sriphrapradaeng. 1999. Diagnostic criteria for diabetes mellitus and other categories of glucose intolerance: 1997 criteria by the Expert Committee on the Diagnosis and Classification of Diabetes Mellitus (ADA), 1998 WHO consultation criteria, and 1985 WHO criteria. *Res Clin Pract* 44 (1):21–26.

Rios, J. L., F. Francini, and G. R. Schinella. 2015. Natural products for the treatment of type 2 diabetes mellitus. *Planta Med* 81 (12–13): 975–994.

Riserus, U., W. C. Willett, and F. B. Hu. 2009. Dietary fats and prevention of type 2 diabetes. *Prog Lipid Res* 48 (1):44–51.

Romaguera, D., Norat, T., Wark, P. A., Vergnaud, A. C., Schulze, M. B., van Woudenbergh, G. J., Drogan, D. et al. 2013. Consumption of sweet beverages and type 2 diabetes incidence in European adults: Results from EPIC-InterAct. *Diabetologia* 56 (7):1520–1530.

Salas-Salvado, J., M. Bullo, N. Babio, M. A. Martinez-Gonzalez, N. Ibarrola-Jurado, J. Basora, R. Estruch et al. 2011. Reduction in the incidence of type 2 diabetes with the Mediterranean diet: Results of the PREDIMED-Reus nutrition intervention randomized trial. *Diabetes Care* 34 (1):14–19.

Salas-Salvado, J., M. Bullo, R. Estruch, E. Ros, M. I. Covas, N. Ibarrola-Jurado, D. Corella et al. 2014. Prevention of diabetes with Mediterranean diets: A subgroup analysis of a randomized trial. *Ann Intern Med* 160 (1):1–10.

Salmeron, J., F. B. Hu, J. E. Manson, M. J. Stampfer, G. A. Colditz, E. B. Rimm, and W. C. Willett. 2001. Dietary fat intake and risk of type 2 diabetes in women. *Am J Clin Nutr* 73 (6):1019–1026.

Schulze, M. B., M. Schulz, C. Heidemann, A. Schienkiewitz, K. Hoffmann, and H. Boeing. 2007. Fiber and magnesium intake and incidence of type 2 diabetes: A prospective study and meta-analysis. *Arch Intern Med* 167 (9):956–965.

Schroder, H. 2007. Protective mechanisms of the Mediterranean diet in obesity and type 2 diabetes. *J Nutr Biochem* 18 (3):149–160.

Skyler, J. S., Bergenstal, R., Bonow, R. O., Buse, J., Deedwania, P., Gale, E. A., Howard, B. V. et al. 2009. Intensive glycemic control and the prevention of cardiovascular events: Implications of the ACCORD, ADVANCE, and VA diabetes trials: A position statement of the American Diabetes Association and a scientific statement of the American College of Cardiology Foundation and the American Heart Association. *Diabetes Care* 32 (1):187–192.

Song, Y., L. Wang, A. G. Pittas, L. C. Del Gobbo, C. Zhang, J. E. Manson, and F. B. Hu. 2013. Blood 25-hydroxy vitamin D levels and incident type 2 diabetes: A meta-analysis of prospective studies. *Diabetes Care* 36 (5):1422–1428.

Sood, N., W. L. Baker, and C. I. Coleman. 2008. Effect of glucomannan on plasma lipid and glucose concentrations, body weight, and blood pressure: Systematic review and meta-analysis. *Am J Clin Nutr* 88 (4):1167–1175.

Sotaniemi, E. A., Haapakoski, E., and Rautio, A. 1995. Ginseng therapy in non-insulin-dependent diabetic patients. *Diabetes Care* 18 (10):1373–1375.

Svensson, E., Berencsi, K., Sander, S., Mor, A., Rungby, J., Nielsen, J. S., Friborg, S. et al. 2016. Association of parental history of type 2 diabetes with age, lifestyle, anthropometric factors, and clinical severity at type 2 diabetes diagnosis: Results from the DD2 study. *Diabetes Metab Res Rev* 32 (3):308–315.

Talaei, M., and A. Pan. 2015. Role of phytoestrogens in prevention and management of type 2 diabetes. *World J Diabetes* 6 (2):271–283.

Thomas, G. N., Jiang, C. Q., Taheri, S., Xiao, Z. H., Tomlinson, B., Cheung, B. M., Lam, T. H., Barnett, A. H., and Cheng, K. K. 2010. A systematic review of lifestyle modification and glucose intolerance in the prevention of type 2 diabetes. *Curr Diabetes Rev* 6 (6):378–387.

Tinker, L. F., Bonds, D. E., Margolis, K. L., Manson, J. E., Howard, B. V., Larson, J., Perri, M. G. et al. 2008. Low-fat dietary pattern and risk of treated diabetes mellitus in postmenopausal women: The Women's Health Initiative randomized controlled dietary modification trial. *Arch Intern Med* 168 (14):1500–1511.

Tonstad, S., Stewart, K., Oda, K., Batech, M., Herring, R. P., and Fraser, G. E. 2013. Vegetarian diets and incidence of diabetes in the Adventist Health Study-2. *Nutr Metab Cardiovasc Dis* 23 (4):292–299.

Tosh, S. M. 2013. Review of human studies investigating the post-prandial blood-glucose lowering ability of oat and barley food products. *Eur J Clin Nutr* 67 (4):310–317.

van Dam, R. M., E. B. Rimm, W. C. Willett, M. J. Stampfer, and F. B. Hu. 2002. Dietary patterns and risk for type 2 diabetes mellitus in U.S. men. *Ann Intern Med* 136 (3):201–209.

Viana, L. V., Gross, J. L., and Azevedo, M. J. 2014. Dietary intervention in patients with gestational diabetes mellitus: A systematic review and meta-analysis of randomized clinical trials on maternal and newborn outcomes. *Diabetes Care* 37 (12):3345–3355.

Vuksan, V., J. L. Sievenpiper, V. Y. Koo, T. Francis, U. Beljan-Zdravkovic, Z. Xu, and E. Vidgen. 2000. American ginseng (*Panax quinquefolius* L.) reduces postprandial glycemia in nondiabetic subjects and subjects with type 2 diabetes mellitus. *Arch Intern Med* 160 (7):1009–1013.

Wang, L. F., H. J. Wang, D. Ao, Z. Liu, Y. Wang, and H. X. Yang. 2015. Influence of pre-pregnancy obesity on the development of macrosomia and large for gestational age in women with or without gestational diabetes mellitus in Chinese population. *J Perinatol* 35 (12):985–990.

Wild, S., G. Roglic, A. Green, R. Sicree, and H. King. 2004. Global prevalence of diabetes: Estimates for the year 2000 and projections for 2030. *Diabetes Care* 27 (5):1047–1053.

Williams, P. G. 2014. The benefits of breakfast cereal consumption: A systematic review of the evidence base. *Adv Nutr* 5 (5):636S–673S.

Wilson, V. 2015. Reversing type 2 diabetes with lifestyle change. *Nurs Times* 111 (12):17–19.

Wu, J. H., R. Micha, F. Imamura, A. Pan, M. L. Biggs, O. Ajaz, L. Djousse, F. B. Hu, and D. Mozaffarian. 2012. Omega-3 fatty acids and incident type 2 diabetes: A systematic review and meta-analysis. *Br J Nutr* 107 (Suppl 2):S214–S227.

Zhang, G., Pan, A., Zong, G., Yu, Z., Wu, H., Chen, X., Tang, L. et al. 2011. Substituting white rice with brown rice for 16 weeks does not substantially affect metabolic risk factors in middle-aged Chinese men and women with diabetes or a high risk for diabetes. *J Nutr* 141 (9):1685–1690.

Zhao, Z., S. Li, G. Liu, F. Yan, X. Ma, Z. Huang, and H. Tian. 2012. Body iron stores and heme-iron intake in relation to risk of type 2 diabetes: A systematic review and meta-analysis. *PLoS One* 7 (7):e41641.

6 HEAL for Heart Diseases

Ioanna Bakogianni, Dimitra Karageorgou,
Muna Ibrahim Atalla Al Baloushi,
and Antonis Zampelas

CONTENTS

6.1   INTRODUCTION

6.1.1   EPIDEMIOLOGY OF CARDIOVASCULAR DISEASE

Among non-communicable disease (NCDs), cardiovascular disease (CVD) is the leading cause of morbidity and mortality in the world (World Health Organization [WHO] 2014). CVD is a class of diseases that involve heart and blood vessels. It includes coronary artery disease (CAD), such as angina and myocardial infarction, also known as acute coronary syndrome (ACS), as well as other CVDs, such as stroke, peripheral artery disease, hypertensive heart disease, rheumatic heart disease, cardiomyopathy, atrial fibrillation, congenital heart disease, endocarditis, aortic aneurysms, and venous thrombosis. Coronary artery disease and stroke account for 80% of CVD deaths in males and 75% of CVD deaths in females. It is noteworthy that of the 17.5 million deaths due to CVD globally in 2012, an estimated 7.4 million were attributed to ischemic heart disease and 6.7 million to stroke (WHO 2014). It has also been projected that the number of people who will die from CVD, mainly from heart disease and stroke, could reach 23.3 million globally by 2030 (Mathers and Loncar 2006; WHO 2014).

6.1.2   ATHEROSCLEROSIS AND BLOOD LIPIDS

Atherosclerosis in the blood vessels is the underlying disease process that results in CAD and stroke. It is a complex pathological process of blood vessel walls and develops progressively over many years. In atherosclerosis, fatty material and cholesterol are deposited inside the lumen of medium- and large-sized blood vessels (arteries). The deposits (plaques) cause the inner surface of the blood vessels to become irregular, resulting in narrower lumen and rigid vessel walls, ultimately blocking blood flow mainly through plaque rupture. The main risk factors of atherosclerosis development include (1) behavioral risk factors (unhealthy diet, tobacco use, physical inactivity, excessive consumption of alcohol), (2) metabolic risk factors (dyslipidemia, hypertension, diabetes), and (3) other risk factors (age, gender, family history).

Lipid metabolism is of great interest, since a raised plasma low-density lipoprotein (LDL) cholesterol level is the main independent risk factor of developing CVD (da Silva et al. 2015). Refer to Chapter 4, Section 4.1 and Figure 4.1 for information on lipoproteins. During the process of atherogenesis, LDL particles enter the arterial wall, either oxidized or enzymatically degraded, and aggregate. Modified LDL particles follow the atherogenic pathway that leads to atherosclerotic plaque formation (Figure 6.1), instead of the pathway followed by native LDL particles, which supplies cholesterol to peripheral cells. Figure 6.1 shows the pathogenesis of atherosclerosis.

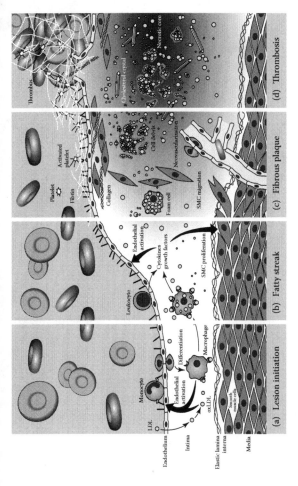

FIGURE 6.1 Pathogenesis of atherosclerosis: (a) In the first stage, low-density lipoprotein (LDL) cholesterol is deposited in the endothelium and undergoes oxidative modification, resulting in oxidized LDL (oxLDL). OxLDL stimulates the endothelial cells to express adhesion molecules (vascular cell adhesion molecule-1 [VCAM-1], P-selectin) and various chemokines (e.g., monocyte chemoattractant protein-1 [MCP-1], interleukin-8 [IL-8]). This leads to a recruitment of monocytes, which transmigrate into the intima and differentiate to proatherogenic macrophages. (b) Macrophages harvest residual oxLDL via their scavenger receptors and add to the endothelial activation and, subsequently, leukocyte recruitment with the secretion of tumor necrosis factor-α (TNF-α) and IL-6. (c) The increasing plaque volume promotes neovascularization. Proliferating smooth-muscle cells (SMCs) stabilize the nascent fibrous plaque. With the deposition of fibrin and activated platelets on the dysfunctional endothelium that expresses tissue factor (TF) and von Willebrand factor (vWF), a prothrombotic milieu is formed. (d) Foam cells can undergo apoptosis and release cell debris and lipids, which will result in the formation of a necrotic core. In addition, proteases secreted from foam cells can destabilize the plaque. This can lead to plaque rupture; in which case, extracellular matrix molecules (e.g., collagens, elastin, TF, vWF) catalyze thrombotic events. (From D. C. Steinl and B. A. Kaufmann, *Int J Mol Sci*, 16, 9749–9769, 2015.)

The atheroprotective mechanism of high-density lipoprotein (HDL) has been debated and is given in detail by others (Rosales et al. 2015). The cholesterol burden of the arterial wall can be reduced by the reverse cholesterol transport, wherein subendothelial foam cells transfer cholesterol to HDL to form larger HDL. These HDL particles diffuse into the plasma compartment, where free cholesterol is esterified and returns to the liver, where it is internalized by liver hepatocytes via the HDL receptor. This dynamic process is influenced by several factors, such as the dietary ingestion of cholesterol, saturated fats, and carbohydrates, and mainly by the insulin resistance of the individual. However, it appears that there are some considerations in this hypothesis. As the cholesterol content of reassembled HDL is increased, the balance of cellular cholesterol shifts from efflux to influx above 15 mol% in the HDL, so the net flux of cholesterol between the cell and HDL shifts from efflux to influx. Concurrent with increased cholesterol influx, intracellular cholesterol biosynthesis is downregulated, while that of cholesterol esterification increases.

Cholesterol efflux is altered in patients with metabolic syndrome (MetS). A recent study compared efflux to the plasma of control subjects with obese MetS patients before and after weight loss (Shaw et al. 2000). Surprisingly, the efflux to MetS patients' plasma was higher than that of the control subjects' plasma, but weight loss among the MetS patients "normalized" efflux by reducing it to control values. The affinity of LDL for cholesterol is greater than that of HDL, so that the rate of cholesterol desorption from HDL is much faster than that from LDL (da Silva et al. 2015). However, the number of HDL particles in human plasma is nearly 10 times greater than that of all other lipoproteins combined. Therefore, based on chemical kinetics, the most likely first encounter of a cholesterol molecule desorbing from a cell membrane will be HDL. Reducing traditional CVD risk factors—hypertension, total cholesterol, LDL, non-HDL cholesterol, Apo B, and HOMA-IR—is atheroprotective, and reducing these by dietary means and weight loss must also be considered a sensible therapeutic strategy despite the attendant decrease in macrophage cholesterol efflux.

6.1.3 ATHEROSCLEROSIS AND IMMUNE CELLS

There is also an interaction between blood lipids, especially LDL, and immune system cells, which is implicated in atherogenesis (Ilhan and Kalkanli 2015). Monocytes have a key role as they migrate from the circulation into the intima of the arterial wall, where they are transformed into foam cells by taking up modified LDL. These cells provoke the production of proinflammatory cytokines such as IL-1, IL-6, IL-12, IL-15, IL-18, and tumor necrosis factor (TNF) family members (Galkina and Ley 2009; de Jager et al. 2011). Both proinflammatory monocytes and TNF are negatively correlated with fibrous cap thickness in patients with coronary artery disease (CAD). Additionally, interferon γ (IFN-γ) may trigger the macrophages to produce reactive oxygen species (ROS) and neopterin, which is connected to acute coronary syndrome (Ilhan et al. 2005). Toll-like receptors (TLRs) regulate the lipid uptake by macrophages, directly influencing the atheroma formation (Funk et al. 1993; Lee et al. 2008). Furthermore, specific T cells are also targeted to the vessel wall in line with macrophages and are responsible for the production of proinflammatory mediators such as IFN-γ, IL-4, IL-13, and so on, and perform the activation of macrophages (George et al. 2012; Ilhan and Kalkanli 2015; Whitman et al. 2002). In general terms, it seems that because both beneficial and inverse effects have been reported in epidemiological studies, oxidized LDL-specific antibody IgG titers are associated with atherosclerosis, whereas oxidized LDL-specific IgM titers are related to atheroprotection (Nilsson et al. 2005; Shaw et al. 2000).

6.1.4 ATHEROSCLEROSIS AND INFLAMMATION

Inflammation governs all stages of atherosclerosis, from its inception through its progression and its final complication of thrombosis (Libby et al. 2010). As already described, blood monocytes adhere to the dysfunctional endothelial surface and enter the intima, a process driven by mediators associated with risk factors such as proinflammatory cytokines, angiotensin II, and oxidized LDL. The fracture of the plaque's fibrous cap, also driven by inflammatory processes, and subsequent thrombosis cause most cases of fatal myocardial infarction, through plaque rupture or surface erosion (Davies and Thomas 1984; Hansson et al. 2015). Plaque rupture and erosions trigger atherothrombosis by exposing thrombogenic material inside the plaque, such as phospholipids, tissue factor, and matrix molecules, to platelets and coagulation factors (Farb et al. 1996). Platelet aggregates precipitating on these exposed surfaces are stabilized by fibrin networks. Tissue factor, expressed by macrophages and by vascular smooth-muscle cells in the atherosclerotic plaque, can initiate the blood coagulation cascade that leads to fibrin formation (Libby et al. 2011; Wilcox et al. 1989). Disturbance of the balance between prothrombotic and fibrinolytic activity on the plaque surface probably plays an important role for precipitating the thrombotic event (Wilcox et al. 1989). Diet plays a pivotal role in atherogenesis, as nutrients and dietary patterns can influence various aspects of this process. Therefore, it is very important, on one hand, to address the nutrients and dietary patterns that could potentially promote atherogenesis and, on the other hand, to overview the dietary means through which CVD can be prevented.

6.2 SPECIFIC NUTRIENTS IN THE PREVENTION AND TREATMENT OF CARDIOVASCULAR DISEASE

6.2.1 DIETARY FATS

6.2.1.1 Saturated Fatty Acids

The main sources of saturated fatty acids (SFAs) are animal foods (meat, dairy products), commercially prepared food, and some plant oils (palm oils, coconut oils, and coconut butter). Recent research indicates that the effects of SFA consumption on CVD risk are not independent, and vary on the replacement nutrient (Michas et al. 2014). Two recent meta-analyses of cohort studies showed that dietary SFA intake is not associated significantly with risk of coronary heart disease (CHD), stroke, or CVD (Mente et al. 2009; Siri-Tarino et al. 2010). However, the effect of SFAs on CVD varies depending on the replacement nutrients (Michas et al. 2014). In particular, when polyunsaturated fatty acids (PUFAs) replaced SFAs, this was associated with reduced CHD risk (Jakobsen et al. 2009). The replacement of SFAs with monounsaturated fatty acids (MUFAs) had no beneficial effect, while SFA replacement with carbohydrates was associated with higher CHD risk (Jakobsen et al. 2009). Finally, a meta-analysis of 48 randomized controlled trials (RCTs) showed that reducing saturated fat by reducing and/or modifying dietary fat can decrease the risk of cardiovascular events (Hooper et al. 2012). The 2013 AHA/ACC Guidelines on Lifestyle Management to Reduce Cardiovascular Risk recommend that adults who would benefit from LDL cholesterol lowering should only consume 5%–6% from SFAs (Eckel et al. 2014).

Table 6.1 shows a summary of nutrient functions and recommendations for the prevention and control of heart diseases.

6.2.1.2 Trans Fatty Acids

Trans fatty acids (TFAs) are associated with increased LDL and lipoprotein-α (Lp[a]) levels, decreased HDL cholesterol levels, increased inflammatory markers levels, and impaired endothelial function (Mozaffarian et al. 2006). Meta-analyses have reported a positive association between the intake of TFA and CHD morbidity and mortality (Mente et al. 2009; Mozaffarian and Clarke 2009). It is therefore suggested that TFA intake should be limited to less than 1% of total daily calories (Perk et al. 2012).

6.2.1.3 n-6 Polyunsaturated Fatty Acids

The n-6 PUFAs most often studied include linoleic acid (LA) and arachidonic acid (AA). A large body of evidence suggests that higher intakes of n-6 PUFAs may result in a reduced risk of CHD (Harris et al. 2009). Findings from the Nurses' Health Study suggested that n-6 PUFAs have a beneficial effect on cardiac death risk (Chiuve et al. 2012b). A meta-analysis of 8 RCTs indicated that for every 5% energy substitution of SFA with n-6 PUFA, there was a 10% reduction in CHD risk (Mozaffarian et al. 2010). In 2009, the AHA Science Advisory after combining data from RCTs, observational studies, and animal experiments suggested that the consumption of at least 5%–10% of energy from n-6 PUFAs results in a reduced risk of CHD compared with lower intakes, while higher intakes seem to remain safe and may also enhance the beneficial effect (Harris et al. 2009).

6.2.1.4 n-3 Polyunsaturated Fatty Acids

Many studies have examined the beneficial effect of n-3 PUFAs in the prevention and treatment of CVD. n-3 PUFAs include α-linolenic acid, eicosapentaenoic acid (EPA), docosahexaenoic acid (DHA), and docosapentaenoic acid (DPA). α-Linolenic acid is mainly found in plant sources and specifically in a limited number of seeds, nuts, and their oils, such as flaxseed oil, rapeseed oil, walnut oil, and soybean oil. EPA and DHA are derived mainly from seafood such as anchovies, salmon, and mackerel. DPA is also derived from seafood but in significantly smaller amounts, and at the same time it is endogenously synthesized from DHA (USDA 2016). There are several mechanisms associated with the beneficial effect of n-3 fatty acids on CVD. Firstly, n-3 PUFAs result in the lowering of plasma triglyceride (TG) synthesis (Harris and Bulchandani 2006). n-3 PUFAs have also been associated with reduced systolic and diastolic blood pressure (Mozaffarian and Wu 2011), have anti-arrhythmic effects (Endo and Arita 2016), result in improved endothelial function

TABLE 6.1
Nutrient Functions and Recommendations for Reducing the Risk of Heart Disease

Nutrient	Nutrient Functions and Recommendations
Saturated fatty acids	Dietary saturated fatty acids intake is not associated significantly with risk of CHD (Siri-Tarino et al. 2010). The effect of saturated fatty acids on CVD risk depends on the replacement nutrient (Michas et al. 2014). It is recommended that SFAs should account for <10% of total energy intake, through replacement by polyunsaturated fatty acids (Montalescot et al. 2013).
Trans fatty acids	Trans fatty acids are associated with increased levels of LDL, blood lipoprotein-α, and inflammatory factors, decreased levels of HDL, and impaired endothelial function (Mozaffarian et al. 2006). They are positively associated with CHD morbidity and mortality. It is recommended that trans-unsaturated fatty acids do not exceed 1% of total energy intake (Montalescot et al. 2013).
n-6 Polyunsaturated fatty acids	n-6 Polyunsaturated fatty acids may have a beneficial effect on cardiac death risk, and intakes of at least 5%–10% energy intake from n-6 PUFAs is associated with a reduced risk of coronary heart disease (Harris et al. 2009).
n-3 Polyunsaturated fatty acids	The consumption of n-3 polyunsaturated fatty acids from fish and fish oils has a cardioprotective effect (Endo and Arita 2016). It is recommended to consume fish at least twice a week (preferably oily fish). It is suggested to consume n-3 PUFAs from fish and fish oils rather than from food supplements (Montalescot et al. 2013).
Monounsaturated fatty acids	MUFAs as a replacement nutrient for carbohydrates and saturated fatty acids have been shown to decrease blood pressure, increase HDL cholesterol levels, and decrease hs-CRP levels (Michas et al. 2014).
Fiber	Fiber intake is inversely associated with CVD mortality (Liu et al. 2015).
Antioxidants	Based on data from intervention controlled trials, it is not recommended to use antioxidant vitamin supplementation to prevent or treat CVD.
Vitamin C	It has been shown that vitamin C has no significant inverse association with cardiovascular events and all cause mortality.
Vitamin A	High plasma levels of carotenoids may be associated with reduced oxidative stress, lower levels of inflammation, improved endothelial function, and higher levels of HDL cholesterol; however, the findings are not consistent. It is not recommended to use β-carotene supplementation in the prevention of cardiovascular disease.
Vitamin E	Vitamin E may have anti-inflammatory and cardioprotective functions. Meta-analyses have failed to support the beneficial effect of vitamin E and its supplementation for the primary prevention of cardiovascular disease is not recommended (Moyer and Force 2014).
Vitamin D	It has been shown that low blood vitamin D levels may be associated with increased risk of CHD (Grandi et al. 2010). The correction of low vitamin D levels may reduce CVD morbidity and mortality (Eilat-Adar et al. 2013). It is not recommended to use vitamin D supplements in order to prevent CVD in people with normal vitamin D levels (Eilat-Adar et al. 2013).
Polyphenolic compounds	Polyphenolic compounds may have antioxidant and cardioprotective function; however, the evidence is limited and further research is required (Rangel-Huerta et al. 2015).
B vitamins	B vitamins (folate, vitamin B_6, and vitamin B_{12}) or folate supplementation can result in lower levels of homocysteine and CHD risk (Muskiet 2005). Folic acid and vitamin B supplements are not effective for the primary or secondary prevention of CVD and stroke.

(Mozaffarian and Wu 2011), and in high doses have anti-inflammatory properties and contribute to the cardioprotective effect (Endo and Arita 2016; Oh et al. 2010).

The consumption of n-3 PUFAs from fish and fish oils has a cardioprotective effect (Endo and Arita 2016). Meta-analyses of RCTs show that the consumption of n-3 PUFAs results in a significant reduction in CHD death (Marik and Varon 2009; Mozaffarian and Wu 2011). At the same time, another meta-analysis indicated that dietary intake of long-chain n-3 PUFAs and circulating long-chain n-3 PUFAs are associated with a significant decrease in coronary risk (Wen et al. 2014). A meta-analysis of cohort studies also suggests that high intake of n-3 PUFAs may augment the prevention of stroke in women but the beneficial effect was not established in men (Larsson et al. 2012). It has been shown that patients with stroke had lower erythrocyte levels of n-3 PUFAs (Park et al. 2009). Another meta-analysis showed an inverse statistically significant association between high fish consumption and the risk of stroke (Larsson and Orsini 2011). Overall, an association between n-3 PUFAs and stroke cannot be established and the evidence cannot support n-3 PUFA supplementation as a means for stroke prevention. Most studies agree that n-3 PUFA consumption at moderate levels could reduce CHD mortality compared with low or no consumption through mechanisms such as membrane modification, the regulation of proinflammatory gene expression, and the production of lipid mediators, which have been recognized to augment the protective role of PUFAs in CHD (Endo and Arita 2016; Mozaffarian and Wu 2011). As far as treatment is concerned, n-3 PUFA supplementation seems to be effective in the treatment of hypertriglyceridemia and heart failure (Nestel et al. 2015).

Guidelines recommend the consumption of fish at least twice a week, with one of the servings as oily fish (McMurray et al. 2012; Montalescot et al. 2013). The recommendation of the European Society of Cardiology is that patients with stable heart disease should increase n-3 PUFA intake through fish consumption, rather than from supplements (Montalescot et al. 2013).

6.2.1.5 Monounsaturated Fatty Acids

The main sources of MUFAs are nuts, olive oil, canola oil, high oleic safflower oil, sunflower oil, and avocado. The replacement of carbohydrates with MUFAs decreases TG, VLDL, hs-CRP, and blood pressure (BP), and increases HDL and Apo A; MUFA consumption also decreases total cholesterol and LDL (Michas et al. 2014). A meta-analysis indicated that high (>12%) MUFA diets are significantly associated with reduced systolic and diastolic BP (Schwingshackl et al. 2011). Based on the available data, the recommendations for the intake of MUFAs remain unclear (Perk et al. 2012). However, it is supported that populations at risk of CVD should continue replacing saturated fatty acids with unsaturated fat, although the type of unsaturated fat is not clear yet (Hooper et al. 2012).

6.2.2 Protein

Several studies have evaluated the effect of low-carbohydrate, high-protein diets on CVD. In a prospective cohort study it has been shown that low-carbohydrate and high-protein diets, regardless of the source of the proteins and the nature of the carbohydrates, are associated with increased risk of CVD (Lagiou et al. 2012). Proteins from plant-based compared with animal-based food sources may have different effects on CVD risk (Richter et al. 2015). Vegetable protein lowers the risk of CVD by decreasing total cholesterol, LDL, and TG levels (Anderson et al. 1995). There is not enough evidence about the effect of protein type on CVD, as there are many complexities regarding the amino acid content and the nonprotein compounds derived from different food sources. However, current evidence supports the idea that CVD risk can be reduced by a dietary pattern that provides more plant sources and also includes animal-based protein foods that are unprocessed and low in saturated fat (Richter et al. 2015).

6.2.3 FIBER

It has been strongly suggested that dietary fiber intake might be protective against CAD (Bernstein et al. 2013; Retelny et al. 2008). Fiber is associated with improved lipid profile by reducing cholesterol, oxidized LDL, and TG levels, resulting in the decreased formation of atherosclerotic plaque. Fiber intake causes a delay in intestinal absorption, effectively reducing blood glucose concentration (Chandalia et al. 2000; Hollaender et al. 2015). Lower blood glucose levels result in improved insulin sensitivity, which reduces inflammation and improves antioxidant processes (Chandalia et al. 2000; Wu et al. 2015). A meta-analysis of population-based cohort studies indicated that higher fiber intake reduces CHD incidence by 7% and CHD mortality by 17% (Wu et al. 2015). The incidence of CHD had a significant inverse association with high fruit, vegetable, and cereal fiber (Mozaffarian and Wu 2011).

6.2.4 ANTIOXIDANTS

It is now well established that oxidative stress and the resultant oxidation of LDL by free radicals increases atherogenesis. Some of the antioxidants of interest are detailed in the following sections.

6.2.4.1 Vitamin C

Vitamin C (ascorbate or ascorbic acid) is a water-soluble vitamin. The main dietary vitamin C sources are citrus fruit, kiwi, mango, and peppers. A meta-analysis of 15 cohort studies indicated that subjects with the highest intake of vitamin C had 16% lower risk of CHD compared with subjects with the lowest vitamin C intake (Ye and Song 2008). A number of clinical trials have found an inverse association between plasma concentration of vitamin C and markers of endothelial dysfunction and/or inflammation; however, recent studies indicate that there is no significant association between vitamin C intake and cardiovascular events (Goszcz et al. 2015). Finally, the Cochrane review on antioxidants concludes that vitamin C has no significant inverse association with all-cause mortality (Bjelakovic et al. 2012).

6.2.4.2 Carotenoids and Vitamin A

Carotenoids are lipid soluble and include more than 600 compounds, but the most common carotenoids in the human diet are α-carotene, β-carotene, β-cryptoxanthin, lycopene, lutein, and zeaxanthin. Vitamin A (retinol) can be synthesized from β-carotene in the gut. Carotenoids are found in fruits and vegetables. High levels of carotenoids in the plasma are associated with reduced oxidative stress, improved endothelial function, and lower levels of inflammation (Hozawa et al. 2007). Higher plasma levels of α-carotene and β-carotene are associated with a lower incidence of atherosclerosis (D'Odorico et al. 2000). Lycopene, which mainly derives from tomato intake, is associated with a reduced risk of myocardial infarction and reduced risk of mortality in subjects with high levels of lycopene in adipose tissue (Kohlmeier et al. 1997). The U.S. Preventive Task Force does not recommend β-carotene supplementation for the prevention of CVD (Montalescot et al. 2013).

6.2.4.3 Vitamin E

Cell cultures and animal studies have shown that vitamin E prevents the oxidative modification of LDL (Negre-Salvayre et al. 1995). Additionally, vitamin E acts as an anti-inflammatory agent, especially at high doses (Bhupathiraju and Tucker 2011). Vitamin E supplementation is associated with lower CHD risk and CHD mortality (Kushi et al. 1996; Meyer et al. 1996). On the contrary, meta-analysis of clinical trials failed to support the role of vitamin E in CVD prevention (Eidelman et al. 2004). Despite the fact that there is a lot of evidence from experimental studies that support that vitamin E has a cardioprotective effect, vitamin E supplementation cannot be incorporated into recommendations for primary CVD prevention (Moyer and Force 2014).

6.2.4.4 Vitamin D

The underlying mechanisms for a potential role of vitamin D in CHD prevention include the inhibition of vascular smooth-muscle proliferation, the suppression of vascular calcification, the downregulation of proinflammatory cytokines, the upregulation of anti-inflammatory cytokines, and the action of vitamin D as a negative endocrine regulator of the renin–angiotensin system (Zittermann et al. 2005). Epidemiological studies clearly support that vitamin D has a protective role in cardiovascular disease (Bhupathiraju and Tucker 2011). However, three large trials have failed to prove the inverse relationship between vitamin D and coronary heart disease risk, blood pressure, and levels of serum lipids (Hsia et al. 2007; Jorde et al. 2010; Trivedi et al. 2003). Meta-analyses have shown significant associations between low vitamin D levels and the risk of CVD and overall mortality (Grandi et al. 2010; Pittas et al. 2010). It has been indicated that patients with CHD were more likely to have vitamin D deficiency (Grandi et al. 2010).

6.2.4.5 Polyphenolic Compounds

Polyphenols are a large group of compounds divided into several subgroups: phenolic acids, flavonoids, lignans, and stilbenes. Cocoa, chocolate, tea, and red wine are foods high in polyphenolic compounds. Polyphenols have been shown to have antioxidant properties (Galleano et al. 2010; Quideau et al. 2011). The Rotterdam Study found a significant inverse relationship between total flavonoid intake from the diet—in particular, black tea—and myocardial infarction incidence (Geleijnse et al. 2002). Supplementation with quercetin, which is one of the most frequent polyphenolic compounds in the human diet, was found to reduce systolic BP and plasma oxidized LDL concentrations in subjects with a high risk of CVD (Egert et al. 2009). To sum up, there is available evidence to support that polyphenolic compounds could have a beneficial effect in the prevention of CVD; however, further research and meta-analyses are required in order to establish this relationship (Rangel-Huerta et al. 2015).

6.2.4.6   Vitamin B

Increased dietary intake of vitamin B (folate, vitamin B_6, and vitamin B_{12}) or folate supplementation can result in lower levels of homocysteine (an independent risk factor for CVD) and CHD risk. (Muskiet 2005). A meta-analysis of prospective studies showed that high folate intake was significantly associated with a 31% decreased risk of CAD, while increased folate intake of 200 ug/day was associated with a 12% decreased risk of CAD (Wang et al. 2012). At the same time, there are also several RCTs and meta-analyses that do not support the beneficial effects of vitamin B intake and supplementation in decreasing the risk of CHD (Bazzano et al. 2006). There is not sufficient evidence to allow the use of supplements as a means of secondary prevention and treatment of CHD, and further research needs to be conducted.

6.3   NUTRITIONAL REMEDIES FOR HEART DISEASE

During the last two decades there has been an increasing interest in developing nutraceutical agents that aim at decreasing CVD risk through the management of CVD risk factors (Rocha et al. 2016; Talati et al. 2010). Plant sterols and stanols, natural compounds occurring in plant-based foods, are a distinctive and well-studied example of such agents. Plant sterols and stanols decrease LDL cholesterol (LDLC) by inhibiting the intestinal absorption of ingested cholesterol (Rocha et al. 2016; Talati et al. 2010). A very recent meta-analysis of RCTs showed that the regular intake of plant sterol–enriched foods resulted in a significant LDLC decrease of 14.3 mg/dL (95% CI −17.3; −11.3), although the impact on atherosclerosis-related inflammatory biomarkers was not significant (Rocha et al. 2016). Similar results were found in a previous meta-analysis of RCTs in which plant sterol or stanol supplements reduced LDLC by 12 mg/dL (Amir Shaghaghi et al. 2013).

Other nutraceutical agents include red wine flavonoids, green tea catechins, and garlic, among others. A large amount of studies have shown that low-to-moderate consumption of red wine decreases CVD incidence and mortality risk; red wine's flavonoids have gained a great amount of interest in relation to their effect against CVD (Lippi et al. 2010). Catechins comprise the vast majority of the polyphenols found in green tea, and it is suggested that the attributed cardioprotective effect of green tea is due to these compounds (Hartley et al. 2013). According to two meta-analyses of RCTs, green tea catechins are associated with a significant decrease in LDLC of 5.3 mg/dL (95% CI −9.99; −0.62) and 11.5 mg/dL (95% CI −13.86; −9.36), while no effect was shown for HDL and triglycerides (Hartley et al. 2013; Kim et al. 2011). Finally, the intake of garlic and garlic supplements seems to be associated with a significant decrease in total cholesterol, but the results are controversial regarding LDLC (Schwingshackl et al. 2015).

Overall, although findings on the cardioprotective role of nutraceutical agents are very encouraging, long-term studies assessing their prolonged intake effect regarding the maintenance of their benefits, the optimal dosage scheme, and the potential harms are necessary.

6.4 DIETARY PATTERNS AND HEART DISEASE PREVENTION

The "diet–heart hypothesis" has been actively investigated in nutritional epidemiology during the past few decades (Mozaffarian et al. 2011), although the traditional approach has been to study the effects of single nutrients or foods on health outcomes. Given that individuals do not consume single nutrients but meals consisting of a variety of foods, the analysis of food patterns, rather than single nutrients and single foods, is considered as the ideal approach to examine the effects of the overall diet (Hu 2002). As a result, there has been increasing interest regarding the association that various diet patterns have on the prevention, development, and treatment of chronic diseases (Ros 2012). Among the different dietary patterns, such as the low-fat diet, the low-carbohydrate diet, the Dietary Approaches to Stop Hypertension (DASH) diet, and the Mediterranean diet, the latter has gained the largest part of the scientific interest in recent decades (Sofi et al. 2010), thus it will be the focus of this section.

6.4.1 MEDITERRANEAN DIETARY PATTERNS

The Mediterranean diet is based on the eating habits observed in the areas of the Mediterranean basin during the early 1960s (Keys et al. 1986). It is characterized by the high consumption of fruits, vegetables, whole-grain cereals, legumes, nuts, and seeds; moderate consumption of fish, poultry, dairy products and wine; and limited consumption of red meats and sweets (Kastorini et al. 2011). Olive oil, which is high in monounsaturated fatty acids, is the main source of fat and a distinctive trait of the Mediterranean diet (Willett et al. 1995). Westernization has had a great impact on the Mediterranean diet, though, which has led to the increased consumption of refined carbohydrates, red meat, and saturated fat, whereas the consumption of whole-grain cereals and legumes has decreased (Martinez-Gonzalez et al. 2011). A variety of indices have been developed as measures of Mediterranean diet adherence, focusing on the identification of the overall dietary pattern, but there is not yet a direct method to assess adherence (Mila-Villarroel et al. 2011). Hence, due to the absence of common criteria defining the Mediterranean diet, each index is based on the available data and the study objectives (Mila-Villarroel et al. 2011). One of the most widely used indices is the Mediterranean dietary score (MDS) developed by Trichopoulou et al. (1995) and later modified for non-Mediterranean populations (Trichopoulou et al. 2005).

6.4.1.1 Prevention and Treatment of Total CVD

In terms of heart health, the Mediterranean diet has been found to have an atheroprotective role and to be associated with CVD risk reduction and the improvement of the attributing risk factors (Sofi et al. 2010, 2014). A recent meta-analysis of 14 prospective studies showed that a 2-point increase in the MDS (Trichopoulou et al. 2003) was associated with significantly higher protection against CVD and, in particular, with a 10% lower risk of CVD incidence and/or mortality (Sofi et al. 2014). This meta-analysis updated a previous one by the same group that had showed a similar result (RR 0.90; 95% CI 0.87–0.93) (Sofi et al. 2010). An even more recent meta-analysis of 20 prospective studies also revealed the inverse association of high Mediterranean diet adherence with a decreased risk of CVD incidence (fatal or nonfatal) (RR 0.71; 95% CI 0.65, 0.78) compared with the lowest adherence (Grosso et al. 2015).

Although dietary patterns receive increased attention compared with single nutrients or food groups, the lack of consistency in the methods used (e.g., variations in definitions, metrics, and statistical approaches) led the 2007 World Cancer Research Fund Report (World Cancer Research Fund and Research 2007) and the 2010 Dietary Guidelines Advisory Committee (USDA 2010) to decide, at the time, that firm conclusions regarding the association of dietary patterns and health outcomes could not be drawn due to insufficient evidence. Following these recommendations, the Dietary Patterns Methods Project (DPMP) was initiated in 2012 by the National Cancer Institute in an attempt to strengthen the already existing evidence (Reedy et al. 2014). The DPMP relates dietary patterns to mortality by conducting simultaneous analyses in three U.S. cohorts that all use identical methods and models (Liese et al. 2015). The assessment of the dietary patterns was performed through the systematic examination of four indices (the Healthy Eating Index 2010 [HEI-2010] [Guenther et al. 2013], the Alternative Healthy Eating Index 2010 [AHEI-2010] [Chiuve et al. 2012a], the Alternate Mediterranean Diet [aMED] score [Fung et al. 2005], and the Dietary Approaches to Stop Hypertension [DASH] score [Fung et al. 2008]) and their associations with all-cause, CVD, and cancer mortality among older adults in the United States (Reedy et al. 2014). The sample consisted of adults between the ages of 50 and 71 that were followed from 1995 through to the end of 2011 (Reedy et al. 2014). During the 15 years of follow-up, 86,419 deaths were documented overall, of which 23,502 were CVD deaths (15,497 for men and 8,005 for women) (Reedy et al. 2014). The DPMP reported that aMED showed significant associations with CVD mortality.

Only a few RCTs have been carried out to assess the effect of the Mediterranean diet on total CVD. It is worth mentioning that the most important is the Prevención con Dieta Mediterránea (PREDIMED) study, a large RCT that assesses the impact of the Mediterranean diet on the primary prevention of CVD, within the frame of the Mediterranean diet (Estruch et al. 2013). The sample of the trial consisted of men and women who did not have CVD at baseline, but had either type 2 diabetes or at least three cardiovascular risk factors (current smoking, hypertension, high LDL or lipid-lowering therapy, low HDL, overweight/obesity, family history of premature CHD). Their results showed that adherence to the Mediterranean diet, with extra supplementation of either extra virgin olive oil (mean consumption at the end of the trial 50 g/day) or nuts (mean consumption at the end of the trial 30 g/day) and no energy restriction compared with a low-fat control diet, resulted in a significant risk reduction of total CVD—a composite of cardiovascular death, myocardial infarction, and stroke (HR 0.70, 95% CI 0.54–0.92 for the olive oil group and HR 0.72,

95% CI 0.54–0.96 for the nuts group) (Estruch et al. 2013). A meta-analysis of four RCTs, including the results of the PREDIMED study, showed that for a total of 12,293 individuals at high CVD risk and 590 composite cases of CVD, the pooled estimated risk of fatal and nonfatal CVD incidence was 0.55 (95% CI 0.39, 0.76) for the Mediterranean diet group compared with the control (Grosso et al. 2015). The interventions among the four studies differed regarding the focus on Mediterranean diet components, while participants in the control groups were given similar dietary advice (Grosso et al. 2015).

Very few studies have been realized for the assessment of the Mediterranean diet on CVD treatment (secondary prevention). Results from the Lyon Diet Heart Study, an RCT that investigated the effect of the Mediterranean diet on the recurrence rate after a first incident of myocardial infarction (de Lorgeril et al. 1999), confirmed its beneficial effects. The hazard ratios between the group of participants that followed the Mediterranean diet and the group of participants that did not receive any dietary recommendation ranged from 0.28 to 0.53 for the various end points (cardiac death and nonfatal myocardial infarction: HR 0.28, 95% CI 0.15–0.53; the preceding plus major secondary end points [unstable angina, stroke, heart failure, etc.]: HR 0.33, 95% CI 0.21–0.52; the preceding plus minor events requiring hospital admission: HR 0.53 95% CI 0.38–0.74) (de Lorgeril et al. 1999). It seems that even variations of the Mediterranean diet can have a beneficial secondary prevention effect as shown by an RCT that assessed the impact of an Indo-Mediterranean diet on total CVD mortality compared with the dietary pattern recommended by Step 1 of the National Cholesterol Education Program (NCEP1) and found that the risk of CVD incidence (fatal or nonfatal) was reduced for the Indo-Mediterranean diet group by 52% (Singh et al. 2002).

6.4.1.2   Prevention and Treatment of Coronary Heart Disease (CHD)

According to a recent meta-analysis of four prospective studies, high adherence to the Mediterranean diet was inversely associated with CHD risk (RR 0.72, 95% CI 0.60–0.86) and myocardial infarction risk (RR 0.67, 95% CI 0.54–0.83) (Grosso et al. 2015). It has been revealed that the Mediterranean diet is the dietary pattern with the strongest causal evidence of protection from CHD, compared with 33 others using a predefined algorithm of the Bradford Hill criteria combined with experimental evidence (Mente et al. 2009). The Spanish EPIC study (European Prospective Investigation into Cancer and Nutrition), including 40,000 participants, showed that higher adherence to the Mediterranean diet was associated significantly with 40% reduced CHD risk (Buckland et al. 2009). Another analysis on the same cohort revealed that the "evolved Mediterranean diet," characterized by the consumption of plant-based foods and olive oil, was associated with a lower CHD incident risk (HR 0.73, 95% CI 0.57–0.94) for the participants with the highest adherence compared with those with the lowest (Guallar-Castillon et al. 2012).

6.4.1.3   Potential Underlying Mechanisms

The antioxidant and anti-inflammatory properties of the individual components of the Mediterranean diet are responsible for its atheroprotective effects. The foods that comprise the basis of the Mediterranean diet, which is by definition plant based, undergo minimal processing, leading to the effective preservation of their nutrients, hence the overall diet exerts higher antioxidants levels. Moreover, given that the main fat source of the Mediterranean diet is olive oil, the amount of saturated and trans fat provided by this dietary pattern is very low (Kastorini et al. 2011). A meta-analysis of seven RCTs assessing the effect of the Mediterranean diet over low-fat diets on cardiovascular risk factors showed that after 2 years of follow-up the Mediterranean diet was more beneficial regarding changes on systolic and diastolic BP, total cholesterol, and hs-CRP (Nordmann et al. 2011). A second meta-analysis of both epidemiological studies and RCTs showed that adherence to the Mediterranean diet is optimal both for the metabolic syndrome overall and for its components related to CVD development (insulin resistance, HDL, TG, and blood pressure levels) (Kastorini et al. 2011; Santaniemi et al. 2013).

6.4.2 THE DASH DIET AND OTHER DIETARY PATTERNS

The Dietary Approaches to Stop Hypertension (DASH) diet refers to a dietary pattern that aims to control hypertension. This pattern is rich in fruit, vegetables, and low-fat dairy products, includes whole grains, poultry, fish, and nuts, and limits saturated fat, red meat, sweets, and sugar-containing beverages (Conlin et al. 2000). The DASH score, which exists in several versions, is used in order to assess adherence to the DASH dietary pattern. The DASH score version most commonly found in the literature with U.S. populations includes eight components (whole grains, vegetables, fruit, nuts and legumes, low-fat dairy, red and processed meat, sugar-sweetened beverages, sodium), each of which scores 5 points for a total of 40 points, while the scoring system is based on sex-specific quintile rankings (Fung et al. 2008).

Other dietary patterns include (1) very low carbohydrate diets (V-LCDs), (2) low-fat diets, (3) hypothesis-driven dietary patterns, and (4) empirically derived dietary patterns.

The V-LCD or ketogenic dietary patterns are considered to have a carbohydrate intake of 20–50 g/day (equivalent to 20% or less of the daily calorie intake from carbohydrates) (Stradling et al. 2014). There are a lot of popular examples of carbohydrate-restricted diets, such as the South Beach, Zone, and Atkins diets. Of these, the Atkins diet is the only ketogenic diet, although it is non-energy restricted, having less than 20% of the daily calorie intake from carbohydrates (Stradling et al. 2014). The South Beach diet is energy restricted and limits carbohydrate intake to approximately 40% of total energy intake, while it encourages the consumption of lower glycemic index carbohydrate foods. The Zone diet, despite the carbohydrate restriction, promotes a balanced intake of carbohydrate, protein, and fat (40:30:30) (Stradling et al. 2014).

Low-fat diets are those in which the energy from fat consumption does not exceed 30% of total energy consumption.

The hypothesis-driven dietary patterns are usually determined by applying an index that assesses adherence to certain guidelines. Specifically, the HEI was developed to quantify adherence to the Dietary Guidelines for Americans (Guenther et al. 2013). It includes 12 components (total vegetables, "greens and beans," total fruit, whole fruit, seafood and plant proteins, total protein foods, whole grains, low-fat dairy, fatty acid ratio [{PUFA + MUFA}:SFA], refined grains, sodium, "empty calories") and it scores for a total out of 100 points (Reedy et al. 2014). The AHEI was developed based on foods and nutrients associated with chronic disease risk and includes 11 components (whole grains, vegetables, fruit, nuts and legumes, trans fat, EPA and DHA, PUFAs, alcohol, red and processed meat, sugar-sweetened beverages and fruit juices, sodium), while it scores for a total out of 110 points (Chiuve et al. 2012a). Dietary patterns can be also derived empirically in order to explore the structure of dietary patterns in the population, either by principal component analysis (PCA) or cluster analysis (Bhupathiraju and Tucker 2011).

6.4.2.1 Prevention of Total CVD and CHD

The adherence to a DASH-like diet, according to a meta-analysis of six cohort studies, was shown to significantly reduce the risk of both total CVD (RR 0.80, 95% CI 0.74–0.86) and CHD (RR 0.79, 95% CI 0.71–0.88) (Salehi-Abargouei et al. 2013). The Nurses' Health Study reported a 14% lower risk of CHD for the highest compared with the lowest quintile of the DASH diet score (Fung et al. 2008). The Iowa Women's Health Study also observed that women showing the highest adherence to the DASH diet had 23% lower risk of CHD mortality; however, that lost its significance after adjustment for other risk factors (Folsom et al. 2007). Results from National Health and Nutrition Examination Survey (NHANES) revealed that a DASH-like diet was not significantly associated with CVD mortality in adults with hypertension (Parikh et al. 2009). Nonetheless, due to the beneficial effect that the DASH diet has on CVD risk factors, it is considered to have an overall protective effect on the development of CVD (Bhupathiraju and Tucker 2011).

In terms of V-LCDs, a systematic review and meta-analysis of 23 RCTs investigating the prolonged effects of V-LCDs on CVD risk factors in obese subjects revealed that a 6- and 12-month weight loss improved major cardiovascular risk factors. However, it was shown that a significant reduction in LDL was only found in subjects adhering to the dietary pattern for over 12 months, suggesting that LDL is reduced if weight loss is sustained for over 12 months (Santos et al. 2012). Nonetheless, V-LCDs are traditionally criticized due to the subsequent increase in fat intake, particularly saturated fats as well as nutritional deficiencies that are related to limiting the intake of healthy foods such as whole grains, fruits, and fiber, all of which contain micronutrients associated with CVD risk reduction (Stradling et al. 2014). Similarly controversial effects seem to be reported for low-fat diets. A meta-analysis of 32 RCTs revealed that low-fat diets resulted in a quantitatively greater reduction of total cholesterol and LDL cholesterol in the long term in comparison with high-fat diets (ranging from high SFA to high unsaturated fat) (Schwingshackl and Hoffmann 2013). However, low-fat diets caused a greater increase of TG and a greater decrease of HDL levels when compared with high-fat diets. A meta-analysis that compared low- with high-fat diets showed that although HDL was improved by low-fat diets, total cholesterol and LDL were also increased (Hu et al. 2012).

Diets of the highest quality, as assessed by the HEI, AHEI, and DASH scores, were associated with a significant reduction in the risk of CVD by 22% (Schwingshackl and Hoffmann 2015). The DPMP project partially answers the question as to whether there is one or multiple approaches to healthful eating associated with reduced CVD mortality, with its findings suggesting that all four indices (HEI, AHEI, DASH, and aMED) capture the essential and common foods and nutrients of a healthy diet (whole grains, vegetables, fruit, and plant-based proteins) (Reedy et al. 2014). A limitation to that, however, is that there are various ways to prepare and cook foods, information that cannot be captured due to the structure of food frequency questionnaires (FFQs) (Liese et al. 2015). In total, the DPMP findings did not clearly indicate that a certain index performed better than another, as the differences in HRs were very small and probably not clinically meaningful. Nonetheless, not all available dietary indices were assessed, thus the uncertainty of whether there are other diet quality measures that might better capture a healthy diet remains (Liese et al. 2015).

Finally, in terms of the empirically derived dietary patterns, the results of such analyses can be proven rather enlightening since they capture and characterize the current dietary patterns of the population. For example, in the Whitehall II study, four clusters were identified ("unhealthy," characterized by white bread, processed meat, French fries, and full-cream milk; "sweet," characterized by white bread, biscuits, cakes, processed meat, and high-fat dairy products; "Mediterranean-like," defined by fruit, vegetables, rice, pasta, and wine; and "healthy," with a high intake of fruit, vegetables, wholemeal bread, and low-fat dairy, and a low intake of alcohol). The healthy cluster, compared with the unhealthy, was associated with a reduced risk of fatal CHD and nonfatal MI by 29% (95% CI 0.51–0.98) (Brunner et al. 2008). A noteworthy finding of the study, though, is that that the Mediterranean-like cluster was characterized by a high intake of butter, which does not align to the traditional Mediterranean diet (Brunner et al. 2008). Several large-scale epidemiological studies have used factor analysis to derive dietary patterns, and the majority focuses on two patterns: the "prudent" pattern, characterized by vegetables, fruit, legumes, fish, poultry, and whole grains, and the "Western" pattern, characterized by red meat, processed meat, refined grains, French fries, and sweets/desserts (Bhupathiraju and Tucker 2011). The first pattern is associated with a reduced risk of CHD and CVD mortality, while the second one is associated with a significantly increased risk (Bhupathiraju and Tucker 2011). Similarly, when PCA is applied to ethnic populations, the patterns of interest are a "traditional" pattern, a healthy, and a Western pattern (Kim 2009; Shimazu et al. 2007). For example, the Japanese pattern, characterized by soybean products, fish, seaweed, vegetables, fruit, and green tea, was not associated with CHD mortality, while the animal food pattern, defined by high intakes of animal-derived products, coffee, and alcohol, was significantly associated with a higher CHD mortality risk (Shimazu et al. 2007).

6.5 NUTRITIONAL COUNSELING FOR CORONARY HEART DISEASE

The WHO has stated that over three-quarters of all CVD mortality may be prevented with lifestyle changes (Perk et al. 2012). The U.S. Preventive Task Force has found that medium- to high-intensity dietary counseling for patients with hyperlipidemia and other risk factors for CVD can result in the patients adopting the core components of a healthy diet (Moyer and Force 2012). At the same time, the data regarding the effect of medium- to high-intensity behavioral counseling interventions on the rates of CVD events are inadequate (Moyer and Force 2012). Although the correlations between a healthy diet, physical activity, and the incidence of CVD are strong, it seems that the initiation of behavioral counseling in the primary care setting to promote a healthy diet and physical activity has a small beneficial effect in the prevention of cardiovascular disease (Moyer and Force 2012). It seems that combining the knowledge and skills of clinicians and nutrition experts into multimodal behavioral interventions could help in the optimization of preventive efforts (Anderson et al. 2013). Dietary habits influence the risk of cardiovascular disease either through their effect on risk factors such as cholesterol, blood pressure, body weight, and diabetes or through an effect independent of these risk factors (Perk et al. 2012). The risk factors of cardiovascular disease could be potential targets for intervention and nutritional counseling (Anderson et al. 2013). Nutrition therapy is a very significant component of health behavior interventions and one of its main goals is the improvement of the lipid profile, which could potentially result in the reduction of cardiovascular events. The characteristics of the dietary patterns that could be suggested for patients with CVD or who are at risk of CVD are that energy intake should be limited to the amount needed to maintain (or obtain) a healthy weight, saturated fatty acids should account for <10% of total energy intake, trans fatty acids should be consumed as little as possible (preferably <1% of total energy intake), and patients should consume <5 g of salt per day, 30–45 g of fiber per day, 2–3 servings of fruit per day, and 2–3 servings of vegetables per day (Perk et al. 2012).

6.6 CASE STUDIES

6.6.1 CASE STUDY 1: PRIMARY PREVENTION

Mrs. A. B. is a 55-year-old African American female who has a family history of hypertension. She has a history of smoking 1.5 packs/day for the last 15 years and she follows a relatively sedentary lifestyle. She has a BMI of 27 and in her last blood test both total cholesterol and LDL levels were elevated. According to her nutritional assessment, it seems that her salt intake is quite high, while her diet is high in fat and very low in fruits and vegetables. Give responses to the following:

1. Suggest lifestyle modifications that would lower Mrs. A. B.'s CVD risk. (*Hint*: Some lifestyle modifications could be smoking cessation, weight loss, regular exercise, the improvement of eating habits.)
2. Suggest the main characteristics of the nutritional plan that Mrs. A. B. should follow in order to lower her blood pressure and improve her CVD risk. (*Hint*: The DASH diet could be suggested.)

6.6.2 CASE STUDY 2: SECONDARY PREVENTION

Mr. S. W., a 57-year-old male, has suffered myocardial infarction (MI) and has been treated with angioplasty. He smokes cigarettes (1.5 packs/day for 35 years). He has family history of CAD. His lab tests showed high total and LDL cholesterol and low HDL cholesterol. He is obese and does not do any kind of physical activity.

According to his nutritional assessment he follows a diet rich in high-fat junk food and high in sodium. Give responses to the following:

1. What risk factors could be addressed through nutrition therapy? (*Hint*: Weight, lipid profile.)
2. What are your recommendations for Mr. S. W.'s nutritional intake both during the hospitalization and afterward? (*Hint*: Consider a liquid diet free of caffeine in the first 24 hours after angioplasty. Consider small meals thereafter. Sodium may need to be restricted. Consider advice on healthier dietary patterns.)
3. What other issues might you consider to support the success of his lifestyle changes? (*Hint*: Smoking cessation, physical activity.)

REFERENCES

Amir Shaghaghi, M., S. S. Abumweis, and P. J. Jones. 2013. Cholesterol-lowering efficacy of plant sterols/stanols provided in capsule and tablet formats: Results of a systematic review and meta-analysis. *J Acad Nutr Diet* 113 (11):1494–1503.

Anderson, T. J., J. Gregoire, R. A. Hegele, P. Couture, G. B. Mancini, R. McPherson, G. A. Francis et al. 2013. 2012 update of the Canadian Cardiovascular Society guidelines for the diagnosis and treatment of dyslipidemia for the prevention of cardiovascular disease in the adult. *Can J Cardiol* 29 (2):151–167.

Anderson, J. W., B. M. Johnstone, and M. E. Cook-Newell. 1995 Meta-analysis of the effects of soy protein intake on serum lipids. *N Engl J Med* 333 (5):276–282.

Bazzano, L. A., K. Reynolds, K. N. Holder, and J. He. 2006. Effect of folic acid supplementation on risk of cardiovascular diseases: A meta-analysis of randomized controlled trials. *JAMA* 296 (22):2720–2726.

Bernstein, A. M., B. Titgemeier, K. Kirkpatrick, M. Golubic, and M. F. Roizen. 2013. Major cereal grain fibers and psyllium in relation to cardiovascular health. *Nutrients* 5 (5):1471–1487.

Bhupathiraju, S. N., and K. L. Tucker. 2011. Coronary heart disease prevention: Nutrients, foods, and dietary patterns. *Clin Chim Acta* 412 (17–18):1493–1514.

Bjelakovic, G., D. Nikolova, L. L. Gluud, R. G. Simonetti, and C. Gluud. 2012. Antioxidant supplements for prevention of mortality in healthy participants and patients with various diseases. *Cochrane Database Syst Rev* 3:CD007176.

Brunner, E. J., A. Mosdol, D. R. Witte, P. Martikainen, M. Stafford, M. J. Shipley, and M. G. Marmot. 2008. Dietary patterns and 15-y risks of major coronary events, diabetes, and mortality. *Am J Clin Nutr* 87 (5):1414–1421.

Buckland, G., C. A. Gonzalez, A. Agudo, M. Vilardell, A. Berenguer, P. Amiano, E. Ardanaz et al. 2009. Adherence to the Mediterranean diet and risk of coronary heart disease in the Spanish EPIC cohort study. *Am J Epidemiol* 170 (12):1518–1529.

Chandalia, M., A. Garg, D. Lutjohann, K. von Bergmann, S. M. Grundy, and L. J. Brinkley. 2000. Beneficial effects of high dietary fiber intake in patients with type 2 diabetes mellitus. *N Engl J Med* 342 (19):1392–1398.

Chiuve, S. E., T. T. Fung, E. B. Rimm, F. B. Hu, M. L. McCullough, M. Wang, M. J. Stampfer, and W. C. Willett. 2012a. Alternative dietary indices both strongly predict risk of chronic disease. *J Nutr* 142 (6):1009–1018.

Chiuve, S. E., E. B. Rimm, R. K. Sandhu, A. M. Bernstein, K. M. Rexrode, J. E. Manson, W. C. Willett, and C. M. Albert. 2012b. Dietary fat quality and risk of sudden cardiac death in women. *Am J Clin Nutr* 96 (3):498–507.

Conlin, P. R., D. Chow, E. R. Miller, 3rd, L. P. Svetkey, P. H. Lin, D. W. Harsha, T. J. Moore, F. M. Sacks, and L. J. Appel. 2000. The effect of dietary patterns on blood pressure control in hypertensive patients: Results from the Dietary Approaches to Stop Hypertension (DASH) trial. *Am J Hypertens* 13 (9):949–955.

da Silva, I. T., B. de Almeida-Pititto, and S. R. Ferreira. 2015. Reassessing lipid metabolism and its potentialities in the prediction of cardiovascular risk. *Arch Endocrinol Metab* 59 (2):171–180.

Davies, M. J., and A. Thomas. 1984. Thrombosis and acute coronary-artery lesions in sudden cardiac ischemic death. *N Engl J Med* 310 (18):1137–1140.

de Jager, S. C., B. Bermudez, I. Bot, R. R. Koenen, M. Bot, A. Kavelaars, V. de Waard et al. 2011. Growth differentiation factor 15 deficiency protects against atherosclerosis by attenuating CCR2-mediated macrophage chemotaxis. *J Exp Med* 208 (2):217–225.

de Lorgeril, M., P. Salen, J. L. Martin, I. Monjaud, J. Delaye, and N. Mamelle. 1999. Mediterranean diet, traditional risk factors, and the rate of cardiovascular complications after myocardial infarction: Final report of the Lyon Diet Heart Study. *Circulation* 99 (6):779–785.

D'Odorico, A., D. Martines, S. Kiechl, G. Egger, F. Oberhollenzer, P. Bonvicini, G. C. Sturniolo, R. Naccarato, and J. Willeit. 2000. High plasma levels of alpha- and beta-carotene are associated with a lower risk of atherosclerosis: Results from the Bruneck study. *Atherosclerosis* 153 (1):231–239.

Eckel, R. H., J. M. Jakicic, J. D. Ard, V. S. Hubbard, J. M. de Jesus, I-M. Lee, A. H. Lichtenstein et al. 2014. 2013 AHA/ACC guideline on lifestyle management to reduce cardiovascular risk: A report of the American College of Cardiology/American Heart Association Task Force on practice guidelines. *Circulation* 129 (25 Suppl 2):S76–S99.

Egert, S., A. Bosy-Westphal, J. Seiberl, C. Kurbitz, U. Settler, S. Plachta-Danielzik, A. E. Wagner et al. 2009. Quercetin reduces systolic blood pressure and plasma oxidised low-density lipoprotein concentrations in overweight subjects with a high-cardiovascular disease risk phenotype: A double-blinded, placebo-controlled cross-over study. *Br J Nutr* 102 (7):1065–1074.

Eidelman, R. S., D. Hollar, P. R. Hebert, G. A. Lamas, and C. H. Hennekens. 2004. Randomized trials of vitamin E in the treatment and prevention of cardiovascular disease. *Arch Intern Med* 164 (14):1552–1556.

Eilat-Adar, S., T. Sinai, C. Yosefy, and Y. Henkin. 2013. Nutritional recommendations for cardiovascular disease prevention. *Nutrients* 5 (9):3646–3683.

Endo, J., and M. Arita. 2016. Cardioprotective mechanism of omega-3 polyunsaturated fatty acids. *J Cardiol* 67 (1):22–27.

Estruch, R., E. Ros, J. Salas-Salvado, M. I. Covas, D. Corella, F. Aros, E. Gomez-Gracia et al. and PREDIMED study investigators. 2013. Primary prevention of cardiovascular disease with a Mediterranean diet. *N Engl J Med* 368 (14):1279–1290.

Farb, Andrew, Allen P. Burke, Anita L. Tang, Youhui Liang, Poonam Mannan, John Smialek, and Renu Virmani. 1996. Coronary plaque erosion without rupture into a lipid core: A frequent cause of coronary thrombosis in sudden coronary death. *Circulation* 93(7): 1354–1363.

Folsom, A. R., E. D. Parker, and L. J. Harnack. 2007. Degree of concordance with DASH diet guidelines and incidence of hypertension and fatal cardiovascular disease. *Am J Hypertens* 20 (3):225–232.

Fung, T. T., S. E. Chiuve, M. L. McCullough, K. M. Rexrode, G. Logroscino, and F. B. Hu. 2008. Adherence to a DASH-style diet and risk of coronary heart disease and stroke in women. *Arch Intern Med* 168 (7):713–720.

Fung, T. T., M. L. McCullough, P. K. Newby, J. E. Manson, J. B. Meigs, N. Rifai, W. C. Willett, and F. B. Hu. 2005. Diet-quality scores and plasma concentrations of markers of inflammation and endothelial dysfunction. *Am J Clin Nutr* 82 (1):163–173.

Funk, J. L., K. R. Feingold, A. H. Moser, and C. Grunfeld. 1993. Lipopolysaccharide stimula-
tion of RAW 264.7 macrophages induces lipid accumulation and foam cell formation.
Atherosclerosis 98 (1):67–82.

Galkina, E., and K. Ley. 2009. Immune and inflammatory mechanisms of atherosclerosis.
Annu Rev Immunol 27:165–197.

Galleano, M., S. V. Verstraeten, P. I. Oteiza, and C. G. Fraga. 2010. Antioxidant actions of
flavonoids: Thermodynamic and kinetic analysis. *Arch Biochem Biophys* 501 (1):23–30.

Geleijnse, J. M., L. J. Launer, D. A. Van der Kuip, A. Hofman, and J. C. Witteman. 2002.
Inverse association of tea and flavonoid intakes with incident myocardial infarction: The
Rotterdam Study. *Am J Clin Nutr* 75 (5):880–886.

George, J., S. Schwartzenberg, D. Medvedovsky, M. Jonas, G. Charach, A. Afek, and
A. Shamiss. 2012. Regulatory T cells and IL-10 levels are reduced in patients with vulnerable coronary plaques. *Atherosclerosis* 222 (2):519–523.

Goszcz, K., S. J. Deakin, G. G. Duthie, D. Stewart, S. J. Leslie, and I. L. Megson. 2015.
Antioxidants in cardiovascular therapy: Panacea or false hope? *Front Cardiovasc Med*
2:29.

Grandi, N. C., L. P. Breitling, and H. Brenner. 2010. Vitamin D and cardiovascular disease:
Systematic review and meta-analysis of prospective studies. *Prev Med* 51 (3–4):228–233.

Grosso, G., S. Marventano, J. Yang, A. Micek, A. Pajak, L. Scalfi, F. Galvano, and S. N. Kales.
2015. A comprehensive meta-analysis on evidence of Mediterranean diet and cardiovascular disease: Are individual components equal? *Crit Rev Food Sci Nutr* 0.

Guallar-Castillón, P., F. Rodríguez-Artalejo, M. J. Tormo, M. J. Sánchez, L. Rodríguez, J. R.
Quirós, C. Navarro et al. 2012. Major dietary patterns and risk of coronary heart disease
in middle-aged persons from a Mediterranean country: The EPIC-Spain cohort study.
Nutr Metab Cardiovasc Dis 22 (3):192–199.

Guenther, P. M., K. O. Casavale, J. Reedy, S. I. Kirkpatrick, H. A. Hiza, K. J. Kuczynski, L.
L. Kahle, and S. M. Krebs-Smith. 2013. Update of the healthy eating index: HEI-2010.
J Acad Nutr Diet 113 (4):569–580.

Hansson, G. K., P. Libby, and I. Tabas. 2015. Inflammation and plaque vulnerability. *J Intern
Med* 278 (5):483–93.

Harris, W. S., and D. Bulchandani. 2006. Why do omega-3 fatty acids lower serum triglycerides? *Curr Opin Lipidol* 17 (4):387–393.

Harris, W. S., D. Mozaffarian, E. Rimm, P. Kris-Etherton, L. L. Rudel, L. J. Appel, M. M.
Engler, M. B. Engler, and F. Sacks. 2009. Omega-6 fatty acids and risk for cardiovascular disease: A science advisory from the American Heart Association Nutrition
Subcommittee of the Council on Nutrition, Physical Activity, and Metabolism; Council
on Cardiovascular Nursing; and Council on Epidemiology and Prevention. *Circulation*
119 (6):902–907.

Hartley, L., N. Flowers, J. Holmes, A. Clarke, S. Stranges, L. Hooper, and K. Rees. 2013.
Green and black tea for the primary prevention of cardiovascular disease. *Cochrane
Database Syst Rev* 6:CD009934.

Hollaender, P. L., A. B. Ross, and M. Kristensen. 2015. Whole-grain and blood lipid changes
in apparently healthy adults: A systematic review and meta-analysis of randomized controlled studies. *Am J Clin Nutr* 102 (3):556–572.

Hooper, L., C. D. Summerbell, R. Thompson, D. Sills, F. G. Roberts, H. J. Moore, and
G. Davey Smith. 2012. Reduced or modified dietary fat for preventing cardiovascular
disease. *Cochrane Database Syst Rev* 5:CD002137.

Hozawa, A., D. R. Jacobs, Jr., M. W. Steffes, M. D. Gross, L. M. Steffen, and D. H. Lee.
2007. Relationships of circulating carotenoid concentrations with several markers of
inflammation, oxidative stress, and endothelial dysfunction: The Coronary Artery
Risk Development in Young Adults (CARDIA)/Young Adult Longitudinal Trends in
Antioxidants (YALTA) Study. *Clin Chem* 53 (3):447–55.

Hsia, J., G. Heiss, H. Ren, M. Allison, N. C. Dolan, P. Greenland, S. R. Heckbert et al. and Investigators Women's Health Initiative. 2007. Calcium/vitamin D supplementation and cardiovascular events. *Circulation* 115 (7):846–854.

Hu, F. B. 2002. Dietary pattern analysis: A new direction in nutritional epidemiology. *Curr Opin Lipidol* 13 (1):3–9.

Hu, T., K. T. Mills, L. Yao, K. Demanelis, M. Eloustaz, W. S. Yancy, Jr., T. N. Kelly, J. He, and L. A. Bazzano. 2012. Effects of low-carbohydrate diets versus low-fat diets on metabolic risk factors: A meta-analysis of randomized controlled clinical trials. *Am J Epidemiol* 176 (Suppl 7):S44–S54.

Ilhan, F., H. Akbulut, I. Karaca, A. Godekmerdan, E. Ilkay, and V. Bulut. 2005. Procalcitonin, C-reactive protein and neopterin levels in patients with coronary atherosclerosis. *Acta Cardiol* 60 (4):361–365.

Ilhan, F., and S. T. Kalkanli. 2015. Atherosclerosis and the role of immune cells. *World J Clin Cases* 3 (4):345–352.

Jakobsen, M. U., E. J. O'Reilly, B. L. Heitmann, M. A. Pereira, K. Balter, G. E. Fraser, U. Goldbourt et al. 2009. Major types of dietary fat and risk of coronary heart disease: A pooled analysis of 11 cohort studies. *Am J Clin Nutr* 89 (5):1425–1432.

Jorde, R., M. Sneve, P. Torjesen, and Y. Figenschau. 2010. No improvement in cardiovascular risk factors in overweight and obese subjects after supplementation with vitamin D3 for 1 year. *J Intern Med* 267 (5):462–472.

Kastorini, C. M., H. J. Milionis, K. Esposito, D. Giugliano, J. A. Goudevenos, and D. B. Panagiotakos. 2011. The effect of Mediterranean diet on metabolic syndrome and its components: A meta-analysis of 50 studies and 534,906 individuals. *J Am Coll Cardiol* 57 (11):1299–1313.

Keys, A., A. Menotti, M. J. Karvonen, C. Aravanis, H. Blackburn, R. Buzina, B. S. Djordjevic et al. 1986. The diet and 15-year death rate in the seven countries study. *Am J Epidemiol* 124 (6):903–915.

Kim, A., A. Chiu, M. K. Barone, D. Avino, F. Wang, C. I. Coleman, and O. J. Phung. 2011. Green tea catechins decrease total and low-density lipoprotein cholesterol: A systematic review and meta-analysis. *J Am Diet Assoc* 111 (11):1720–1729.

Kim, Y. O. 2009. Dietary patterns associated with hypertension among Korean males. *Nutr Res Pract* 3 (2):162–166.

Kohlmeier, L., J. D. Kark, E. Gomez-Gracia, B. C. Martin, S. E. Steck, A. F. Kardinaal, J. Ringstad et al. 1997. Lycopene and myocardial infarction risk in the EURAMIC study. *Am J Epidemiol* 146 (8):618–626.

Kushi, L. H., A. R. Folsom, R. J. Prineas, P. J. Mink, Y. Wu, and R. M. Bostick. 1996. Dietary antioxidant vitamins and death from coronary heart disease in postmenopausal women. *N Engl J Med* 334 (18):1156–1162.

Lagiou, P., S. Sandin, M. Lof, D. Trichopoulos, H. O. Adami, and E. Weiderpass. 2012. Low carbohydrate-high protein diet and incidence of cardiovascular diseases in Swedish women: Prospective cohort study. *BMJ* 344:e4026.

Larsson, S. C., and N. Orsini. 2011. Fish consumption and the risk of stroke: A dose-response meta-analysis. *Stroke* 42 (12):3621–3623.

Larsson, S. C., N. Orsini, and A. Wolk. 2012. Long-chain omega-3 polyunsaturated fatty acids and risk of stroke: A meta-analysis. *Eur J Epidemiol* 27 (12):895–901.

Lee, J. G., E. J. Lim, D. W. Park, S. H. Lee, J. R. Kim, and S. H. Baek. 2008. A combination of Lox-1 and Nox1 regulates TLR9-mediated foam cell formation. *Cell Signal* 20 (12):2266–2275.

Libby, P., Y. Okamoto, V. Z. Rocha, and E. Folco. 2010. Inflammation in atherosclerosis: Transition from theory to practice. *Circ J* 74 (2):213–220.

Libby, P., P. M. Ridker, and G. K. Hansson. 2011. Progress and challenges in translating the biology of atherosclerosis. *Nature* 473 (7347):317–325.

Liese, A. D., S. M. Krebs-Smith, A. F. Subar, S. M. George, B. E. Harmon, M. L. Neuhouser, C. J. Boushey, T. E. Schap, and J. Reedy. 2015. The dietary patterns methods project: Synthesis of findings across cohorts and relevance to dietary guidance. *J Nutr* 145 (3):393–402.

Lippi, G., M. Franchini, E. J. Favaloro, and G. Targher. 2010. Moderate red wine consumption and cardiovascular disease risk: Beyond the "French paradox." *Semin Thromb Hemost* 36 (1):59–70.

Liu, Lihua, Shan Wang, and Jianchao Liu. 2015. Fiber consumption and all-cause, cardiovascular, and cancer mortalities: A systematic review and meta-analysis of cohort studies. *Molecular nutrition & food research* 59(1): 139–146.

Marik, P. E., and J. Varon. 2009. Omega-3 dietary supplements and the risk of cardiovascular events: A systematic review. *Clin Cardiol* 32 (7):365–372.

Martinez-Gonzalez, M. A., M. Garcia-Lopez, M. Bes-Rastrollo, E. Toledo, E. H. Martinez-Lapiscina, M. Delgado-Rodriguez, Z. Vazquez, S. Benito, and J. J. Beunza. 2011. Mediterranean diet and the incidence of cardiovascular disease: A Spanish cohort. *Nutr Metab Cardiovasc Dis* 21 (4):237–244.

Mathers, C. D., and D. Loncar. 2006. Projections of global mortality and burden of disease from 2002 to 2030. *PLoS Med* 3 (11):e442.

McMurray, J. J., S. Adamopoulos, S. D. Anker, A. Auricchio, M. Bohm, K. Dickstein, V. Falk et al. and ESC Committee for Practice Guidelines. 2012. ESC guidelines for the diagnosis and treatment of acute and chronic heart failure 2012: The Task Force for the Diagnosis and Treatment of Acute and Chronic Heart Failure 2012 of the European Society of Cardiology; Developed in collaboration with the Heart Failure Association *(HFA) of the ESC. Eur Heart J* 33 (14):1787–1847.

Mente, A., L. de Koning, H. S. Shannon, and S. S. Anand. 2009. A systematic review of the evidence supporting a causal link between dietary factors and coronary heart disease. *Arch Intern Med* 169 (7):659–669.

Meyer, F., I. Bairati, and G. R. Dagenais. 1996. Lower ischemic heart disease incidence and mortality among vitamin supplement users. *Can J Cardiol* 12 (10):930–934.

Michas, G., R. Micha, and A. Zampelas. 2014. Dietary fats and cardiovascular disease: Putting together the pieces of a complicated puzzle. *Atherosclerosis* 234 (2):320–328.

Mila-Villarroel, R., A. Bach-Faig, J. Puig, A. Puchal, A. Farran, L. Serra-Majem, and J. L. Carrasco. 2011. Comparison and evaluation of the reliability of indexes of adherence to the Mediterranean diet. *Public Health Nutr* 14 (12A):2338–2345.

Montalescot, G., U. Sechtem, S. Achenbach, F. Andreotti, C. Arden, A. Budaj, R. Bugiardini et al. 2013. 2013 ESC guidelines on the management of stable coronary artery disease: The Task Force on the Management of Stable Coronary Artery Disease of the European Society of Cardiology. *Eur Heart J* 34 (38):2949–3003.

Moyer, V. A., and U.S. Preventive Services Task Force. 2012. Behavioral counseling interventions to promote a healthful diet and physical activity for cardiovascular disease prevention in adults: U.S. Preventive Services Task Force recommendation statement. *Ann Intern Med* 157 (5):367–3671.

Moyer, V. A., and U.S. Preventive Services Task Force. 2014. Vitamin, mineral, and multivitamin supplements for the primary prevention of cardiovascular disease and cancer: U.S. Preventive Services Task Force recommendation statement. *Ann Intern Med* 160 (8):558–564.

Mozaffarian, D., L. J. Appel, and L. Van Horn. 2011. Components of a cardioprotective diet: New insights. *Circulation* 23 (24):2870–2891.

Mozaffarian, D., and R. Clarke. 2009. Quantitative effects on cardiovascular risk factors and coronary heart disease risk of replacing partially hydrogenated vegetable oils with other fats and oils. *Eur J Clin Nutr* 63 (Suppl 2):S22–33.

Mozaffarian, D., M. B. Katan, A. Ascherio, M. J. Stampfer, and W. C. Willett. 2006. Trans fatty acids and cardiovascular disease. *N Engl J Med* 354 (15):1601–1613.

Mozaffarian, D., R. Micha, and S. Wallace. 2010. Effects on coronary heart disease of increasing polyunsaturated fat in place of saturated fat: A systematic review and meta-analysis of randomized controlled trials. *PLoS Med* 7 (3):e1000252.

Mozaffarian, D., and J. H. Wu. 2011. Omega-3 fatty acids and cardiovascular disease: Effects on risk factors, molecular pathways, and clinical events. *J Am Coll Cardiol* 58 (20):2047–2067.

Muskiet, F. A. 2005. The importance of (early) folate status to primary and secondary coronary artery disease prevention. *Reprod Toxicol* 20 (3):403–410.

Negre-Salvayre, A., L. Mabile, J. Delchambre, and R. Salvayre. 1995. α-Tocopherol, ascorbic acid, and rutin inhibit synergistically the copper-promoted LDL oxidation and the cytotoxicity of oxidized LDL to cultured endothelial cells. *Biol Trace Elem Res* 47 (1–3):81–91.

Nestel, P., P. Clifton, D. Colquhoun, M. Noakes, T. A. Mori, D. Sullivan, and B. Thomas. 2015. Indications for omega-3 long chain polyunsaturated fatty acid in the prevention and treatment of cardiovascular disease. *Heart Lung Circ* 24 (8):769–779.

Nilsson, J., G. K. Hansson, and P. K. Shah. 2005. Immunomodulation of atherosclerosis: Implications for vaccine development. *Arterioscler Thromb Vasc Biol* 25 (1):18–28.

Nordmann, A. J., K. Suter-Zimmermann, H. C. Bucher, I. Shai, K. R. Tuttle, R. Estruch, and M. Briel. 2011. Meta-analysis comparing Mediterranean to low-fat diets for modification of cardiovascular risk factors. *Am J Med* 124 (9):841–851 e2.

Oh, D. Y., S. Talukdar, E. J. Bae, T. Imamura, H. Morinaga, W. Fan, P. Li, W. J. Lu, S. M. Watkins, and J. M. Olefsky. 2010. GPR120 is an omega-3 fatty acid receptor mediating potent anti-inflammatory and insulin-sensitizing effects. *Cell* 142 (5):687–698.

Parikh, A., S. R. Lipsitz, and S. Natarajan. 2009. Association between a DASH-like diet and mortality in adults with hypertension: Findings from a population-based follow-up study. *Am J Hypertens* 22 (4):409–416.

Park, Y., S. Park, H. Yi, H. Y. Kim, S. J. Kang, J. Kim, and H. Ahn. 2009. Low level of n-3 polyunsaturated fatty acids in erythrocytes is a risk factor for both acute ischemic and hemorrhagic stroke in Koreans. *Nutr Res* 29 (12):825–830.

Perk, J., G. De Backer, H. Gohlke, I. Graham, Ž. Reiner, M. Verschuren, C. Albus et al. 2012. European guidelines on cardiovascular disease prevention in clinical practice (version 2012). *Eur Heart J* 33 (13):1635–1701.

Pittas, A. G., M. Chung, T. Trikalinos, J. Mitri, M. Brendel, K. Patel, A. H. Lichtenstein, J. Lau, and E. M. Balk. 2010. Systematic review: Vitamin D and cardiometabolic outcomes. *Ann Intern Med* 152 (5):307–314.

Quideau, S., D. Deffieux, C. Douat-Casassus, and L. Pouysegu. 2011. Plant polyphenols: Chemical properties, biological activities, and synthesis. *Angew Chem Int Ed Engl* 50 (3):586–621.

Rangel-Huerta, O. D., B. Pastor-Villaescusa, C. M. Aguilera, and A. Gil. 2015. A systematic review of the efficacy of bioactive compounds in cardiovascular disease: Phenolic compounds. *Nutrients* 7 (7):5177–5216.

Reedy, J., S. M. Krebs-Smith, P. E. Miller, A. D. Liese, L. L. Kahle, Y. Park, and A. F. Subar. 2014. Higher diet quality is associated with decreased risk of all-cause, cardiovascular disease, and cancer mortality among older adults. *J Nutr* 144 (6):881–889.

Retelny, V. S., A. Neuendorf, and J. L. Roth. 2008. Nutrition protocols for the prevention of cardiovascular disease. *Nutr Clin Pract* 23 (5):468–476.

Richter, C. K., A. C. Skulas-Ray, C. M. Champagne, and P. M. Kris-Etherton. 2015. Plant protein and animal proteins: Do they differentially affect cardiovascular disease risk? *Adv Nutr* 6 (6):712–728.

Rocha, Z. Viviane, Rouyanne T. Ras, Ana C. Gagliardi, Leonardo C. Mangili, Elke A. Trautwein, and Raul D. Santos. 2016. Effects of phytosterols on markers of inflammation: A systematic review and meta-analysis. *Atherosclerosis* 248: 76–83.

Ros, E. 2012. Olive oil and CVD: Accruing evidence of a protective effect. *Br J Nutr* 108 (11):1931–1933.

Rosales, C., B. K. Gillard, A. M. Gotto, Jr., and H. J. Pownall. 2015. High-density lipoprotein processing and premature cardiovascular disease. *Methodist Debakey Cardiovasc J* 11 (3):181–185.

Salehi-Abargouei, A., Z. Maghsoudi, F. Shirani, and L. Azadbakht. 2013. Effects of Dietary Approaches to Stop Hypertension (DASH)-style diet on fatal or nonfatal cardiovascular diseases incidence: A systematic review and meta-analysis on observational prospective studies. *Nutrition* 29 (4):611–618.

Santaniemi, M., O. Ukkola, E. Malo, R. Bloigu, and Y. A. Kesaniemi. 2013. Metabolic syndrome in the prediction of cardiovascular events: The potential additive role of hsCRP and adiponectin. *Eur J Prev Cardiol* 21(10):1242–8.

Santos, F. L., S. S. Esteves, A. da Costa Pereira, W. S. Yancy, Jr., and J. P. Nunes. 2012. Systematic review and meta-analysis of clinical trials of the effects of low carbohydrate diets on cardiovascular risk factors. *Obes Rev* 13 (11):1048–1066.

Schwingshackl, L., and G. Hoffmann. 2013. Comparison of effects of long-term low-fat vs high-fat diets on blood lipid levels in overweight or obese patients: A systematic review and meta-analysis. *J Acad Nutr Diet* 113 (12):1640–1661.

Schwingshackl, L., and G. Hoffmann. 2015. Diet quality as assessed by the Healthy Eating Index, the Alternate Healthy Eating Index, the Dietary Approaches to Stop Hypertension score, and health outcomes: A systematic review and meta-analysis of cohort studies. *J Acad Nutr Diet* 115 (5):780–800 e5.

Schwingshackl, L., B. Missbach, and G. Hoffmann. 2015. An umbrella review of garlic intake and risk of cardiovascular disease. *Phytomedicine* pii: S0944-7113(15)00335-9

Schwingshackl, L., B. Strasser, and G. Hoffmann. 2011. Effects of monounsaturated fatty acids on cardiovascular risk factors: A systematic review and meta-analysis. *Ann Nutr Metab* 59 (2–4):176–186.

Shaw, P. X., S. Horkko, M. K. Chang, L. K. Curtiss, W. Palinski, G. J. Silverman, and J. L. Witztum. 2000. Natural antibodies with the T15 idiotype may act in atherosclerosis, apoptotic clearance, and protective immunity. *J Clin Invest* 105 (12):1731–1740.

Shimazu, T., S. Kuriyama, A. Hozawa, K. Ohmori, Y. Sato, N. Nakaya, Y. Nishino, Y. Tsubono, and I. Tsuji. 2007. Dietary patterns and cardiovascular disease mortality in Japan: A prospective cohort study. *Int J Epidemiol* 36 (3):600–609.

Singh, R. B., G. Dubnov, M. A. Niaz, S. Ghosh, R. Singh, S. S. Rastogi, O. Manor, D. Pella, and E. M. Berry. 2002. Effect of an Indo-Mediterranean diet on progression of coronary artery disease in high risk patients (Indo-Mediterranean Diet Heart Study): A randomised single-blind trial. *Lancet* 360 (9344):1455–1461.

Siri-Tarino, P. W., Q. Sun, F. B. Hu, and R. M. Krauss. 2010. Meta-analysis of prospective cohort studies evaluating the association of saturated fat with cardiovascular disease. *Am J Clin Nutr* 91 (3):535–546.

Sofi, F., R. Abbate, G. F. Gensini, and A. Casini. 2010. Accruing evidence on benefits of adherence to the Mediterranean diet on health: An updated systematic review and meta-analysis. *Am J Clin Nutr* 92 (5):1189–1196.

Sofi, F., C. Macchi, R. Abbate, G. F. Gensini, and A. Casini. 2014. Mediterranean diet and health status: An updated meta-analysis and a proposal for a literature-based adherence score. *Public Health Nutr* 17 (12):2769–2782.

Stradling, C., M. Hamid, S. Taheri, and G. N. Thomas. 2014. A review of dietary influences on cardiovascular health, Part 2: Dietary patterns. *Cardiovasc Hematol Disord Drug Targets* 14 (1):50–63.

Talati, R., D. M. Sobieraj, S. S. Makanji, O. J. Phung, and C. I. Coleman. 2010. The comparative efficacy of plant sterols and stanols on serum lipids: A systematic review and meta-analysis. *J Am Diet Assoc* 110 (5):719–726.

Trichopoulou, A., T. Costacou, C. Bamia, and D. Trichopoulos. 2003. Adherence to a Mediterranean diet and survival in a Greek population. *N Engl J Med* 348 (26):2599–2608.

Trichopoulou, A., A. Kouris-Blazos, M. L. Wahlqvist, C. Gnardellis, P. Lagiou, E. Polychronopoulos, T. Vassilakou, L. Lipworth, and D. Trichopoulos. 1995. Diet and overall survival in elderly people. *BMJ* 311 (7018):1457–1460.

Trichopoulou, A., P. Orfanos, T. Norat, B. Bueno-de-Mesquita, M. C. Ocké, P. H. M Peeters, Y. T. van der Schouw et al. 2005. Modified Mediterranean diet and survival: EPIC-elderly prospective cohort study. *BMJ* 330 (7498):991.

Trivedi, D. P., R. Doll, and K. T. Khaw. 2003. Effect of four monthly oral vitamin D3 (cholecalciferol) supplementation on fractures and mortality in men and women living in the community: Randomised double blind controlled trial. *BMJ* 326 (7387):469.

USDA. 2010. *U.S. Department of Health and Human Services. Dietary guidelines for Americans,* 2010. Washington, DC: U.S. Government Printing Office.

USDA, Agricultural Research Service. 2016. USDA National Nutrient Database for Standard Reference. Accessed January 3, 2016. http://www.ars.usda.gov/ba/bhnrc/ndl.

Wang, Z. M., B. Zhou, Z. L. Nie, W. Gao, Y. S. Wang, H. Zhao, J. Zhu, J. J. Yan, Z. J. Yang, and L. S. Wang. 2012. Folate and risk of coronary heart disease: A meta-analysis of prospective studies. *Nutr Metab Cardiovasc Dis* 22 (10):890–899.

Wen, Y. T., J. H. Dai, and Q. Gao. 2014. Effects of omega-3 fatty acid on major cardiovascular events and mortality in patients with coronary heart disease: A meta-analysis of randomized controlled trials. *Nutr Metab Cardiovasc Dis* 24 (5):470–475.

Whitman, S. C., P. Ravisankar, and A. Daugherty. 2002. IFN-gamma deficiency exerts gender-specific effects on atherogenesis in apolipoprotein E−/− mice. *J Interferon Cytokine Res* 22 (6):661–670.

WHO. 2014. Global status report on noncommunicable diseases. Geneva, Switzerland: World Health Orgnization.

Wilcox, J. N., K. M. Smith, S. M. Schwartz, and D. Gordon. 1989. Localization of tissue factor in the normal vessel wall and in the atherosclerotic plaque. *Proc Natl Acad Sci USA* 86 (8):2839–2843.

Willett, W. C., F. Sacks, A. Trichopoulou, G. Drescher, A. Ferro-Luzzi, E. Helsing, and D. Trichopoulos. 1995. Mediterranean diet pyramid: A cultural model for healthy eating. *Am J Clin Nutr* 61 (6 Suppl):1402S–1406S.

World Cancer Research Fund and American Institute for Cancer Research. 2007. *Food, Nutrition, Physical Activity, and the Prevention of Cancer: A Global Perspective.* Washington, DC: AICR.

Wu, Y., Y. Qian, Y. Pan, P. Li, J. Yang, X. Ye, and G. Xu. 2015. Association between dietary fiber intake and risk of coronary heart disease: A meta-analysis. *Clin Nutr* 34 (4):603–611.

Ye, Z., and H. Song. 2008. Antioxidant vitamins intake and the risk of coronary heart disease: Meta-analysis of cohort studies. *Eur J Cardiovasc Prev Rehabil* 15 (1):26–34.

Zittermann, A., S. S. Schleithoff, and R. Koerfer. 2005. Putting cardiovascular disease and vitamin D insufficiency into perspective. *Br J Nutr* 94 (4):483–492.

7 HEAL for Stroke

Claudia Stefani Marcilio, Antonio Cordeiro Mattos, Gustavo B.F. Oliveira, and Álvaro Avezum

CONTENTS

7.1 STROKE EPIDEMIOLOGY

7.1.1 BURDEN OF STROKE

Stroke is one of the major public health concerns. It is a significant contributor of disability and mortality, being the second-most common cause of death and the third-most common cause of disability-adjusted life years (Feigin et al. 2014; Krishnamurthi et al. 2013; O'Donnell et al. 2010).

7.1.2 RISK FACTORS FOR STROKE

The classical risk factors of coronary heart disease (CHD) are very important in preventing stroke overall, although the impact of these factors could be different in each region and for each type of stroke. Despite the relevance in terms of public health of the mortality and disability associated with stroke, only recently have we identified the risk factors associated with stroke and their respective population attributable risk (PAR) worldwide. Indeed, the current burden of stroke may be less explained by nonmodifiable risk factors (age, sex, race/ethnicity, and family history) compared with modifiable factors such as hypertension, smoking, and hypercholes-terolemia. Five modifiable risk factors (hypertension, current smoking, abdominal obesity, poor diet, and a lack of physical activity) account for more than 80% of the PAR for stroke (ischemic and intracerebral hemorrhagic strokes) (O'Donnell et al. 2010).

- *Hypertension*: Hypertension is the main risk factor for all types of stroke, the PAR being 51.8% (95% confidence interval [CI] 47.7–55.8) for all types of stroke, 45.2% (95% CI 40.3–50.0) for ischemic stroke, and 73.6% (95% CI 67.0–79.3) for hemorrhagic stroke. Hence, effective blood pressure (BP) control is clinically relevant for populations concerning stroke prevention (Meschia et al. 2014; O'Donnell et al. 2010).
- *Tobacco smoking*: The higher the frequency of tobacco smoking, the higher the risk of all categories of stroke. This association has been found in many studies, has being mandatory to quit smoking for primary and secondary stroke prevention because the risk of stroke is significantly lower in non-smokers and former smokers as compared to current smokers (Kwon et al. 2016; Lucke-Wold et al. 2012; Meschia et al. 2014; O'Donnell et al. 2010; Shah and Cole 2010).
- *Abdominal obesity*: Waist-to-hip ratio or abdominal obesity is a better pre-dictor of stroke than body mass index. The higher the waist-to-hip ratio, the higher the risk of all categories of stroke.
- *Poor diet*: Cultural and social behaviors that impact eating habits are com-plex and difficult to analyze in most clinical studies. It is known that a balanced diet with low salt intake and reduced fat consumption can prevent stroke (Haheim et al. 1993; Meschia et al. 2014; O'Donnell et al. 2010; Yusuf et al. 2004).
- *Lack of physical activity*: Being physically active is crucial for stroke prevention. For cardiovascular diseases (CVDs), 29% of strokes can be attributed to physical inactivity compared with 12% for acute myocar-dial infarction, as evidenced by the INTERSTROKE and INTERHEART population-based case control studies (O'Donnell et al. 2010). The mech-anism of physical activity in stroke prevention remains unclear, though many researchers recognize that physical activity plays an important role in controlling risk factors for stroke such as diabetes and hypertension, and also affects metabolism and inflammatory processes (Haheim et al. 1993; Meschia et al. 2014; Yusuf et al. 2004).

7.2 STROKE CLASSIFICATION

In general, strokes can be classified as ischemic or hemorrhagic, which in turn are further subdivided into distinct subtypes. Establishing this primary distinction clearly has important implications for management in both primary and secondary prevention.

- *Ischemic stroke* accounts for approximately 85% of all strokes in high-income countries. It may be further subtyped into large-vessel, cardio-embolic, small-vessel (lacunar), or cryptogenic stroke based on the Trial of ORG 10172 in Acute Stroke Treatment (TOAST) criteria. Such stroke subtypes are likely to have varying etiologies and prognoses, requiring different treatment and prevention strategies. Ischemic stroke may also be subcategorized based on the location of injury within the brain. Such categorization, utilizing the Oxfordshire Community Stroke Project (OCSP) criteria, may be established utilizing clinical history and physical examination (Hsia and Tong 2003; Jackson and Sudlow 2005). Combined with basic neuroimaging (noncontrast CT of the brain), categories include total anterior circulation infarct (TACI), partial anterior circulation infarct (PACI), lacunar infarct (LACI), and posterior circulation infarct (POCI).
- *Hemorrhagic stroke* accounts for 15% of all strokes in high-income countries, may be further subtyped into subarachnoid hemorrhage (SAH) and intracerebral hemorrhage (ICH). Their contribution to the burden of stroke disease appears to vary considerably between countries, with evidence suggesting that hemorrhagic stroke accounts for a greater proportion of all strokes in many low-income countries. In most cases (~80%), SAH results from the rupture of an intracranial saccular aneurysm. ICH results in bleeding directly into the brain tissue and is most often caused by severe hypertension, amyloid angiopathy, or vascular anomalies, although it has been suggested that etiologies may differ between high- and low-income countries (Adams et al. 1993; Bamford et al. 1991; Ferro 2003; Tolonen et al. 2002).

7.3 DIETARY HABITS AND RISK OF STROKE

The proportion of the estimated 100 million individuals worldwide who have vascular disease, especially from lower-income countries, living in rural areas, and who adopt healthy lifestyle behaviors, is not known (Teo et al. 2013; Yusuf et al. 2001). Modernization, excessive calorie intake, and the increased prevalence of obesity, metabolic syndrome, and type 2 diabetes mellitus threaten to halt the decline of stroke incidence in high-income countries and to accelerate the increase in stroke incidence in low- and middle-income countries (Finucane et al. 2011; Swinburn et al. 2011). Accurately assessing and understanding the role of nutrition in the causes and course of the consequences of stroke will be crucial in developing and implementing strategies to reduce the global burden of stroke (Franklin and Cushman 2011; Goldstein et al. 2011).

The American Heart Association (AHA) supports that maintaining a healthy diet is one of "the best weapons for fighting CVD" and a significant contributor to stroke reduction (American Heart Association 2015; Spence 2006). In fact, research has found that those maintaining a "healthy lifestyle have an 80% lower risk of a first stroke compared with those who do not" (Chiuve et al. 2008). Maintaining a healthy diet is a critical determinant of health overall and of stroke at the individual and population level (Jacobs and Steffen 2003). Dietary research and intervention development, including the collection and validation of dietary intake, are both multifaceted and complex. There are many levels of complexity to understanding the interaction of nutrients (i.e., nutrients are never eaten in isolation) and accounting for the influence of access, economics, culture, and environment on diet/dietary patterns (Kontogianni and Panagiotakos 2014). Despite the obstacles, there is a growing body of literature examining individual nutrient intake, including sodium, fat, cholesterol, vitamins, minerals, and other supplements, along with dietary factors such as fruit/ vegetable intake, animal protein, and beverage consumption (Ding and Mozaffarian 2006).

Unfortunately, much of the research findings are mixed and often inconclusive. Ding and Mozaffarian (2006) conclude that the "optimal diet to reduce the incidence of stroke is not well established [and] further investigation of specific effects on stroke incidence is warranted." Furthermore, only a few dietary interventions investigating the effect of diet/dietary patterns and risk of stroke have been initiated (Ding and Mozaffarian 2006).

A large and diverse body of evidence has implicated several aspects of diet in the pathogenesis of high BP, the major modifiable risk factor for ischemic stroke. African Americans are especially sensitive to the BP-raising effects of high salt intake, low potassium intake, and suboptimal diet. In this setting, dietary changes have the potential to substantially reduce racial disparities in BP and stroke (Appel et al. 2006). A meta-analysis found a strong, inverse relationship between servings of fruits and vegetables and subsequent stroke. Compared with persons who consumed 3 servings of fruits and vegetables per day, the relative risk of ischemic stroke was lower in those who consumed 3–5 servings/day (RR 0.88, 95% CI 0.79–0.98) and those who consumed 5 servings/day (RR 0.72, 95% CI 0.66–0.79). The dose-responsive relationship extends into the higher ranges of intake, specifically in the analyses of the Nurses' Health Study (NHS) and the Health Professionals' Follow-Up Study; the relative risk of incident stroke was 0.69 (95% CI 0.52–0.92) for persons in the highest versus lowest quintiles of fruit and vegetable intake (Joshipura et al. 1999). Median intake in the highest quintile was 10.2 servings of fruits and vegetables in men and 9.2 servings in women. Risk of stroke was reduced by 6% (95% CI 1%–10%) for each serving/day increment in intake of fruits and vegetables.

In ecological and some prospective studies, a higher level of sodium intake is associated with an increased risk of stroke (He et al. 1999; Nagata et al. 2004). A higher level of potassium intake is also associated with a reduced risk of stroke in prospective studies (Ascherio et al. 1998; Khaw and Barrett-Connor 1987). It should be emphasized that a plethora of methodological limitations, particularly difficulties in estimating dietary electrolyte intake, hinder risk assessment and may lead to false negative or even paradoxical results in observational studies (Goldstein et al. 2011). One trial tested the effects of replacing regular salt (sodium chloride) with a potassium-enriched salt in elderly Taiwanese men (Chang et al. 2006). In addition to increased overall survivorship and reduced costs, the potassium-enriched salt reduced the risk of death from cerebrovascular disease by 50%. This trial did not present follow-up BP measurements; hence, it is unclear whether BP reduction accounted for the beneficial effects of the intervention. In a Women's Health Initiative (WHI) study, a low-fat diet that emphasized the consumption of whole grains, fruits, and vegetables did not reduce stroke incidence; however, the intervention did not achieve a substantial difference in fruit and vegetable consumption (a mean difference of only 1.1 servings/day) and did not reduce BP substantially (a mean difference of 0.5 mm Hg for both systolic and diastolic BP) (Howard et al. 2006). Diets rich in fruits and vegetables, including those based on the Dietary Approaches to Stop Hypertension (DASH) diet (rich in fruits, vegetables, and low-fat dairy products and reduced in saturated and total fat), lower BP (Appel et al. 2006) and hence may reduce stroke risk. Other dietary factors may affect the risk of stroke, but the evidence is insufficient to make specific recommendations. In Asian countries, a low intake of animal protein, saturated fat, and cholesterol has been associated with a decreased risk of stroke, but such relationships have been less apparent in Western countries (Goldstein et al. 2011).

7.4   KEY SCIENTIFIC EVIDENCE DOCUMENTING FOOD GROUPS/DIETARY PATTERNS AND RISK OF STROKE

Numerous reviews and meta-analyses have summarized the evidence for food groups and risk of stroke (Hankey 2012; Hu et al. 2014; Medeiros et al. 2012; Sherzai et al. 2012; Tracy 2013). The majority of the evidence pertains to the primary prevention of stroke in large cohort studies, and focuses on micronutrients, food groups, and dietary patterns. Two key points emerge: (1) increased fruit and vegetable consumption reduce stroke risk and (2) low fat is not better for reducing the rates of stroke and may be a harmful risk reduction strategy (Dearborn et al. 2015).

Globally, the low adoption of healthy diets has been reported, particularly among individuals with prior coronary heart disease and/or stroke. Moreover, the lowest prevalence of eating healthy diets has been observed in lower-income countries (Teo et al. 2013). Prospective cohorts, such as the Nurses' Health Study, the Danish Diet, Cancer and Health Study, and the Framingham cohort among others add to the compelling evidence that increasing fruit and vegetable consumption is associated with the reduced burden of stroke (Dauchet et al. 2005; Gillman et al. 1995; He et al. 2006; Johnsen et al. 2003; Joshipura et al. 1999; Mizrahi et al. 2009). The INTERSTROKE study also demonstrated that fruit was associated with a lower risk of ischemic stroke. Across diverse populations with unique dietary patterns, mounting evidence is indicating that a higher consumption of plant-based food items is associated with a reduced risk of stroke (O'Donnell et al. 2010). The evidence is not as consistent for other food groups (such as meat, dairy, and eggs) and incident stroke, but fish consumption seems to be beneficial. Overall, evidence suggests a modest protective effect of fish consumption and incident stroke, although some studies found no association. This may depend on the way fish is eaten, as in many cultures fish is salted, which may negate its beneficial effects. One meta-analysis of prospective studies reported a 6% reduction in stroke by consuming an increment of 3 or more servings of fish per week (Larsson and Orsini 2011). A cohort in Japan, which has a much lower consumption of animal products and higher fish consumption than Western countries, has seen the increasing consumption of meat, dairy, and eggs since the 1960s and an associated reduction in cerebrovascular mortality during this time. It is unclear if the increased consumption of animal products is truly protective or if other dietary changes, such as a reduction in sodium, could account for this difference. In other populations, total meat consumption may be associated with a higher risk of ischemic stroke; however, as meat consumption increases, it is likely that consumption of other beneficial food groups (such as fruits and vegetables) decreases (Micha et al. 2010).

There is increasing evidence that processed foods and not meats contribute to cardiovascular risk. The preservation of processed meats, such as ham, cold cuts, and bacon, occurs by smoking, curing, salting, or the addition of chemical preservatives. Although all studies do not share positive associations with stroke incidence and the consumption of processed meats, the newest evidences suggest an association (Micha et al. 2010). The link between dairy foods, such as milk, cheese, and butter, and stroke is unclear, as no associations have been reproducibly demonstrated.

The association between dietary fat and the risk of stroke is complex. Dietary fat is discussed in terms of total fat; saturated, monounsaturated, or polyunsaturated fat; or trans fat. Saturated fats are found primarily in animal products, such as meat and dairy. Mono- or polyunsaturated fats are found in vegetable oils and fish. Trans fats are synthetic and found in margarine and other processed foods. Total fat, or other types of fat, was not associated with incident stroke in a 14-year follow-up study of U.S. male health-care professionals (He et al. 2003). The U.S. Department of Agriculture released the food pyramid in 1992 to emphasize that "fat is bad," largely ignoring epidemiologic data about different types of fat. Nutrition science has moved beyond the pyramid, but its iconic message continues to influence public perceptions of "healthy eating." One large meta-analysis suggested that saturated fat, previously recommended for lower intake to reduce cardiovascular disease incidence, was not associated with stroke (Cheng et al. 2016). Evidence suggests that the increased consumption of certain types of polyunsaturated fats, such as long-chain omega-3 polyunsaturated fatty acids, may lower stroke risk (Katan et al. 2010). Trans fats, on the other hand, may be associated with increased rates of stroke, at least in men. The effect of fat replacement (i.e., replacing saturated fats in the diet with polyunsaturated fats) has not been evaluated in stroke. My Plate, the new initiative by the U.S. Department of Agriculture, has replaced the pyramid and shifts the emphasis from lowering fat consumption to increasing relative consumption of fruits, vegetables, and whole grains (Estruch et al. 2013). With the existing data, it is difficult to make firm recommendations about fat consumption in stroke patients, and the best data will likely come from studies that incorporate whole dietary patterns.

Dietary patterns look at food groups consumed together, rather than examining associations between individual foods and outcomes. Observational studies suggest that Mediterranean-style diets that are rich in fruits/vegetables, low in red meat, with moderate alcohol intake, and the use of olive oil or nonhydrogenated fats may have the most potential as a dietary intervention to prevent stroke (Estruch et al. 2013). Prospective cohorts, including the Nurses' Health Study, the Northern Manhattan Study, and the European Investigation into Cancer, all demonstrate reduced stroke risk with this pattern. The Dietary Approaches to Stop Hypertension (DASH) diet, which is similar to the Mediterranean diet and emphasizes fruits and vegetables as well as the low intake of red meat and sweets, has also shown the benefits of stroke risk reduction (Fung et al. 2008).

Examining key epidemiologic research surrounding stroke and diet provides a foundation for the development of dietary interventions. The Framingham Heart Study (FHS) and the Nurses' Health Study (NHS) are the first longitudinal epidemiological studies to identify common factors and characteristics contributing to cardiovascular disease (CVD) and stroke incidence. The FHS was groundbreaking, as it was the first to document long-term dietary patterns with a risk of stroke using a 20-year follow-up period (Boden-Albala et al. 2015). The FHS, using a food frequency questionnaire (FFQ), a validated questionnaire, found that those who increased fruit and vegetable consumption had a lower CVD risk ratio across all quintiles (p trend = .01). Every increment of 3 daily servings of fruits and vegetables was correlated with a 22% decrease in the risk of all types of stroke and transient ischemic attack (TIA). Participants who ate more fat, including more saturated fat, were less likely than those with lower-fat diets to develop ischemic stroke. The FHS study had two noteworthy limitations, a homogenous population and limited exploration of possible confounding variables in analyses. Despite the limitations of the FHS, it set a precedent for future diet and CVD research.

A decade after the FHS, the Nurses' Health Study (NHS) began to better understand women's health, with a primary focus on cancer prevention. Over time, the NHS became the largest and longest ongoing observational cohort study. The NHS examined many lifestyle factors, including assessing diet/dietary patterns prospectively and biannually. Study participants completed a 136-item FFQ. NHS findings identified two key dietary patterns, "prudent" and "Western." The prudent diet consists of a high intake of vegetables, fruit, legumes, fish, poultry, and whole grains, while the Western diet consists of a high consumption of red meat, processed meat, refined grains, and sweets (Colditz et al. 1997). When comparing the highest and lowest quintiles of the Western pattern, the NHS reported a greater than 50% increased risk (RR 1.58, 95% CI 1.15–2.15) for total strokes and 1.56 (95% CI 1.05–2.33) for ischemic strokes. The "prudent" dietary intake was associated with a 22% and 26% reduction in total and ischemic strokes, respectively. Both the FHS and NHS triggered a shift in how researchers explore the relationship between diet/dietary patterns relating to CVD and the risk of stroke.

The Northern Manhattan Study (NOMAS) recruited 3183 participants prospectively to explore stroke risk factors in a multiethnic population in northern Manhattan in New York City. NOMAS is the first study of its kind to examine stroke risk factors in a racially diverse population living in the same community. NOMAS conducted multiple substudies and secondary analyses to explore the association between various dietary factors and patterns with stroke risk, incidence, and mortality (Boden-Albala et al. 2009). In a substudy, NOMAS examined the relationship between fat intake and risk of ischemic stroke. On average, NOMAS participants consumed 1565 cal and 61 g of fat daily. Consuming above 65 g total fat daily significantly increased the risk of ischemic stroke (HR 1.6, 95% CI 1.0–2.7). In another analysis, NOMAS participants who consumed high sodium diets had an increased risk of stroke (a rise of 17%/500 mg increase in sodium) independent of vascular risk factors. Consuming >4000 mg/day sodium was associated with a 2.6-fold increase in stroke risk versus <1500 mg/day. Despite the NOMAS findings, recent research has found that salt intake might not be as deleterious as previously documented (Gardener et al. 2012).

The Prospective Urban Rural Epidemiology (PURE) study is a large-scale epidemiologic cohort study that enrolled and followed 156,424 persons, 35–70 years of age, residing in 628 urban and rural communities in 17 low-, middle-, and high-income countries, in which sodium intake was estimated on the basis of measured urinary excretion. An estimated sodium intake of 3–6 g/day was associated with a lower risk of death and cardiovascular events than was either a higher or lower estimated level of intake. Both higher and lower levels of estimated sodium excretion were associated with increased risk, resulting in a J-shaped association curve (Mente et al. 2014a; O'Donnell et al. 2014). Similar results were reported by the ONTARGET and TRANSCEND trials (the Kawasaki formula). Compared with baseline sodium excretion of 4.00–5.99 g/day, sodium excretion of greater than 7 g/day was associated with an increased risk of all CV events, and a sodium excretion of less than 3 g/day was associated with an increased risk of CV mortality. Higher estimated potassium excretion was associated with a reduced risk of stroke (O'Donnell et al. 2011).

An inverse association between coffee consumption and morbidity and mortality due to overall CVD, an effect on stroke, has also been suggested, yet evidence is limited and inconsistent (Gardener et al. 2013). In NOMAS, individuals who drank diet soda every day had a 61% higher risk of vascular events than those who did not drink soda. Alcohol consumption proved to be an interesting finding; moderate alcohol consumption, up to two drinks per day, was significantly protective for ischemic stroke after adjustment for cardiac disease, hypertension, diabetes, current smoking, body mass index, and education (OR 0.51, 95% CI 0.39–0.67). Heavy alcohol consumption, consuming seven or more drinks per day, showed a statistically significant increased risk of ischemic stroke (OR 2.96, 95% CI 1.05–8.29) (Elkind et al. 2006). The INTERSTROKE study reported that, within food groupings (adjusted for age, sex, and region; tertile 3 vs. tertile 1), the increased consumption of fish (OR 0.78, 99% CI 0.66–0.91) and fruit (OR 0.61, 99% CI 0.50–0.73) were associated with reduced risk of stroke.

Table 7.1 gives a description of the effects of dietary patterns on the risk of stroke (Hankey et al. 2012).

There is almost no data on what stroke patients eat either before or after their stroke. The majority of studies in post-stroke diet and nutrition have focused on measures of malnutrition or undernutrition, rather than diet quality, diet composition, or eating habits. In the absence of this information, it is difficult to identify potential opportunities for improvement. We do know that stroke may result in neurological complications (e.g., loss of motor control, dysphagia, and depression) that may increase the risk of malnutrition. Aphasic patients may not be able to communicate when they are hungry or what they want to eat, and prolonged hospitalization may alter metabolic function and metabolic needs. Designing a nutritional intervention must take into account these complications for individual patients. In a literature review of relevant meta-analyses, it was shown that the combination of dietary modification, exercise, aspirin, antihypertensives, and statins may offer a relative risk reduction of 80% for vascular events after a stroke (Apostolopoulou et al. 2012).

Unhealthy diet has a high prevalence overall, but among individuals, after cardiovascular events, the diet quality seemed to be especially poor. In high-income

TABLE 7.1
Effects of Dietary Patterns on the Risk of Stroke

Dietary Patterns	Effects
Healthy diet	High intake of a healthy diet is associated with a reduced risk of stroke in observational studies.[a,b]
Unhealthy diet	High intake of an unhealthy diet is associated with an increased risk of stroke and a population attributable risk of stroke of 19% (99% CI 11–30).[c]
Prudent diet	In women, high intake of a prudent diet is associated with a lower risk of stroke.[d]
Western diet	In women, high intake of a Western diet is associated with a higher risk of stroke.[d]
DASH-style diet	In women, high intake of a DASH-style diet is associated with a lower risk of stroke.[e]
Mediterranean diet	In women, high intake of a Mediterranean diet is associated with a lower risk of stroke, cardiovascular mortality, and all-cause mortality.[f]
Vegetarian diet	Effect on stroke risk is unknown.
Japanese diet	Effect on stroke risk is unknown.

Source: Modified from Hankey et al. Nutrition and the risk of stroke. *Lancet Neurol* 11 (1) (2012): 66–81.

[a] Kurth T. et al. Healthy lifestyle and the risk of stroke in women. *Arch Intern Med* 166 (2006): 1403–1409.
[b] Chiuve S. E. et al. Primary prevention of stroke by healthy lifestyle. *Circulation* 118 (2008): 947–954.
[c] O'Donnell M. J. et al. Risk factors for ischaemic and intracerebral haemorrhagic stroke in 22 countries (The INTERSTROKE Study): A case-control study. *Lancet* 376 (9735) (2010):112–123.
[d] Fung T. T. et al. Prospective study of major dietary patterns an stroke risk in women. *Stroke* 35 (2004): 2014–2019.
[e] Fung T. T. et al. Adherence to a Dash-style diet and risk of coronary heart disease and stroke in women. *Arch Intern Med* 168 (2008): 713–720.
[f] Sofi F. et al. Accruing evidence on benefits of adherence to the Mediterranean diet on health: An update systematic review and meta-analysis. *Am J Clin Nutr* 92 (2010): 1189–1196.

countries the affordability of red meats and fried foods are more common, whereas in poorer countries, healthy foods such as fruits and vegetables may be less so, suggesting that both socioeconomic aspects and behavior have important impacts on the type of diet (Teo et al. 2013).

7.5   NUTRITIONAL COUNSELING AND DIETARY RECOMMENDATIONS

The following recommendations should be considered in nutritional counseling for the primary and secondary prevention of stroke:

- The reduced intake of sodium and increased intake of potassium as indicated in the Dietary Guidelines for Americans report are recommended to lower BP (class I, level of evidence A). The Dietary Guidelines for Americans report recommends a sodium intake of 2.3 g/day (100 mmol/day) for the general population. In blacks, persons with hypertension, and middle- and older-aged persons, a lower level of intake is recommended because these groups are especially sensitive to the BP-lowering effects of a reduced sodium diet. The Dietary Guidelines for Americans recommend a potassium intake of at least 4.7 g/day (120 mmol/day) (U.S. Department of Health and Human Services 2005).

- A DASH-style diet, which emphasizes the consumption of fruits, vegetables, and low-fat dairy products and is reduced in saturated fat, also lowers BP and is recommended (class I, level of evidence A).
- A diet that is rich in fruits and vegetables and thereby high in potassium is beneficial and may lower the risk of stroke (class I, level of evidence B).

Table 7.2 shows the general measures for the primary and secondary prevention of stroke (Goldstein et al. 2010).

The importance of multidisciplinary care must be highlighted, including medical, nutritional and psychological counseling on healthy behavioral change, advising all patients to face the obstacle of personal habit. But it seems that national awareness campaigns would provide additional and sufficient support for all patients and to persuade them to modify their lifestyles (Luz et al. 2011).

7.6 ADHERENCE TO GUIDELINES

Patient adherence to lifestyle modification is obviously crucial, as reflected in the substantial decrease in the occurrence of a second stroke among those who do adhere. In a study in which all the patients who had had a stroke declared the same readiness and willingness to adjust to a healthier lifestyle, only those receiving enhanced secondary prevention, motivation, and surveillance were capable of following a "strict" modification, principal to diet behaviors; patients in the supervised group were able to consume up to 10 portions of fruit and vegetables per week, compared with 1 or 2 portions a week for the control group (Hackam and Spence 2007). Kastorini et al. found differences between sufferers of a first and a second stroke in terms of adherence to a Mediterranean diet. It was observed that for each 1-point increase in the Mediterranean diet score (with increasing scores indicating greater adherence to the Mediterranean diet), the corresponding odds ratio for having a stroke was 0.88 (95% CI 0.82–0.94) (Kastorini et al. 2011).

7.7 FUTURE DIRECTIONS AND CONCLUSION

- A healthy diet may have a similar effect size for secondary prevention in stroke patients. Prudent, Mediterranean, or healthy diets are efficient for stroke prevention and there is no evidence showing that any specific diet is better than another (Goldstein et al. 2011; Yusuf et al. 2016).
- Most stroke patients eat poorly, so any intervention efforts might gain attention. It is common to find adverse dietary practices in stroke patients within the same geographic region. Therefore, effective community-based interventions or strategies might carefully be designed and implemented after identifying barriers for optimal nutrition.

TABLE 7.2

Measures for the Primary and Secondary Prevention of Stroke

General Goals and Recommendations

Stop Smoking

It is mandatory for the patient to avoid environmental tobacco smoke; strongly encourage patient and family to stop smoking. Provide counseling, nicotine replacement, and formal programs as available. Consider all cardiovascular diseases.

Diabetes: Improve Glucose Control

As diabetes has a high prevalence overall, glucose control must be followed closely. Consider the guidelines and recommendations on diet and medical treatments. Keep up additional efforts to treat hypertension and consider the use of statins, based on evidence.

Treat Sleep-Disordered Breathing

Recommend sleep laboratory evaluation for patients with snoring, excessive sleepiness, and recurrent sleep apnea. Control obesity, resistant hypertension, and accumulated cardiovascular risk factors.

Oral Contraceptive Use: Avoid If Risk of Stroke Is High

Inform patients who smoke cigarettes, have migraines (especially with older age or smoking), are >35 years of age, or have had prior thromboembolic events about stroke risk and encourage alternative forms of birth control.

Poor Diet/Nutrition: Eat a Well-Balanced Diet

The diet has to contain as least 5 servings of fruits and vegetables per day, which may reduce stroke risk. Encourage patients to consume a healthy diet and to consider a variety of vegetables, legumes, and fruits in more than 1 serving.

Physical Inactivity: Engage in ≥30 Min of Moderate-Intensity Activity Daily

Encourage moderate exercise (e.g., brisk walking, jogging, cycling, or other aerobic activities). For those that resist adhering to a routine of exercise, incentivize small changes in lifestyle to motivate them at the beginning. Recommend supervised programs for high-risk patients (e.g., cardiac disease) and adaptive programs depending on physical/neurologic deficits on secondary prevention.

Limit Alcohol Consumption

Patients should limit their alcohol consumption to no more than two drinks/day for men and no more than one drink/day for women. For pregnant women, cessation is mandatory until the end of breast-feeding.

Stop Drug Abuse

Include an in-depth history of substance abuse as part of a complete health evaluation for all patients. Deter children and youths from starting the use of legal drugs and developing the risk of changing to hard drugs.

Source: Modified from L. B. Goldstein et al. *Stroke* 42 (2): 517–584, 2011.

- Hypertension is the most important independent risk factor for stroke. Hence, salt restriction should be considered for stroke prevention.
- Obesity, physical inactivity, smoking, alcohol abuse, and stress/depression also are important risk factors and associated with unhealthy lifestyles, so they need special attention and campaigns to control them in the community setting (O'Donnell et al. 2014; Mente et al. 2014b).
- The use of risk scores for more accurate assessments should be encouraged in clinical practice, in order to better control risk factors. They are also

crucial to guide interventions, whether through medication or changes in lifestyle, but mainly in dietary pattern changes.

- Finally, even with adequate knowledge and support, patients have great difficulty in adopting new dietary patterns. The challenges to increasing adherence to a healthy lifestyle are not insurmountable, but overcoming them will require research on nutritional epidemiology in stroke, the comparative effectiveness of various diets, and implementation. It is fundamental to improve the knowledge and resources of health professionals, nonprofit organizations, and governmental institutions globally (Dearborn et al. 2015; Perel et al. 2015).

7.8 CASE STUDIES

Based on the information given in this chapter, try to analyze the following case studies and respond to the questions accordingly.

7.8.1 CASE STUDY 1

A 65-year-old African American male is an auxiliary warehouse professional, has a sedentary lifestyle, has been a smoker for 10 years, and has a family history of coronary artery disease and hypertension (father with a fatal hemorrhagic stroke, mother and one brother with sudden death). He was referred to a nutritionist after examinations requested by the occupational health department, where he had complained of lower back pain. *On examination*: BMI 30 kg/m²;waist circumference 102 cm; hip circumference 90 cm; systolic pressure 130 mm Hg and diastolic blood pressure 90 mm Hg. *Biochemical tests*: Fasting blood glucose 98 mg/dL; total cholesterol 169 mg/dL; LDL 98 mg/dL; HDL 40 mg/dL; triglyceride 350 mg/dL; elevated liver enzymes. *Dietary history revealed*: At breakfast, the patient consumes one large cup of coffee with milk (full cream), two and a half slices of bread with butter, ham, and cheese (four slices each); lunch (usually self-service) is composed of 3 tbsp white rice, two bean shells, two steaks or barbecued meat or two chicken wings, potato salad with vinaigrette, one pastel (cheese, ham and cheese, or meat), corn flour and pepper, Coke Zero or flavored water, gelatin and milk pudding as dessert; for dinner, two slices of bread with ham and cheese, two cups of milk with chocolate powder, or one large cheese pizza or sandwich (burger with fries) with Coke Zero. On Wednesday, the patient consumes beer with snacks (watching football); on average he consumes five cans.

Give responses to the following:

1. Using the information in this chapter, which of the risk factors you have identified in this patient modifiable for stroke and which are not modifiable?
2. Analyzing the dietary survey of this patient, which dietary pattern can you identify and what is its effect on the risk of stroke?
3. According to the risk factors of this patient, what recommendations would you make to reduce the risk of stroke?

7.8.2 CASE STUDY 2

A 35-year-old black female has a sedentary lifestyle, depression, and hypertension, has never smoked, uses oral contraceptives, and has had a first ischemic stroke without sequelae (diagnosed 2 years ago). She consults a nutritionist at the insistence of her husband because she has gained weight regularly over the last 4 or 5 years (about 8 kg). She drinks beer only on weekends (3–5 drinks on Saturdays and Sundays). She has no spontaneous complaints or questions. She refuses to take the medications prescribed by her doctor (atenolol, losartan, aspirin) and has not returned to the doctor in the last year. Family history: Her father died of a heart attack at age 54 (diseases not known); her mother, 71 years, has high blood pressure. Her brother became diabetic after 50 years and underwent coronary artery bypass surgery at 54 years. On examination: height 178 cm, weight 89.0 kg, waist circumference 98 cm. Hydrated, systolic blood pressure 140 mm Hg and diastolic blood pressure 95 mm Hg. Biochemical examination last month: glucose 104 mg/dL; creatinine 1.0 mg/dL; uric acid 7.8 mg/dL; total cholesterol 220 mg/dL; triglycerides 210 mg/dL, HDL 36 mg/dL, LDL 142 mg/dL.

Give responses to the following:

1. Using the information in this chapter, what are the risk factors of this patient and the odds for stroke?
2. What questions would you like to ask her for nutritional assessment?
3. Based on the reported information, what would you recommend for the secondary prevention of stroke?

REFERENCES

Adams, H. P., Jr, B. H. Bendixen, L. J. Kappelle, J. Biller, B. B. Love, D. L. Gordon, and E. E. Marsh, 3rd. 1993. Classification of subtype of acute ischemic stroke: Definitions for use in a multicenter clinical trial; TOAST; Trial of Org 10172 in Acute Stroke Treatment. *Stroke* 24 (1):35–41.

American Heart Association. 2015. The American Heart Association's diet and lifestyle recommendations. Accessed January 15, 2016. http://www.heart.org/HEARTORG/HealthyLiving/HealthyEating/Nutrition/The-American-Heart-Associations-Diet-and-Lifestyle-Recommendations_UCM_305855_Article.jsp#.VtXtO-Ywplo.

Apostolopoulou, M., K. Michalakis, A. Miras, A. Hatzitolios, and C. Savopoulos. 2012. Nutrition in the primary and secondary prevention of stroke. *Maturitas* 72 (1):29–34.

Appel, L. J., M. W. Brands, S. R. Daniels, N. Karanja, P. J. Elmer, and F. M. Sacks. 2006. Dietary approaches to prevent and treat hypertension: A scientific statement from the American Heart Association. *Hypertension* 47 (2):296–308.

Ascherio, A., E. B. Rimm, M. A. Hernan, E. L. Giovannucci, I. Kawachi, M. J. Stampfer, and W. C. Willett. 1998. Intake of potassium, magnesium, calcium, and fiber and risk of stroke among U.S. men. *Circulation* 98 (12):1198–1204.

Bamford, J., P. Sanderock, M. Dennis, J. Burn, and C. Warlow. 1991. Classification and natural history of clinically identifiable subtypes of cerebral infarction. *Lancet* 337 (8756):1521–1526.

Boden-Albala, B., M. S. Elkind, H. White, A. Szumski, M. C. Paik, and R. L. Sacco. 2009. Dietary total fat intake and ischemic stroke risk: The Northern Manhattan Study. *Neuroepidemiology* 32 (4):296–301.

Boden-Albala, B., L. Southwick, and H. Carman. 2015. Dietary interventions to lower the risk of stroke. *Curr Neurol Neurosci Rep* 15 (4):15.

Chang, H. Y., Y. W. Hu, C. S. Yue, Y. W. Wen, W. T. Yeh, L. S. Hsu, S. Y. Tsai, and W. H. Pan. 2006. Effect of potassium-enriched salt on cardiovascular mortality and medical expenses of elderly men. *Am J Clin Nutr* 83 (6):1289–1296.

Cheng, P., J. Wang, W. Shao, M. Liu, and H. Zhang. 2016. Can dietary saturated fat be beneficial in prevention of stroke risk? A meta-analysis. *Neurol Sci* 37 (7):1089–1098.

Chiuve, S. E., K. M. Rexrode, D. Spiegelman, G. Logroscino, J. E. Manson, and E. B. Rimm. 2008. Primary prevention of stroke by healthy lifestyle. *Circulation* 118 (9):947–954.

Colditz, G. A., J. E. Manson, and S. E. Hankinson. 1997. The Nurses' Health Study: 20-year contribution to the understanding of health among women. *J Womens Health* 6 (1):49–62.

Dauchet, L., P. Amouyel, and J. Dallongeville. 2005. Fruit and vegetable consumption and risk of stroke: A meta-analysis of cohort studies. *Neurology* 65 (8):1193–1197.

Dearborn, J. L., V. C. Urrutia, and W. N. Kernan. 2015. The case for diet: A safe and efficacious strategy for secondary stroke prevention. *Front Neurol* 6:1.

Ding, E. L., and D. Mozaffarian. 2006. Optimal dietary habits for the prevention of stroke. *Semin Neurol* 26 (1):11–23.

Elkind, M. S., R. Sciacca, B. Boden-Albala, T. Rundek, M. C. Paik, and R. L. Sacco. 2006. Moderate alcohol consumption reduces risk of ischemic stroke: The Northern Manhattan Study. *Stroke* 37 (1):13–19.

Estruch, R., E. Ros, J. Salas-Salvadó, M.-I. Covas, D. Corella, F. Arós, E. Gómez-Gracia et al. 2013. Primary prevention of cardiovascular disease with a Mediterranean diet. *N Engl J Med* 368 (14):1279–1290.

Feigin, V. L., M. H. Forouzanfar, R. Krishnamurthi, G. A. Mensah, M. Connor, D. A. Bennett, A. E. Moran et al. 2014. Global and regional burden of stroke during 1990–2010: Findings from the Global Burden of Disease Study 2010. *Lancet* 383 (9913):245–254.

Ferro, J. M. 2003. Cardioembolic stroke: An update. *Lancet Neurol* 2 (3):177–188.

Finucane, M. M., G. A. Stevens, M. J. Cowan, G. Danaei, J. K. Lin, C. J. Paciorek, G. M. Singh et al. 2011. National, regional, and global trends in body-mass index since 1980: Systematic analysis of health examination surveys and epidemiological studies with 960 country-years and 9.1 million participants. *Lancet* 377 (9765):557–567.

Franklin, B. A., and M. Cushman. 2011. Recent advances in preventive cardiology and lifestyle medicine: A themed series. *Circulation* 123 (20):2274–2283.

Fung, T. T., S. E. Chiuve, M. L. McCullough, K. M. Rexrode, G. Logroscino, and F. B. Hu. 2008. Adherence to a DASH-style diet and risk of coronary heart disease and stroke in women. *Arch Intern Med* 168 (7):713–720.

Gardener, H., T. Rundek, C. B. Wright, M. S. Elkind, and R. L. Sacco. 2012. Dietary sodium and risk of stroke in the Northern Manhattan Study. *Stroke* 43 (5):1200–1205.

Gardener, H., T. Rundek, C. B. Wright, M. S. V. Elkind, and R. L. Sacco. 2013. Coffee and tea consumption are inversely associated with mortality in a multiethnic urban population. *J Nutr* 143 (8):1299–1308.

Gillman, M. W., L. A. Cupples, D. Gagnon, B. M. Posner, R. C. Ellison, W. P. Castelli, and P. A. Wolf. 1995. Protective effect of fruits and vegetables on development of stroke in men. *JAMA* 273 (14):1113–1117.

Goldstein, L. B., C. D. Bushnell, R. J. Adams, L. J. Appel, L. T. Braun, S. Chaturvedi, M. A. Creager et al. 2011. Guidelines for the primary prevention of stroke: A guideline for healthcare professionals from the American Heart Association/American Stroke Association. *Stroke* 42 (2):517–584.

Hackam, D. G., and J. D. Spence. 2007. Combining multiple approaches for the secondary prevention of vascular events after stroke: A quantitative modeling study. *Stroke* 38 (6):1881–1885.

Haheim, L. L., I. Holme, I. Hjermann, and P. Leren. 1993. Risk factors of stroke incidence and mortality. A 12-year follow-up of the Oslo Study. *Stroke* 24 (10):1484–1489.

Hankey, G. J. 2012. Nutrition and the risk of stroke. *Lancet Neurol* 11 (1):66–81.

He, F. J., C. A. Nowson, and G. A. MacGregor. 2006. Fruit and vegetable consumption and stroke: Meta-analysis of cohort studies. *Lancet* 367 (9507):320–326.

He, J., L. G. Ogden, S. Vupputuri, L. A. Bazzano, C. Loria, and P. K. Whelton. 1999. Dietary sodium intake and subsequent risk of cardiovascular disease in overweight adults. *JAMA* 282 (21):2027–2034.

He, K., A. Merchant, E. B. Rimm, B. A. Rosner, M. J. Stampfer, W. C. Willett, and A. Ascherio. 2003. Dietary fat intake and risk of stroke in male U.S. healthcare professionals: 14 year prospective cohort study. *BMJ* 327 (7418):777–782.

Howard, B. V., J. E. Manson, M. L. Stefanick, S. A. Beresford, G. Frank, B. Jones, R. J. Rodabough et al. 2006. Low-fat dietary pattern and weight change over 7 years: The Women's Health Initiative dietary modification trial. *JAMA* 295 (1):39–49.

Hsia, A. W., and D. C. Tong. 2003. New magnetic resonance imaging and computed tomography techniques for imaging of acute stroke. *Curr Atheroscler Rep* 5 (4):252–259.

Hu, D., J. Huang, Y. Wang, D. Zhang, and Y. Qu. 2014. Fruits and vegetables consumption and risk of stroke: A meta-analysis of prospective cohort studies. *Stroke* 45 (6):1613–1619.

Jackson, C., and C. Sudlow. 2005. Are lacunar strokes really different? A systematic review of differences in risk factor profiles between lacunar and nonlacunar infarcts. *Stroke* 36 (4):891–901.

Jacobs, D. R., Jr, and L. M. Steffen. 2003. Nutrients, foods, and dietary patterns as exposures in research: A framework for food synergy. *Am J Clin Nutr* 78 (3 Suppl):508S–513S.

Johnsen, S. P., K. Overvad, C. Stripp, A. Tjonneland, S. E. Husted, and H. T. Sorensen. 2003. Intake of fruit and vegetables and the risk of ischemic stroke in a cohort of Danish men and women. *Am J Clin Nutr* 78 (1):57–64.

Joshipura, K. J., A. Ascherio, J. E. Manson, M. J. Stampfer, E. B. Rimm, F. E. Speizer, C. H. Hennekens, D. Spiegelman, and W. C. Willett. 1999. Fruit and vegetable intake in relation to risk of ischemic stroke. *JAMA* 282 (13):1233–1239.

Kastorini, C. M., H. J. Milionis, A. Ioannidi, K. Kalantzi, V. Nikolaou, K. N. Vemmos, J. A. Goudevenos, and D. B. Panagiotakos. 2011. Adherence to the Mediterranean diet in relation to acute coronary syndrome or stroke nonfatal events: A comparative analysis of a case/case-control study. *Am Heart J* 162 (4):717–724.

Katan, M. B., I. A. Brouwer, R. Clarke, J. M. Geleijnse, and R. P. Mensink. 2010. Saturated fat and heart disease. *Am J Clin Nutr* 92 (2):459–460; author reply 460–461.

Khaw, K. T., and E. Barrett-Connor. 1987. Dietary potassium and stroke-associated mortality. A 12-year prospective population study. *N Engl J Med* 316 (5):235–240.

Kontogianni, M. D., and D. B. Panagiotakos. 2014. Dietary patterns and stroke: A systematic review and re-meta-analysis. *Maturitas* 79 (1):41–47.

Krishnamurthi, R. V., V. L. Feigin, M. H. Forouzanfar, G. A. Mensah, M. Connor, D. A. Bennett, A. E. Moran et al. 2013. Global and regional burden of first-ever ischaemic and haemorrhagic stroke during 1990–2010: Findings from the Global Burden of Disease Study 2010. *Lancet Glob Health* 1 (5):e259–e281.

Kwon, Y., F. L. Norby, P. N. Jensen, S. K. Agarwal, E. Z. Soliman, G. Y. Lip, W. T. Longstreth, Jr, A. Alonso, S. R. Heckbert, and L. Y. Chen. 2016. Association of smoking, alcohol, and obesity with cardiovascular death and ischemic stroke in atrial fibrillation: The Atherosclerosis Risk in Communities (ARIC) study and Cardiovascular Health Study (CHS). *PLoS One* 11 (1):e0147065.

Larsson, S. C., and N. Orsini. 2011. Fish consumption and the risk of stroke: A dose-response meta-analysis. *Stroke* 42 (12):3621–3623.

Lucke-Wold, B. P., R. C. Turner, A. Noelle Lucke-Wold, C. L. Rosen, and J. D. Huber. 2012. Age and the metabolic syndrome as risk factors for ischemic stroke: Improving preclinical models of ischemic stroke. *Yale J Biol Med* 85 (4):523–539.

Luz, P. L., M. Nishiyama, and A. C. Chagas. 2011. Drugs and lifestyle for the treatment and prevention of coronary artery disease: Comparative analysis of the scientific basis. *Braz J Med Biol Res* 44 (10):973–991.

Medeiros, F., M. de Abreu Casanova, J. C. Fraulob, and M. Trindade. 2012. How can diet influence the risk of stroke? *Int J Hypertens* 2012:763507.

Mente, A., M. J. O'Donnell, G. Dagenais, A. Wielgosz, S. A. Lear, M. J. McQueen, Y. Jiang et al. 2014a. Validation and comparison of three formulae to estimate sodium and potassium excretion from a single morning fasting urine compared to 24-h measures in 11 countries. *J Hypertens* 32 (5): 1005–1014;discussion 1015.

Mente, A., M. J. O'Donnell, S. Rangarajan, M. J. McQueen, P. Poirier, A. Wielgosz, H. Morrison et al. 2014b. Association of urinary sodium and potassium excretion with blood pressure. *N Engl J Med* 371 (7):601–611.

Meschia, J. F., C. Bushnell, B. Boden-Albala, L. T. Braun, D. M. Bravata, S. Chaturvedi, M. A. Creager et al. 2014. Guidelines for the primary prevention of stroke: A statement for healthcare professionals from the American Heart Association/American Stroke Association. *Stroke* 45 (12):3754–3832.

Micha, R., S. K. Wallace, and D. Mozaffarian. 2010. Red and processed meat consumption and risk of incident coronary heart disease, stroke, and diabetes mellitus: A systematic review and meta-analysis. *Circulation* 121 (21):2271–2283.

Mizrahi, A., P. Knekt, J. Montonen, M. A. Laaksonen, M. Heliovaara, and R. Jarvinen. 2009. Plant foods and the risk of cerebrovascular diseases: A potential protection of fruit consumption. *Br J Nutr* 102 (7):1075–1083.

Nagata, C., N. Takatsuka, N. Shimizu, and H. Shimizu. 2004. Sodium intake and risk of death from stroke in Japanese men and women. *Stroke* 35 (7):1543–1547.

O'Donnell, M., A. Mente, S. Rangarajan, M. J. McQueen, X. Wang, L. Liu, H. Yan et al. 2014. Urinary sodium and potassium excretion, mortality, and cardiovascular events. *N Engl J Med* 371 (7):612–623.

O'Donnell, M. J., D. Xavier, L. Liu, H. Zhang, S. L. Chin, P. Rao-Melacini, S. Rangarajan et al. 2010. Risk factors for ischaemic and intracerebral haemorrhagic stroke in 22 countries (the INTERSTROKE study): A case-control study. *Lancet* 376 (9735):112–123.

O'Donnell, M. J., S. Yusuf, A. Mente, P. Gao, J. F. Mann, K. Teo, M. McQueen et al. 2011. Urinary sodium and potassium excretion and risk of cardiovascular events. *JAMA* 306 (20):2229–2238.

Perel, P., A. Avezum, M. Huffman, P. Pais, A. Rodgers, R. Vedanthan, D. Wood, and S. Yusuf. 2015. Reducing premature cardiovascular morbidity and mortality in people with atherosclerotic vascular disease: The World Heart Federation Roadmap for Secondary Prevention of Cardiovascular Disease. *Glob Heart* 10 (2):99–110.

Shah, R. S., and J. W. Cole. 2010. Smoking and stroke: The more you smoke the more you stroke. *Expert Rev Cardiovasc Ther* 8 (7):917–932.

Sherzai, A., L. T. Heim, C. Boothby, and A. D. Sherzai. 2012. Stroke, food groups, and dietary patterns: A systematic review. *Nutr Rev* 70 (8):423–435.

Spence, J. D. 2006. Nutrition and stroke prevention. *Stroke* 37 (9):2430–2435.

Swinburn, B. A., G. Sacks, K. D. Hall, K. McPherson, D. T. Finegood, M. L. Moodie, and S. L. Gortmaker. 2011. The global obesity pandemic: Shaped by global drivers and local environments. *Lancet* 378 (9793):804–814.

Teo, K., S. Lear, S. Islam, P. Mony, M. Dehghan, W. Li, A. Rosengren et al. 2013. Prevalence of a healthy lifestyle among individuals with cardiovascular disease in high-, middle- and low-income countries: The Prospective Urban Rural Epidemiology (PURE) study. *JAMA* 309 (15):1613–1621.

Tolonen, H., M. Mahonen, K. Asplund, D. Rastenyte, K. Kuulasmaa, D. Vanuzzo, and J. Tuomilehto. 2002. Do trends in population levels of blood pressure and other cardiovascular risk factors explain trends in stroke event rates? Comparisons of 15 populations in 9 countries within the WHO MONICA stroke project. World Health Organization Monitoring of Trends and Determinants in Cardiovascular Disease. *Stroke* 33 (10):2367–2375.

Tracy, S. W. 2013. Something new under the sun? The Mediterranean diet and cardiovascular health. *N Engl J Med* 368 (14):1274–1276.

U.S. Department of Health and Human Services. 2005. *Dietary Guidelines for Americans, 2005*. Washington, DC: Government Printing Office.

Yusuf, S., J. Bosch, G. Dagenais, J. Zhu, D. Xavier, L. Liu, P. Pais et al. 2016. Cholesterol lowering in intermediate-risk persons without cardiovascular disease. *N Engl J Med* 374(21), 2021–2031.

Yusuf, S., S. Hawken, S. Ounpuu, T. Dans, A. Avezum, F. Lanas, M. McQueen et al. 2004. Effect of potentially modifiable risk factors associated with myocardial infarction in 52 countries (the INTERHEART study): Case-control study. *Lancet* 364 (9438):937–952.

Yusuf, S., S. Reddy, S. Ounpuu, and S. Anand. 2001. Global burden of cardiovascular diseases, Part 1: General considerations, the epidemiologic transition, risk factors, and impact of urbanization. *Circulation* 104 (22):2746–2753.

8 HEAL for Asthma

Zaid Kajani, Sivakumar Sudhakaran,
and Salim Surani

CONTENTS

8.1 WHAT IS ASTHMA?

8.1.1 INTRODUCTION

This chapter provides an outline of dietary habits that have been shown to aid in reducing asthma symptoms or preventing the development of asthma altogether. While there is no doubt in the scientific community that healthy eating leads to a more productive lifestyle, most patients underestimate the power of proper nutrition, especially when it comes to asthma treatment. However, to understand how certain food groups positively or negatively affect asthmatics, we must first discuss asthma as a condition and the pathophysiology behind it.

8.1.2 CLINICAL DEFINITION

In 1991, the National Heart, Lung, and Blood Institute (NHLBI) and the National Asthma Education and Prevention Program (NAEPP) published the first of three Expert Panel Reports outlining the "Guidelines for the Diagnosis and Treatment of Asthma" (NAEPP 1991). The third and most recent Expert Panel Report (EPR-3), published in 2007, defines asthma as "a common chronic disorder of the airways that is complex and characterized by variable and recurring symptoms, airflow obstruction, bronchial hyper responsiveness, and an underlying inflammation. The interaction of these features of asthma determines the clinical manifestations and severity of asthma and the response to treatment" (NAEPP 2007). The symptoms referred to in this definition include recurrent episodes of wheezing or high-pitched whistling sounds when exhaling, coughing, difficulty breathing or shortness of breath, and chest tightness (NAEPP 2007). These symptoms are usually a result of inflammation and significantly reduced airflow.

It is also important to note that asthma is caused by both genetic and environmental factors (Busse and Lemanske 2001). Thus, a patient with a predisposition for developing asthma may never develop it because the environmental triggers are not present. On the other hand, a patient with no familial history of asthma may develop the condition due to the presence of environmental allergens.

The NHLBI classifies the severity of asthma symptoms into two main categories, "intermittent" and "persistent," based on the frequency of symptoms (NAEPP 2007). Persistent asthma is further split into mild, moderate, and severe subcategories (NAEPP 2007). While the definitions of these categories vary slightly between age groups, symptom frequency is fairly well defined. Patients with intermittent asthma experience symptoms 2 days/week or less, while patients with mild persistent asthma experience symptoms more than 2 days/week, but not daily (NAEPP 2007). Furthermore, patients with moderate persistent asthma experience symptoms daily, and patients with severe persistent asthma experience symptoms multiple times throughout each day (NAEPP 2007).

The exacerbation of asthma symptoms on a daily basis depends on a number of factors, the main one being the presence of triggering agents (Baxi and Phipatanakul 2010). Common asthma triggers include environmental allergens such as house dust mites, animals with fur or hair, cockroaches, mice, pollen, and mold (Baxi and Phipatanakul 2010; NAEPP 2007). Additionally, asthma symptoms can worsen due to air pollution, airborne chemicals or dusts, or smoking (NAEPP 2007). Even strong emotional expressions, such as laughing and crying, or psychological stress can affect asthma (Chen and Miller 2007; NAEPP 2007). Finally, diet, food allergies, changes in weather, and viral infections can also worsen symptoms (NAEPP 2007).

8.1.3 EPIDEMIOLOGY

The Global Initiative for Asthma (GINA) conservatively estimates that as many as 300 million people worldwide are affected by asthma (Masoli et al. 2004). A chronic disease that crosses all ethnic, social, and economic boundaries, asthma is a burden to patients, families, health-care systems, and governments everywhere (Masoli et al. 2004). While asthma rates vary from 1% to 18% between countries, asthma is much more prevalent in developed countries than developing countries (Global Initiative for Asthma 2011). It is estimated that the world's asthmatic population may increase by an additional 100 million by 2025 (World Health Organization 2007). GINA estimates that approximately 250,000 people die each year as a result of asthma (Global Initiative for Asthma 2011), corresponding to about one in every 250 deaths (Masoli et al. 2004). Developing countries account for the vast majority of the mortality—approximately 80% (Lugogo and Kraft 2006). This discrepancy is most likely due to differences in the quality of care, access to resources, and frequency of proper diagnoses. Additionally, in developed countries, asthma is more common among the economically disadvantaged, while in developing countries, it is more common among the affluent (Global Initiative for Asthma 2011).

In 2012, the National Center for Health Statistics (NCHS) reported that more than 22 million Americans were affected by asthma, including more than six million children (Adams et al. 2013). Asthma accounted for more than 440,000 hospitalizations in the United States in 2006, making it the third leading cause of hospitalization among children (Buie et al. 2010). The average asthma-related hospitalization in America in 2010 cost USD 3600 for children and USD 6600 for adults, prices that could quite possibly be avoided by adhering to a lifestyle of healthy eating (Barrett et al. 2006).

Asthma prevalence differs by race and ethnicity. In the United States, asthma rates vary drastically between ethnic populations, with the highest rates in the Puerto Rican, African American, and Filipino populations, and the lowest rates in the Korean and Mexican populations (Davis et al. 2006; Gold and Wright 2005; Lara et al. 2006). These differences could potentially be due to either genetics or environmental factors.

Finally, gender and age can also impact asthma prevalence. In children, asthma is twice as common in boys as it is in girls, and in adults, women are subject to a higher prevalence than men (Global Initiative for Asthma 2011).

8.1.4 Pathophysiology

The pathophysiology of asthma is complex and is a product of the interplay between several factors. In broad terms, inflammation will trigger a state of airway hyper responsiveness as well as airway obstruction. These two factors ultimately combine to create the clinical symptoms that are observed in asthmatic patients. It is also important to note that airway hyperresponsiveness and obstruction may also have cumulative synergistic effects (Cohn et al. 2004). Additionally, there are a number of notable changes that occur in the airway secondary to the prolonged effects of asthma. In acute asthmatic attacks, bronchial smooth-muscle contraction occurs rapidly and essentially narrows the airway in response to a given stimuli (allergens, irritants, etc.) (Busse and Lemanske 2001).

Finally, the last commonly noted change in asthma is airway remodeling. The remodeling (including inflammation, mucous hypersecretion, subepithelial fibrosis, airway smooth-muscle hypertrophy, and angiogenesis) of the airway involves a number of different cells and ultimately causes irreversible changes, rendering patients less responsive to a number of therapeutic strategies (Holgate and Polosa 2006). Also, several inflammatory markers such as C-reactive protein (CRP), interleukin-6 (IL-6), tumor necrosis factor-α (TNF-α), adiponectin, and neuropeptide-Y (NPY) are independently associated with asthma (Lu et al. 2015). A more detailed discussion of these markers is beyond the scope of this text.

8.1.5 TREATMENT

Asthma medications can be categorized into two main groups: long-term medications and quick-relief medications (NAEPP 2007). The difference is fairly intuitive. Long-term medications attempt to control persistent asthma by reducing the frequency and severity of attacks and improving overall pulmonary function, while quick-relief medications respond to acute symptoms immediately (NAEPP 2007). Inhaled corticosteroids, which fall into the long-term category, are by far the most effective anti-inflammatory agents used to control the symptoms of asthma and to improve long-term pulmonary function (Busse and Lemanske 2001). Alternative and adjunctive therapies for the long-term treatment of asthma include cromolyn sodium, nedocromil, immunomodulators, leukotriene modifiers, methylxanthines, and long-acting beta agonists (LABAs) (NAEPP 2007). Within the quick-relief category, short-acting beta agonists (SABAs), which also qualify as bronchodilators, are the therapy of choice. SABAs, such as albuterol, provide temporary relief in the case of exacerbation or bronchospasm, whether it occurs as a result of exercise, exposure to allergens, or any other asthma trigger. Other quick-relief medications include anticholinergic and systemic corticosteroids (NAEPP 2007).

Anti-inflammatory drugs have been shown to reverse some of the symptoms of asthma, but a positive response to therapy often takes weeks to achieve and may be incomplete, especially if airway remodeling has occurred (Bateman et al. 2004). Thus, dietary adjustments may provide an additional benefit when combined with the proper medication.

8.2 FOOD GROUPS AND DIETARY PATTERNS TO PREVENT ASTHMA

As a chronic condition, asthma is incredibly difficult to prevent before its onset, especially because many asthma patients develop the condition during childhood. Despite the difficulty of preventing asthma as a whole, there are some dietary patterns that can be followed to decrease the probability of developing asthma.

8.2.1 NEONATAL BREAST-FEEDING

One of the earliest forms of potential asthma prevention must actually take place immediately after birth. While some of the studies conducted on the link between asthma and neonatal breast-feeding are not completely conclusive, there is significant evidence to suggest that breast-feeding might provide a protective effect against asthma. In fact, a 2001 review and meta-analysis of 12 studies concluded that "exclusive breast-feeding during the first months after birth is associated with lower asthma rates during childhood," and its effects are attributed to the "immunomodulatory qualities of breast milk, avoidance of allergens, or a combination of these and other factors" (Gdalevich et al. 2001). They also specify that the advantage of breast-feeding is strengthened if the patient has a family history of atopy, a syndrome denoted by hypersensitive allergic reactions. A number of other studies have come to the same conclusion about the protective effect of breast-feeding (Chandra 1997; Oddy et al. 1999).

8.2.2 OBESITY

For years now, climbing asthma rates have paralleled climbing obesity rates (Ford 2005). While many studies indicate that obesity might increase a patient's chance of developing asthma, the results are controversial because of the limitations inherent to the methodologies of these studies (Ford 2005). Continued work must be conducted in this area, but since obesity is a potential risk factor for asthma, it would be in the patient's best interests to make lifestyle changes designed to lose excess weight. This effort to prevent asthma development is especially important if the patient has a genetic predisposition for the disorder. A number of studies do suggest that obesity increases the difficulty of controlling asthma symptoms that have already presented (Sutherland 2014). Studies have shown that a sedentary lifestyle among adolescents can lead to asthma (Chen et al. 2015; Groth et al. 2015). They have also shown that levels of inflammatory cytokines (IL-6, hs-CRP, and TNF-α) are increased at extremes of weight. Additionally, the investigators have demonstrated that maintaining a healthy weight among children may decrease the inflammatory cytokines and henceforth decrease the risk of asthma (Chen et al. 2015). Another study has shown that women with asthma tend to weigh more than women without asthma. The data also revealed that all classes of obesity (class 1 of body mass index [BMI] 30–34.9, class 2 of BMI 35–39.9, and class 3 of BMI >40) are associated with an increased risk of asthma among women (Wang et al. 2015). Finally, studies have also shown that airway obstruction increases with obesity (Strunk et al. 2015) and pulmonary function improves after weight loss (Stenius-Aarniala et al. 2000; Weiss 2005). It is imperative that measures be undertaken to exercise regularly and maintain a healthy dietary regimen to optimize weight, especially among female patients.

8.2.3 GENERAL DIET RECOMMENDATIONS

While it is very difficult to prevent the development of asthma because so many uncontrollable factors are at play, the Expert Panel Report 3 (EPR-3) recommends "a varied diet consistent with the Dietary Guidelines for Americans" (NAEPP 2007). In other words, patients need "to consume diets with more fruits, vegetables, and whole grains, and eat less solid fats (saturated fat, trans fat), salt, and added sugars" (NAEPP 2007). This ensures a healthier lifestyle that may make patients less susceptible to developing asthma and other diseases.

8.3 FOOD GROUPS AND DIETARY PATTERNS IN ASTHMA MANAGEMENT

The dietary patterns described in this section may help patients treat their asthma by preventing or reducing the intensity of asthmatic episodes among other symptoms.

8.3.1 Food Groups to Consider Avoiding or Limiting

- *Omega-6 fatty acids*: Omega-6 fatty acids are high in several oils, including corn oil, soybean oil, grape seed oil, margarine oil, and sunflower oil, to name a few. The increased global asthma burden has been partly blamed on an increase in the consumption of omega-6 fatty acids and the decreased consumption of omega-3 fatty acids (Black and Sharpe 1997). In addition, studies have shown that high omega-6 fatty acid intake is associated with increased allergies (Miles and Calder 2014).
- *Dairy products and eggs*: Food allergies affect almost 10% of school-going children and their prevalence is on the rise (Turner and Boyle 2014). Eggs and dairy products have been associated with asthma and milk allergy. Egg allergy is the second-most common allergy, next to cow milk allergy. It is mediated by immunoglobulin E (IgE) and most children outgrow this allergy by the age of 16 years (Hasan et al. 2013). Forty-two allergens found in egg yolk may play an important role in this allergy. Egg allergy can cause asthma, urticaria, rhinitis, and atopic dermatitis among other conditions (Dhanapala et al. 2015). Cow milk allergy is also very prevalent worldwide. In the event of a severe allergic reaction to dairy products, especially anaphylaxis, immunotherapy has been beneficial as a treatment (Elizur et al. 2015). Also, early life exposure to unpasteurized milk has been shown to have a protective affect against atopy and asthma and should be considered (Sozanska et al. 2013, 2014).
- *Salt*: There is wide variation in the use of salt among different ethnic groups. A higher salt intake has been associated with asthma. Dietary salt has also been shown to increase airway inflammation, especially following exercise (Mickleborough et al. 2005). Attempts have been focused toward reducing dietary sodium; however, in a Cochrane meta-analysis, researchers failed to find evidence that dietary sodium reduction can reduce asthma (Pogson and McKeever 2011). Despite the unclear data, it is still suggested that patients consume salt in moderation to avoid cardiovascular disease complications such as hypertension.
- *Food additives and preservatives*: Asthma often occurs in 5% of the people who have food allergies and many food allergies are caused by food additives (Ozol and Mete 2008). There are several preservatives and additives used in frozen and canned foods. Patients with a history of allergies and asthma should be especially cautious when consuming frozen and canned foods, because the preservatives and additives may make their symptoms worse. Sulfites have been widely used as preservatives in the food and pharmaceutical industries. Any form of sulfite exposure has been shown

to cause allergic reactions and worsen asthma. Though the sensitivity may vary, patients with severe asthma are generally affected more than others (Vally et al. 2009). A reaction to food additives should always be suspected in patients with severe or uncontrollable asthma, or in patients with a history of worsening asthma symptoms after consuming certain commercially prepared foods as opposed to home-prepared organic food. Testing has not been shown to be effective in diagnosing reactions to food preservatives. If the index of suspicion is high, avoidance can help identify the harmful additive products more effectively (Wilson and Bahna 2005).

- *Soda*: A recent study by Park and coworkers on 15,960 high school children showed the link between regular soda intake and asthma. The odds of having asthma were higher among students who drank more than two sodas per day when compared with those who did not drink soda (Park et al. 2013).

In addition to the agents discussed earlier, which can possibly exacerbate asthma, it is advisable to avoid any food products that can worsen an individual's asthma symptoms.

8.3.2 FOODS WITH POTENTIALLY BENEFICIAL EFFECTS

- *Flavonoids*: Shaheen and coworkers found that after controlling for confounding factors, selenium and red wine consumption were negatively associated with asthma. The beneficial effects of selenium (found in apples) and red wine may point toward the role of flavonoids in asthma treatment (Shaheen et al. 2001). Resveratrol, a compound found in red wine, may be responsible for helping patients with asthma due to its antioxidant and anti-inflammatory properties (Kamholz 2006).
- *Omega-3 fatty acids*: These compounds are found in fish oil and have been postulated to have a beneficial role in asthma due to their anti-inflammatory properties, but the exact mechanism of the effect is unknown (Miyata and Arita 2015). Several studies have shown the beneficial effects of fish oil consumption during pregnancy and lactation by decreasing allergy and atopy, as well as its protective role in early childhood (Antova et al. 2003; Hoppu et al. 2005; Kim et al. 2005; Sausenthaler et al. 2007). On the other hand, a case control study showed that dietary omega-3 fatty acids do not have protective effects, whereas a higher level of erythrocyte membrane linoleic acid was associated with reduced asthma risk (Broadfield et al. 2004). In addition, several other studies have shown inconsistent effects of fish oil on asthma (Burns et al. 2007; Miyata and Arita 2015; Woods et al. 2004). For example, Kitz and colleagues (2010) demonstrated that a low level of omega-3 fatty acid intake was associated with increased respiratory symptoms. Thus, no conclusion can be drawn from the data in the literature on the beneficial effects of omega-3 fatty acids, although some of the data suggests that if a patient is deficient in omega-3 fatty acids, their risk of asthma increases. Omega-3 fatty acids possess anti-inflammatory properties by virtue of docosahexaenoic acid (DHA) and eicosapentaenoic acid

(EPA), which have shown to be beneficial for asthma patients (Han et al. 2015; Miyata and Arita 2015). For practical purposes, it can be said that an adequate dietary requirement should be met for omega-3 fatty acids to avoid an increased risk of allergies or asthma.

- *Caffeine*: Caffeine has been shown to have a weak bronchodilatory effect on respiratory muscles (Welsh et al. 2010). A Cochrane database analysis of all available studies concluded that caffeine does modestly improve airway function (up to 4 h) in patients with asthma (Welsh et al. 2010).

- *Vitamin B_6*: Vitamin B_6 is found in sunflower seeds, pistachio nuts, bananas, avocados, energy drinks, cooked tuna, sirloin, pork, turkey, and chicken, to name a few sources. Vitamin B_6 plays an important role in homocysteine metabolism. An increase in homocysteine levels has been shown to be associated with asthma (Ubbink et al. 1996). Consuming foods rich in vitamin B_6 leads to an increase in vitamin B levels and a decrease in homocysteine levels (Tucker et al. 2004).

- *Vitamins C and E*: Several fruits and vegetables are rich in vitamins C and E. They are found in several foods, plants, and vegetables, such as kiwi, garlic, endives, sunflower seeds, sweet potatoes, carrot, mustard greens, and avocados. In an Italian study, investigators found that the intake of kiwi fruit and citrus fruit offered a protective effect against asthma, especially in children with history of asthma (Forastiere et al. 2000). In addition, sunflower seeds, which have significant amounts of vitamin E, have been shown to be beneficial for asthma sufferers in a mouse model, though further studies are needed (Heo et al. 2008). Sweet potatoes have also been recommended for asthma due to their high content of vitamin C and potassium. Pink, orange, and yellow varieties also have beta-carotene, which has a protective effect, but no controlled studies have demonstrated its benefit. Kale or borecole belongs to the plant species *Brassica oleracea*. It is commonly consumed as a vegetable and has been postulated to have a protective effect against asthma. Studies in an animal model have confirmed its benefit (Kabiri Rad et al. 2013). Avocado has been postulated to have many functions, from softening skin to alleviating asthma symptoms. It has a very high concentration of glutathione and vitamin E. Glutathione has been shown to have a protective effect against free radical damage and it is helpful in preventing bronchoconstriction (Blonder et al. 2014; Fatani 2014; Khatri et al. 2014). It is suggested that patients with severe latex allergies avoid avocado, kiwi, and banana, as allergic reactions and anaphylaxis have been seen in those situations (Abrams et al. 2011; Gawchik 2011; Isola et al. 2003).

- *Quercetin*: Eating apples or drinking apple juice has been shown to have a protective effect against asthma due to the bioflavonoid component quercetin. Quercetin has been shown to have a protective effect both in animal models (Oliveira et al. 2015) and humans (Sakai-Kashiwabara and Asano 2013; Townsend and Emala 2013). In addition, quercetin has also been able to suppress eosinophil counts, suggesting an important role in eosinophil-mediated allergic asthma (Sakai-Kashiwabara and Asano 2013).

- *Carotenoids*: Carotenoids are red, orange, and yellow plant pigments occurring naturally in several plants (fruits and vegetables), such as endives, sweet potatoes, tomatoes, kale, cantaloupes, and carrots to name a few. Beta-carotene, lycopene, and lutein are all different varieties of carotenoids. Carotenoids have a large amount of vitamin A. The protective effect of vitamin A against asthma has been controversial. It is thought to have an effect via its antioxidant properties (Ferreira et al. 2014; McKeever and Britton 2004).
- *Magnesium*: Magnesium has been used as a treatment for severe asthma. Some studies have shown it to be beneficial, whereas other randomized trials have found no benefit in the treatment of severe asthma (Alansari et al. 2015; Petrov et al. 2014; Singhi et al. 2014). The discussion of these studies is beyond the scope of this chapter. However, magnesium has been shown to have a bronchodilatory effect and an anti-inflammatory effect. It also stimulates nitric oxide and prostacyclin production, which may help to reduce asthma symptoms (Bichara 2009). Magnesium is found in a number of common foods, such as spinach, squash, pumpkin, fish, soy beans, avocado, dried fruit, brown rice, and so on.
- *Lycopene*: Lycopene is found in abundance in tomatoes. It is also found in guava, pink grapefruit, and watermelon. It acts by virtue of its antioxidant and anti-inflammatory properties. Lycopene was found to be beneficial in asthma through the use of an animal model. It was shown to decrease Th2 responses (Hazlewood et al. 2011). In the PLAVA trial in humans, lycopene- and vitamin A–containing foods were found to be beneficial among patients with asthma (Riccioni et al. 2007).

Table 8.1 summarizes the possible food groups, their nutritional roles in asthma, and their modes of action.

Table 8.2 summarizes the foods and nutrients that should be limited as well as the ones that should be consumed in relation to asthma.

8.3.3 Dietary Patterns That May Improve Symptoms

- *Western diet*: A number of studies have been conducted with the goal of determining the effect of a standard Western diet on asthma incidence, prevalence, and morbidity. One review, conducted by Brigham and colleagues, discusses 10 observational studies from North America, Europe, and Asia (Brigham et al. 2015). This review, which characterizes the Western diet as a "high intake of processed meats and refined grains, high-fat dairy products, and sugary desserts and drinks," concludes that "current evidence does not support an association between a Western diet and incident or prevalent adult asthma but does suggest a possible link between a Western diet pattern and adult asthma morbidity" (Brigham et al. 2015). Another observational study conducted on a large group of French females by Varraso and coworkers (2009) concluded that the Western diet, defined similarly, is associated with an increased frequency of asthma attacks

TABLE 8.1
Role of Food Groups and Nutrients in Asthma and Their Mechanisms of Action

Magnesium	Bronchodilator and anti-inflammatory effect; stabilizes T cells; inhibits mast cell degranulation; stimulates nitric oxide and prostacyclin
Vitamin A	Antioxidant
Vitamin C	Antioxidant; prostaglandin inhibitor
Vitamin E	Antioxidant; inhibition of IgE; membrane stabilization
Vitamin B_6	Increase in homocysteine level; maintenance of red cell membrane
Lycopene	Antioxidant and anti-inflammatory
Quercetin	Immunomodulatory and anti-inflammatory
Rosmarinic acid	Decreases proinflammatory mediators such as myeloperoxidase, adenosine deaminase, nitrate, and IL-17A; increases the anti-inflammatory IL-10
Ginger	Anti-inflammation by inhibiting Th2 mediator; decreases inflammatory mediator IL-4 and IL-5; also inhibits phosphodiesterase PDE4D and cytoskeletal protein
Turmeric	Anti-inflammatory and antifibrotic; blocks Notch 1 and 2 receptors
Zinc	Antioxidant; action on superoxide dismutase
Omega-3 fatty acid	Anti-inflammatory via docosahexaenoic acid and eicosapentaenoic acid
Flavonoids	Antioxidants; mast cell stabilization
Carotenoids	Antioxidants

TABLE 8.2
Foods and Nutrients: Their Effect on Asthma

Food Groups/Nutrients to Consider Avoiding or Limiting	Food Groups with Potential Benefits
Omega-6 fatty acid	Omega-3 fatty acid
Dairy products and eggs	Vitamin A, C, E, B_6
Avocado/banana/kiwi in patients with latex allergy	Lycopene
Salt	Quercetin
Food additives *and* preservatives (sulfites)	Rosemary (rosmarinic acid)
Soda	Ginger and turmeric
Western diet	Zinc
	Magnesium-containing foods
	Carotenoids
	Fruits and vegetables
	Mediterranean diet

(OR 1.79, 95% CI 1.11–3.73) but not with an increased incidence of asthma. While there is obviously still some uncertainty, it is fairly safe to conclude that an unhealthy Western diet probably exacerbates asthma symptoms and is thus not beneficial with regard to managing them.

- *Nuts, wine, fish, fruit, and vegetables*: Patients who adhered to a dietary pattern involving high quantities of nuts and wine showed a decreased risk of reporting frequent asthma attacks (OR 0.65, 95% CI 0.31–0.96) (Varraso et al. 2009). A recent 2015 study by Barros and colleagues confirms the detrimental effect of high-fat, high-sugar, and high-salt diets and proposes the beneficial effects of diets high in fish, fruit, and vegetables both for patients with current asthma symptoms (OR 0.84, 95% CI 0.73–0.98) and for patients currently taking asthma medication (OR 0.84, 95% CI 0.72–0.98) (Barros et al. 2015).

- *Mediterranean diet*: The classic Mediterranean diet has also been a source of great interest due to its potential protective effect against asthma symptoms. Chatzi and colleagues (2007) conducted the first study on the association between a Mediterranean diet and the occurrence of asthma among children in Crete in 2007. The study defined a Mediterranean diet as "characterized by an increased intake of plant foods, such as fruits and vegetables, bread and cereals (primarily whole grain), legumes and nuts," with olive oil as the primary source of fat, and found that strict adherence to this diet protected strongly against allergic rhinitis (OR 0.34, 95% CI 0.18–0.64) but only modestly against wheezing and atopy (Chatzi et al. 2007). Also of interest, the researchers concluded that increased consumption of nuts decreased the reported amount of wheezing (OR 0.46, 95% CI 0.20–0.98), while increased consumption of margarine had the opposite effect with regard to wheezing (OR 2.19, 95% CI 1.01–4.82) as well as rhinitis (OR 2.10, 95% CI 1.31–3.37) (Chatzi et al. 2007). De Batlle and collaborators (2008) conducted a very similar study on a group of Mexican children. It was found that the consumption of a Mediterranean diet was inversely associated with asthma, wheezing, rhinitis, sneezing, and watery eyes (de Batlle et al. 2008). The results of these studies all demonstrate the necessity for the increased reliance on diet-based intervention for asthma patients.

A meta-analysis by Nurmatov and colleagues (2011), which conducted a search through 11 databases, coming up with 62 studies, mainly case control or cohort design, concluded that the evidence, though weak, was supportive of a diet containing vitamins A, D, and E, zinc, fruits, vegetables, and also a Mediterranean diet for use in asthma prevention.

8.4 HOME REMEDIES FOR ASTHMA

Some of the foods that can be considered as remedies for asthma are

- *Garlic*: Garlic has been shown to help in allergy-mediated asthma. The effect is thought to be due to diallyl disulfide (DADS), one of the major compounds in garlic. DADS has been shown to decrease the expression of proinflammatory proteins and enhance the expression of antioxidant proteins (Shin et al. 2013).
- *Ginger*: Ginger has been implicated to have a beneficial role in asthma due to its anti-inflammatory properties. It inhibits the Th2-mediated immune response, which is evident by a decrease in IL-4 and IL-5 levels in

bronchoalveolar fluid (Khan et al. 2015). Another study has shown that the components of ginger can potentiate the effects of beta agonists by causing the relaxation of the airway smooth muscle (Townsend et al. 2014).

- *Turmeric*: Turmeric (*Curcuma longa*) is known for its anti-inflammatory and anti-fibrotic properties. It blocks Notch 1 and Notch 2 receptors, which play an important role in inflammation. It has been shown to be of benefit in asthma (Chong et al. 2014). In addition, it also decreases the inflammation in asthma by blocking the Nrf2/HO-1 pathway (Liu et al. 2015). Studies have also shown curcumin (which is a principal component in turmeric) to be helpful as an adjunct therapy to medication and to improve the forced expiratory volume one second (FEV1) (Abidi et al. 2014; Glickman-Simon and Lindsay 2013; Jang et al. 2014).

- *Rosmarinic acid*: Rosemary has been used to flavor fish, meat, and even bread. It is especially native to the Indian and Mediterranean regions. It has been shown to have anti-inflammatory properties. It decreases proinflammatory mediators such as myeloperoxidase, adenosine-deaminase, nitrite, interleukin (IL) 17A and has been shown to increase anti-inflammatory markers such as IL-10 (da Rosa et al. 2013). In addition, it has been shown that rosemary and its constituents, specifically caffeic acid, can have a role in the prevention and treatment of asthma (al-Sereiti et al. 1999).

8.5   NUTRITIONAL COUNSELING

In terms of asthma as it relates to nutrition, it is imperative that a good nutritional history is taken. To achieve this, physicians should ask detailed questions about the composition of a patient's daily caloric intake. Patients should be asked about the number of meals and snacks they consume over 24 hours, how often they eat out (and where they go), as well as the frequency of consumption of meats, poultry, fish, fruits, vegetables, dairy, water, and sweets. Finally, as part of a nutritional history, it is critical to ask about the intake of herbal products, vitamins, or exogenous supplements of any kind (Hark and Deen 1999).

The diagnosis of asthma is generally made using a number of tools. The initial investigation may often start with a detailed family and past medical history. From here, physical exam features such as wheezing, allergic skin conditions, runny nose, or swollen nasal passages may all indicate a diagnosis of asthma. Various diagnostic tests such as spirometry, bronchoprovocation, and allergy testing may be used to confirm asthma. There are also a number of other tests that may be completed to rule out diseases such as gastroesophageal reflux disease (GERD) or obstructive sleep apnea (OSA), which may present with similar symptoms as asthma.

Nutritional management is important; physicians should take a detailed nutritional history and seek to optimize a given patient's diet to insure long-term health. Diet plans can be modified according to recommendations from the American Heart Association (Krauss et al. 1996). Finally, patients with acute or chronic diseases that require complex dietary requirements should consult with a registered dietician (Hark and Deen 1999).

8.6 CASE STUDIES

8.6.1 CASE STUDY 1

A 31-year-old female and her 5-year-old son visit a physician at the clinic for a well-child examination. The boy is growing well and has been consistently meeting all of his developmental milestones; additionally, his past medical/surgical history is unremarkable. After addressing activity, diet, sleep, and safety concerns for the patient, a physical exam is completed. Finally, near the end of the visit the patient's mother brings up some questions she has about asthma. She claims there is a strong history of asthma on her side of the family, and was wondering if any alterations in her son's diet may prevent him from developing asthma. As a health-care professional, what information can you provide to the patient's mother about nutrition and asthma?

Discussion: Asthma is defined as a chronic disorder of the lungs associated with hyper-reactive airway responsiveness and a variable pattern of upper-airway obstruction. Clinical features of asthma include wheezing, breathlessness, persistent cough, chest tightness, and shortness of breath. Asthma as a whole is a relatively common chronic disease, with upward of 300 million people affected worldwide. By 2025 there may be an additional 100 million cases (Masoli et al. 2004). Between the years 2001–2003 there was an average of 20 million people with asthma living in the United States each year, 6.2 million of them being children (Moorman et al. 2007). As no curative therapy currently exists, clinical management of asthma is currently done through a combination of bronchodilators, steroids, and anti-inflammatory therapies. The connection between asthma and nutrition has remained a topic of clinical research interest for many years. The observational and limited intervention data suggests that while there are associations between diet and asthma, the nature, timing, and therapeutic potential of these associations are not very clear (NAEPP 2007). In fact, any and all observed associations may simply be due to confounding external variables. However, from the available data, it appears that the supplementation of one's diet with vitamin C, vitamin E, selenium, and n-3-polyunsaturated fatty acid (n-3-PUFA) may have minimal clinical benefits in preventing asthma. In relation to this case study, currently it is believed that manipulating the levels of n-3-PUFA intake during pregnancy can reduce the chance of childhood asthma and other allergies (Allan and Devereux 2011). Additionally, several cohort studies have reported low maternal vitamin E, vitamin D, and zinc intake during pregnancy tend to be associated with increased likelihood of childhood wheezing and asthma (Devereux et al. 2006; Litonjua et al. 2006; Miyake et al. 2010). Generally, vitamin E is consumed in foods that also contain other nutrients. In fact, any decrease in the incidence of childhood asthma may be due to the interactions of the various nutrients consumed more so than the effects of vitamin E alone (Allan and Devereux 2011). A Mediterranean diet has also been shown to be beneficial in asthma. Ultimately, the role of dietary interventions to prevent childhood asthma can only be understood through further intervention studies. Following the advice discussed above, may marginally improve the prevention of asthma during childhood, but these results remain largely variable.

8.6.2 CASE STUDY 2

You are talking to a 14-year-old male and his father about how well his asthma is currently managed using his prescribed medications. Aside from asthma, the patient's past medical/surgical history is unremarkable. His only prescribed medications are for asthma control. During the exam, the patient has many questions regarding his asthma, including how common it is, what causes it, how his current medications prevent asthmatic flare-ups, and what foods he should avoid to control them. What general information can be provided to answer the patient's questions regarding asthma, specifically regarding medications used and foods to be avoided for asthmatic control?

Discussion: Asthma affects people of all ages and ethnicities; however, the prevalence of asthma has steadily increased over several decades in both Westernized and less developed countries. These favorable trends have generally been attributed to the more widespread use of inhaled corticosteroids as well as a host of other highly effective medications used to control asthma. Asthma is generally due to a combination of reactive airway smooth-muscle contraction and bronchial irritation/inflammation that causes secondary tightening of the chest, shortness of breath, coughing, and wheezing (Shore 2004). Therapeutic strategies essentially revolve around controlling each of these different variables to prevent asthma attacks. As a whole, drugs used to prevent asthma attacks are generally classified according to their predominant effect. Examples include medications that cause airway smooth-muscle relaxation (bronchodilators) or that decrease airway inflammation (anti-inflammatory agents). There exists a relative hierarchy in terms of medications prescribed for asthma control, with increasing strength/coverage as an asthmatic pattern becomes more unpredictable. At the lowest level (the most benign cases of asthma) are SABAs; slightly above this are inhaled steroids or leukotriene receptor antagonists. If a patient's asthma still remains aggressive, combination therapy may be required. An inhaled steroid with a LABA or leukotriene modifier is a common combination. If at this point, the asthma is still uncontrolled, triple therapy in the form of an inhaled steroid, a LABA, and a leukotriene modifier is recommended (Fanta 2009). Finally, in rare cases omalizumab, an anti-IgE monoclonal antibody, is approved for patients over 12 years of age, especially those who have elevated levels of IgE (Fanta 2009). Treatment with omalizumab has been shown to decrease asthmatic exacerbations, even among patients who may already be taking medications to control their asthma (Humbert et al. 2005). The greatest drawback to this drug, however, is its price, as its cost is in the neighborhood of USD 10,000–30,000 annually (Bousquet et al. 2007). Information about foods that should be considered limiting for asthma control are detailed in Section 8.3.1 and Table 8.2.

REFERENCES

Abidi, A., Gupta, S., Agarwal, M., Bhalla, H. L., and Saluja, M. 2014. Evaluation of efficacy of curcumin as an add-on therapy in patients of bronchial asthma. *J Clin Diagn Res* 8(8): HC19-24.

Abrams, E. M., Becker, A. B., and Gerstner, T. V. 2011. Anaphylaxis related to avocado ingestion: A case and review. *Allergy Asthma Clin Immunol* 7(1): 12.

Adams, P. F., Kirzinger, W. K., and Martinez, M. 2013. Summary health statistics for the U.S. population: National Health Interview Survey, 2012. *Vital Health Stat* 10(259): 1–95.

Alansari, K., Ahmed, W., Davidson, B. L., Alamri, M., Zakaria, I., and Alrifaai, M. 2015. Nebulized magnesium for moderate and severe pediatric asthma: A randomized trial. *Pediatr Pulmonol* 50(12): 1191–1199.

Allan, K., and Devereux, G. 2011. Diet and asthma: Nutrition implications from prevention to treatment. *J Am Diet Assoc* 111(2): 258–268.

al-Sereiti, M. R., Abu-Amer, K. M., and Sen, P. 1999. Pharmacology of rosemary (*Rosmarinus officinalis* Linn.) and its therapeutic potentials. *Indian J Exp Biol* 37(2): 124–130.

Antova, T., S. Pattenden, B. Nikiforov, G. S. Leonardi, B. Boeva, T. Fletcher, P. Rudnai et al. (2003). Nutrition and respiratory health in children in six Central and Eastern European countries. *Thoraxn* 58(3): 231–236.

Barrett, M. L., Wier, L. M., and Washington, R. 2006. Trends in pediatric and adult hospital stays for Asthma, 2000–2010. Healthcare Cost and Utilization Project (HCUP) Statistical Briefs, Statistical Brief #169. Rockville, MD: Department of Health and Human Services, Public Health Service, Agency for Health Care Policy and Research.

Barros, R., A. Moreira, P. Padrão, V. H. Teixeira, P. Carvalho, L. Delgado, C. Lopes, M. Severo, and P. Moreira. 2015. Dietary patterns and asthma prevalence, incidence and control. *Clin Exp Allergy* 45(11): 1673–1680.

Bateman, E. D., Boushey, H. A., Bousquet, J., Busse, W. W., Clark, T. J. H., Pauwels, R. A., and Pedersen, S. E. 2004. Can guideline-defined asthma control be achieved? The Gaining Optimal Asthma Control study. *Am J Respir Crit Care Med* 170(8): 836–844.

Baxi, S. N., and Phipatanakul, W. 2010. The role of allergen exposure and avoidance in asthma. *Adolesc Med State Art Rev* 21(1): 57–71, viii–ix.

Bichara, M. D., and Goldman, R. D. 2009. Magnesium for treatment of asthma in children. *Can Fam Physician* 55(9): 887–889.

Black, P. N., and Sharpe, S. 1997. Dietary fat and asthma: Is there a connection? *Eur Respir J* 10(1): 6–12.

Blonder, J. P., Mutka, S. C., Sun, X., Qiu, J., Green, L. H., Mehra, N. K., Boyanapalli, R. et al. 2014. Pharmacologic inhibition of S-nitrosoglutathione reductase protects against experimental asthma in BALB/c mice through attenuation of both bronchoconstriction and inflammation. *BMC Pulm Med* 14: 3.

Bousquet, J., Rabe, K., Humbert, M., Chung, K. F., Berger, W., Fox, H., Ayre, G. et al. 2007. Predicting and evaluating response to omalizumab in patients with severe allergic asthma. *Respir Med* 101(7): 1483–1492.

Brigham, E. P., Kolahdooz, F., Hansel, N., Breysse, P. N., Davis, M., Sharma, S., Matsui, E. C., Diette, G., and McCormack, M. C. 2015. Association between Western diet pattern and adult asthma: A focused review. *Ann Allergy Asthma Immunol* 114(4): 273–280.

Broadfield, E. C., McKeever, T. M., Whitehurst, A., Lewis, S. A., Lawson, N., Britton, J., and Fogarty, A. 2004. A case-control study of dietary and erythrocyte membrane fatty acids in asthma. *Clin Exp Allergy* 34(8): 1232–1236.

Buie, V. C., Owings, M. F., DeFrances, C. J., and Golosinskiy, A. 2010. National hospital discharge survey: 2006 annual summary. *Vital Health Stat* 13(168): 1–79.

Burns, J. S., Dockery, D. W., Neas, L. M., Schwartz, J., Coull, B. A., Raizenne, M., and Speizer, F. E. 2007. Low dietary nutrient intakes and respiratory health in adolescents. *Chest* 132(1): 238–245.

Busse, W. W., and Lemanske, R. F., Jr. 2001. Asthma. *N Engl J Med* 344(5): 350–362.

Chandra, R. K. 1997. Five-year follow-up of high-risk infants with family history of allergy who were exclusively breast-fed or fed partial whey hydrolysate, soy, and conventional cow's milk formulas. *J Pediatr Gastroenterol Nutr* 24(4): 380–388.

Chatzi, L., Apostolaki, G., Bibakis, I., Skypala, I., Bibaki-Liakou, V., Tzanakis, N., Kogevinas, M., and Cullinan, P. 2007. Protective effect of fruits, vegetables and the Mediterranean diet on asthma and allergies among children in Crete. *Thorax* 62(8): 677–683.

Chen, E., and Miller, G. E. 2007. Stress and inflammation in exacerbations of asthma. *Brain Behav Immun* 21(8): 993–999.

Chen, X. J., Zhang, Y. H., Wang, D. H., and Liu, Y. L. 2015. Effects of body mass index and serum inflammatory cytokines on asthma control in children with asthma. *Zhongguo Dang Dai Er Ke Za Zhi* 17(7): 698–701.

Chong, L., Zhang, W., Nie, Y., Yu, G., Liu, L., Lin, L., Wen, S., Zhu, L., and Li, C. 2014. Protective effect of curcumin on acute airway inflammation of allergic asthma in mice through Notch1-GATA3 signaling pathway. *Inflammation* 37(5): 1476–1485.

Cohn, L., Elias, J. A., and Chupp, G. L. 2004. Asthma: Mechanisms of disease persistence and progression. *Annu Rev Immunol* 22: 789–815.

da Rosa, J. S., Facchin, B. M., Bastos, J., Siqueira, M. A., Micke, G. A., Dalmarco, E. M., Pizzolatti, M. G., and Fröde, T. S. (2013). Systemic administration of *Rosmarinus officinalis* attenuates the inflammatory response induced by carrageenan in the mouse model of pleurisy. *Planta Med* 79(17): 1605–1614.

Davis, A. M., Kreutzer, R., Lipsett, M., King, G., and Shaikh, N. 2006. Asthma prevalence in Hispanic and Asian American ethnic subgroups: Results from the California Healthy Kids Survey. *Pediatrics* 118(2): e363–370.

de Batlle, J., Garcia-Aymerich, J., Barraza-Villarreal, A., Anto, J. M., and Romieu, I. 2008. Mediterranean diet is associated with reduced asthma and rhinitis in Mexican children. *Allergy* 63(10): 1310–1316.

Devereux, G., Turner, S. W., Craig, L. C. A., McNeill, G., Martindale, S., Harbour, P. J., Helms, P. J., and Seaton, A. 2006. Low maternal vitamin E intake during pregnancy is associated with asthma in 5-year-old children. *Am J Respir Crit Care Med* 174(5): 499–507.

Dhanapala, P., De Silva, C., Doran, T., and Suphioglu, C. 2015. Cracking the egg: An insight into egg hypersensitivity. *Mol Immunol* 66(2): 375–383.

Elizur, A., Goldberg, M. R., Levy, M. B., Nachshon, L., and Katz, Y. 2015. Oral immunotherapy in cow's milk allergic patients: Course and long-term outcome according to asthma status. *Ann Allergy Asthma Immunol* 114(3): 240–244 e241.

Fanta, C. H. 2009. Asthma. *N Engl J Med* 360(10): 1002–1014.

Fatani, S. H. 2014. Biomarkers of oxidative stress in acute and chronic bronchial asthma. *J Asthma* 51(6): 578–584.

Ferreira, C. A., de Souza, F. I., Melges, A. P., Fonseca, F. A., Sole, D., and Sarni, R. O. 2014. Retinol, beta-carotene, oxidative stress, and metabolic syndrome components in obese asthmatic children. *Pediatr Allergy Immunol* 25(3): 292–294.

Forastiere, F., Pistelli, R., Sestini, P., Fortes, C., Renzoni, E., Rusconi, F., Dell'Orco, V., Ciccone, G., Bisanti, L., and SIDRIA Collaborative Group. 2000. Consumption of fresh fruit rich in vitamin C and wheezing symptoms in children. *Thorax* 55(4): 283–288.

Ford, E. S. 2005. The epidemiology of obesity and asthma. *J Allergy Clin Immunol* 115(5): 897–909.

Gawchik, S. M. 2011. Latex allergy. *Mt Sinai J Med* 78(5): 759–772.

Gdalevich, M., Mimouni, D., and Mimouni, M. 2001. Breast-feeding and the risk of bronchial asthma in childhood: A systematic review with meta-analysis of prospective studies. *J Pediatr* 139(2): 261–266.

Glickman-Simon, R., and Lindsay, T. 2013. Yoga for back pain, cranberry for cystitis prevention, soy isoflavones for hot flashes, curcumin for pre-diabetes, and breathing retraining for asthma. *Explore (NY)* 9(4): 251–254.

Global Initiative for Asthma. 2011. *Global Strategy for Asthma Management and Prevention.* Global Initiative for Asthma. www.globalasthmanetwork.org.

Gold, D. R., and Wright, R. 2005. Population disparities in asthma. *Annu Rev Public Health* 26: 89–113.

Groth, S. W., Rhee, H., and Kitzman, H. 2015. Relationships among obesity, physical activity and sedentary behavior in young adolescents with and without lifetime asthma. *J Asthma* 53(1):19–24.

Han, Y. Y., Forno, E., Holguin, F., and Celedon, J. C. 2015. Diet and asthma: An update. *Curr Opin Allergy Clin Immunol* 15(4): 369–374.

Hark, L., and Deen, D., Jr. 1999. Taking a nutrition history: A practical approach for family physicians. *Am Fam Physician* 59(6):1521–1528, 1531–1522.

Hasan, S. A., Wells, R. D., and Davis, C. M. 2013. Egg hypersensitivity in review. *Allergy Asthma Proc* 34(1): 26–32.

Hazlewood, L. C., Wood, L. G., Hansbro, P. M., and Foster, P. S. 2011. Dietary lycopene supplementation suppresses Th2 responses and lung eosinophilia in a mouse model of allergic asthma. *J Nutr Biochem* 22(1): 95–100.

Heo, J.-C., Woo, S.-U., Kweon, M., Park, J.-Y., Lee, H. K., Son, M., Rho, J.-R., and Lee, S.-H. 2008. Aqueous extract of the *Helianthus annuus* seed alleviates asthmatic symptoms *in vivo*. *Int J Mol Med* 21(1): 57–61.

Holgate, S. T., and Polosa, R. 2006. The mechanisms, diagnosis, and management of severe asthma in adults. *Lancet* 368(9537): 780–793.

Hoppu, U., Rinne, M., Lampi, A. M., and Isolauri, E. 2005. Breast milk fatty acid composition is associated with development of atopic dermatitis in the infant. *J Pediatr Gastroenterol Nutr* 41(3): 335–338.

Humbert, M., Beasley, R., Ayres, J., Slavin, R., Hebert, J., Bousquet, J., Beeh, K.-M. et al. 2005. Benefits of omalizumab as add-on therapy in patients with severe persistent asthma who are inadequately controlled despite best available therapy (GINA 2002 step 4 treatment): INNOVATE. *Allergy* 60(3): 309–316.

Isola, S., Ricciardi, L., Saitta, S., Fedele, R., Mazzeo, L., Fogliani, O., Gangemi, S., and Purello-D'Ambrosio, F. 2003. Latex allergy and fruit cross-reaction in subjects who are nonatopic. *Allergy Asthma Proc* 24(3): 193–197.

Jang, D. J., Kim, S. T., Oh, E., and Lee, K. 2014. Enhanced oral bioavailability and antiasthmatic efficacy of curcumin using redispersible dry emulsion. *Biomed Mater Eng* 24(1): 917–930.

Kabiri Rad, M., Neamati, A., Boskabady, M. H., Mahdavi-Shahri, N., and Mahmoudabady, M. (2013). The preventive effect of *Brassica napus* L. oil on pathophysiological changes of respiratory system in experimental asthmatic rat. *Avicenna J Phytomed* 3(1): 56–63.

Kamholz, S. L. 2006. Wine, spirits and the lung: Good, bad or indifferent? *Trans Am Clin Climatol Assoc* 117: 129–145; discussion 145.

Khan, A. M., Shahzad, M., Raza Asim, M. B., Imran, M., and Shabbir, A. 2015. *Zingiber officinale* ameliorates allergic asthma via suppression of Th2-mediated immune response. *Pharm Biol* 53(3): 359–367.

Khatri, S. B., Peabody, J., Burwell, L., Harris, F., and Brown, L. S. 2014. Systemic antioxidants and lung function in asthmatics during high ozone season: A closer look at albumin, glutathione, and associations with lung function. *Clin Transl Sci* 7(4): 314–318.

Kim, J. L., Elfman, L., Mi, Y., Johansson, M., Smedje, G., and Norback, D. 2005. Current asthma and respiratory symptoms among pupils in relation to dietary factors and allergens in the school environment. *Indoor Air* 15(3): 170–182.

Kitz, R., Rose, M. A., Schubert, R., Beermann, C., Kaufmann, A., Böhles, H. J., Schulze, J., and Zielen, S. 2010. Omega-3 polyunsaturated fatty acids and bronchial inflammation in grass pollen allergy after allergen challenge. *Respir Med* 104(12): 1793–1798.

Krauss, R. M., Deckelbaum, R. J., Ernst, N., Fisher, E., Howard, B. V., Knopp, R. H., Kotchen, T. et al. 1996. Dietary guidelines for healthy American adults: A statement for health professionals from the Nutrition Committee, American Heart Association. *Circulation* 94(7): 1795–1800.

Lara, M., Akinbami, L., Flores, G., and Morgenstern, H. 2006. Heterogeneity of childhood asthma among Hispanic children: Puerto Rican children bear a disproportionate burden. *Pediatrics* 117(1): 43–53.

Litonjua, A. A., Rifas-Shiman, S. L., Ly, N. P., Tantisira, K. G., Rich-Edwards, J. W., Camargo, C. A., Weiss, S. T., Gillman, M. W., and Gold, D. R. 2006. Maternal antioxidant intake in pregnancy and wheezing illnesses in children at 2 y of age. *Am J Clin Nutr* 84(4): 903–911.

Liu, L., Shang, Y., Li, M., Han, X., Wang, J., and Wang, J. 2015. Curcumin ameliorates asthmatic airway inflammation by activating nuclear factor-E2-related factor 2/haem oxygenase (HO)-1 signalling pathway. *Clin Exp Pharmacol Physiol* 42(5): 520–529.

Lu, Y., Van Bever, H. P. S., Lim, T. K., Kuan, W. S., Thiam Goh, D. Y., Mahadevan, M., Sim, T. B., Ho, R., Larbi, A., and Ng, T. P. 2015. Obesity, asthma prevalence and IL-4: Roles of inflammatory cytokines, adiponectin and neuropeptide Y. *Pediatr Allergy Immunol* 26(6): 530–536.

Lugogo, N. L., and Kraft, M. 2006. Epidemiology of asthma. *Clin Chest Med* 27(1):1–15, v.

Masoli, M., Fabian, D., Holt, S., Beasley, R., and Global Initiative for Asthma. 2004. The global burden of asthma: Executive summary of the GINA Dissemination Committee report. *Allergy* 59(5): 469–478.

McKeever, T. M., and Britton, J. 2004. Diet and asthma. *Am J Respir Crit Care Med* 170(7): 725–729.

Mickleborough, T. D., Lindley, M. R., and Ray, S. 2005. Dietary salt, airway inflammation, and diffusion capacity in exercise-induced asthma. *Med Sci Sports Exerc* 37(6): 904–914.

Miles, E. A., and Calder, P. C. 2014. Omega-6 and omega-3 polyunsaturated fatty acids and allergic diseases in infancy and childhood. *Curr Pharm Des* 20(6): 946–953.

Miyake, Y., Sasaki, S., Tanaka, K., and Hirota, Y. 2010. Consumption of vegetables, fruit, and antioxidants during pregnancy and wheeze and eczema in infants. *Allergy* 65(6): 758–765.

Miyata, J., and Arita, M. 2015. Role of omega-3 fatty acids and their metabolites in asthma and allergic diseases. *Allergol Int* 64(1): 27–34.

Moorman, J. E., Rudd, R. A., Johnson, C. A., King, M., Minor, P., and Bailey, C. 2007. National surveillance for asthma: United States, 1980–2004. *MMWR Surveill Summ* 56(8): 1–54.

NAEPP. 1991. Guidelines for the diagnosis and management of asthma: National Heart, Lung, and Blood Institute; National Asthma Education Program; Expert Panel Report. *J Allergy Clin Immunol* 88(3 Pt 2): 425–534.

NAEPP. 2007. Expert Panel Report 3 (EPR-3): Guidelines for the diagnosis and management of asthma: Summary report 2007. *J Allergy Clin Immunol* 120(5 Suppl): S94–S138.

Nurmatov, U., Devereux, G., and Sheikh, A. 2011. Nutrients and foods for the primary prevention of asthma and allergy: Systematic review and meta-analysis. *J Allergy Clin Immunol* 127(3): 724–733 e721–730.

Oddy, W. H., Holt, P. G., Sly, P. D., Read, A. W., Landau, L. I., Stanley, F. J., Kendall, G. E., and Burton, P. R. 1999. Association between breast feeding and asthma in 6 year old children: Findings of a prospective birth cohort study. *BMJ* 319(7213): 815–819.

Oliveira, T. T., Campos, K. M., Cerqueira-Lima, A. T., Brasil Carneiro, T. C., da Silva Velozo, E., Melo, I. C. A. R., Figueiredo, E. A. et al. 2015. Potential therapeutic effect of *Allium cepa* L. and quercetin in a murine model of *Blomia tropicalis* induced asthma. *Daru* 23: 18.

Ozol, D., and Mete, E. 2008. Asthma and food allergy. *Curr Opin Pulm Med* 14(1): 9–12.

Park, S., Blanck, H. M., Sherry, B., Jones, S. E., and Pan, L. 2013. Regular-soda intake independent of weight status is associated with asthma among U.S. high school students. *J Acad Nutr Diet* 113(1): 106–111.

Petrov, V. I., Shishimorov, I. N., Perminov, A. A., and Nefedov, I. V. 2014. Influence of magnesium deficiency correction on the effectiveness of bronchial asthma pharmacotherapy in children. *Eksp Klin Farmakol* 77(8): 23–27.

Pogson, Z., and McKeever, T. 2011. Dietary sodium manipulation and asthma. *Cochrane Database Syst Rev* (3), CD000436.

Riccioni, G., Bucciarelli, T., Mancini, B., Di Ilio, C., Della Vecchia, R., and D'Orazio, N. 2007. Plasma lycopene and antioxidant vitamins in asthma: The PLAVA study. *J Asthma* 44(6): 429–432.

Sakai-Kashiwabara, M., and Asano, K. 2013. Inhibitory action of quercetin on eosinophil activation in vitro. *Evid Based Complement Alternat Med* 2013: 127105.

Sausenthaler, S., Koletzko, S., Schaaf, B., Lehmann, I., Borte, M., Herbarth, O., von Berg, A., Wichmann, H. E., Heinrich, J., and LISA Study Group. 2007. Maternal diet during pregnancy in relation to eczema and allergic sensitization in the offspring at 2 y of age. *Am J Clin Nutr* 85(2): 530–537.

Shaheen, S. O., Sterne, J. A., Thompson, R. L., Songhurst, C. E., Margetts, B. M., and Burney, P. G. 2001. Dietary antioxidants and asthma in adults: Population-based case-control study. *Am J Respir Crit Care Med* 164(10 Pt 1): 1823–1828.

Shin, I.-S., Hong, J., Jeon, C.-M., Shin, N.-R., Kwon, O.-K., Kim, H.-S., Kim, J.-C., Oh, S.-R., and Ahn, K.-S. 2013. Diallyl-disulfide, an organosulfur compound of garlic, attenuates airway inflammation via activation of the Nrf-2/HO-1 pathway and NF-kappaB suppression. *Food Chem Toxicol* 62: 506–513.

Shore, S. A. 2004. Airway smooth muscle in asthma: Not just more of the same. *N Engl J Med* 351(6): 531–532.

Singhi, S., Grover, S., Bansal, A., and Chopra, K. 2014. Randomised comparison of intravenous magnesium sulphate, terbutaline and aminophylline for children with acute severe asthma. *Acta Paediatr* 103(12): 1301–1306.

Sozanska, B., Blaszczyk, M., Pearce, N., and Cullinan, P. 2014. Atopy and allergic respiratory disease in rural Poland before and after accession to the European Union. *J Allergy Clin Immunol* 133(5): 1347–1353.

Sozanska, B., Pearce, N., Dudek, K., and Cullinan, P. 2013. Consumption of unpasteurized milk and its effects on atopy and asthma in children and adult inhabitants in rural Poland. *Allergy* 68(5): 644–650.

Stenius-Aarniala, B., Poussa, T., Kvarnstrom, J., Gronlund, E. L., Ylikahri, M., and Mustajoki, P. 2000. Immediate and long-term effects of weight reduction in obese people with asthma: Randomised controlled study. *BMJ* 320(7238): 827–832.

Strunk, R. C., Colvin, R., Bacharier, L. B., Fuhlbrigge, A., Forno, E., Arbelaez, A. M., Tantisira, K. G., and Childhood Asthma Management Program Research Group. 2015. Airway obstruction worsens in young adults with asthma who become obese. *J Allergy Clin Immunol Pract* 3(5): 765–771.

Sutherland, E. R. 2014. Linking obesity and asthma. *Ann N Y Acad Sci* 1311: 31–41.

Townsend, E. A., and Emala, C. W., Sr. 2013. Quercetin acutely relaxes airway smooth muscle and potentiates β-agonist-induced relaxation via dual phosphodiesterase inhibition of PLCβ and PDE4. *Am J Physiol Lung Cell Mol Physiol* 305(5): L396–403.

Townsend, E. A., Zhang, Y., Xu, C., Wakita, R., and Emala, C. W. (2014). Active components of ginger potentiate beta-agonist-induced relaxation of airway smooth muscle by modulating cytoskeletal regulatory proteins. *Am J Respir Cell Mol Biol* 50(1): 115–124.

Tucker, K. L., Olson, B., Bakun, P., Dallal, G. E., Selhub, J., and Rosenberg, I. H. 2004. Breakfast cereal fortified with folic acid, vitamin B-6, and vitamin B-12 increases vitamin concentrations and reduces homocysteine concentrations: A randomized trial. *Am J Clin Nutr* 79(5): 805–811.

Turner, P. J., and Boyle, R. J. (2014). Food allergy in children: What is new? *Curr Opin Clin Nutr Metab Care* 17(3): 285–293.

Ubbink, J. B., van der Merwe, A., Delport, R., Allen, R. H., Stabler, S. P., Riezler, R., and Vermaak, W. J. 1996. The effect of a subnormal vitamin B-6 status on homocysteine metabolism. *J Clin Invest* 98(1): 177–184.

Vally, H., Misso, N. L., and Madan, V. 2009. Clinical effects of sulphite additives. *Clin Exp Allergy* 39(11): 1643–1651.

Varraso, R., Kauffmann, F., Leynaert, B., Le Moual, N., Boutron-Ruault, M. C., Clavel-Chapelon, F., and Romieu, I. 2009. Dietary patterns and asthma in the E3N study. *Eur Respir J* 33(1): 33–41.

Wang, L., Wang, K., Gao, X., Paul, T. K., Cai, J., and Wang, Y. 2015. Sex difference in the association between obesity and asthma in U.S. adults: Findings from a national study. *Respir Med* 109(8): 955–962.

Weiss, S. T. 2005. Obesity: Insight into the origins of asthma. *Nat Immunol* 6(6): 537–539.

Welsh, E. J., Bara, A., Barley, E., and Cates, C. J. 2010. Caffeine for asthma. *Cochrane Database Syst Rev* (1): CD001112.

Wilson, B. G., and Bahna, S. L. 2005. Adverse reactions to food additives. *Ann Allergy Asthma Immunol* 95(6): 499–507; quiz 507, 570.

Woods, R. K., Raven, J. M., Walters, E. H., Abramson, M. J., and Thien, F. C. 2004. Fatty acid levels and risk of asthma in young adults. *Thorax* 59(2): 105–110.

World Health Organization. 2007. *Global Surveillance, Prevention and Control of Chronic Respiratory Diseases: A Comprehensive Approach*. Geneva: World Health Organization.

9 HEAL for Cancers

Shirin Anil and Redhwan Al Naggar

CONTENTS

9.1 INTRODUCTION TO CANCER

According to the U.S. National Library of Medicine, "cancer" is defined as a group of diseases in which an abnormal cell in any part of the body grows uncontrollably, invading the surrounding tissues. It can also spread to other parts of the body through the blood or lymphatic system (NIH—National Cancer Institute 2015), a process called "metastasis." The main types of cancers are

- *Carcinoma*: Originates in the skin or the lining of the internal organs.
- *Sarcoma*: Cancer of the bone, cartilage, muscles, blood vessels, fat, and other supportive and connective tissue.
- *Lymphoma and multiple myeloma*: Arises in the cells of the immune system.
- *Leukemia*: Starts from the blood-forming organs, such as bone marrow. The abnormal blood cells then enter into the bloodstream.
- *Cancer of the nervous system*: Originates in the tissue of the brain or spinal cord.

The history of cancer dates back to the ancient Egyptian era (3000 BC), when eight breast tumors were removed by cauterization with the help of a tool called a "fire drill". Later, the Greek physician Hippocrates (460–370 BC) coined the terms "carcinos" and "carcinoma" to refer to non-ulcer-forming and ulcer-forming tumors, respectively. In Greek, these words mean "crab" and may have been used for tumors due to their finger-like projections, giving them the appearance of a crab. The Roman physician Celsus (28–50 BC) modified Hippocrates's terminologies to the word "cancer," which is the Latin word for crab. The Greek physician Galen (130–200 AD) used the word "oncos" to describe tumors. Today, the study of cancers is called oncology and the physicians who treat cancers are called oncologists (American Cancer Society 2014a).

9.2 CANCER EPIDEMIOLOGY

The World Health Organization (WHO) reports that there are more than 100 types of cancers taking the lives of 8.2 million people annually, which accounts for 13% of all deaths globally, and 70% of these occur in Africa, Asia, and Central and South America. Approximately 14 million new cases of cancers are detected every year, 60% of which are diagnosed in these four regions of the world. The numbers of new cases are expected to rise by 70% in the next 20 years (WHO 2015a).

In 2012, 32.6 million people were living with cancer (within 5 years of diagnosis), the most common cancers in men being lung, prostate, colorectal, stomach, and liver; while in women these were breast, colorectal, lung, cervix uteri, and stomach cancers. The risk of getting cancer before the age of 75 years is 21% in males and 16.4% in females. The age-standardized incidence rate of cancers is 25% higher in males compared with females: 205 versus 165 per 100,000 persons per year (International Agency for Research on Cancer 2015).

9.3 WHAT CAUSES CANCER?

The transformation from a normal to an abnormal cancer-causing cell requires multiple stages, starting from a precancerous lesion and ending in a malignant tumor. Two main mechanisms have been postulated in cancer causation (Trichopoulos et al. 1996). The first is a mutation in certain types of genes called proto-oncogenes and tumor suppressor genes. Proto-oncogenes encourage cell growth and proliferation, while tumor suppressor genes inhibit it (Weinberg 1996). Mutations in proto-oncogenes convert them into carcinogenic oncogenes, which leads to uncontrolled cell growth and proliferation, while mutations in tumor suppressor genes inactivate their inhibitory capacity (Weinberg 1996). The second mechanism is the selective enhancement of the growth of tumor cells or their precursors (Trichopoulos et al. 1996). These mechanisms are triggered by substances or agents called "carcinogens" (National Library of Medicine 2015). There are three main categories of carcinogens (WHO 2015a).

- *Chemical carcinogens*: For example, the components of tobacco smoke and cigarettes, asbestos, aflatoxin (a food contaminant), certain types of food preservatives, and arsenic

- *Physical carcinogens*: For example, ionizing and ultraviolet radiation
- *Biological carcinogens*: For example, infections from bacteria, viruses, or parasites

Aging is also a factor related to cancer and the incidence of certain cancers increases with age. This may be due to the increase in risk accumulation combined with the inhibition or lack of cell repair mechanisms (WHO 2015a).

As a result of the theories mentioned above, for cancer causation, the abnormal cells and tumors acquire biological hallmarks during the steps to malignancy (Hanahan and Weinberg 2011). These are sustained proliferative signaling, the evasion of growth suppressors, invasion activation and metastasis, the enabling of replicative immortality, angiogenesis, resisting cell death, the reprogramming of energy metabolism, and the invasion of the immune system.

Underlying these cancer hallmarks is the genomic instability giving way to genetic diversity, which accelerates their acquisition. Inflammation also promotes them (Hanahan and Weinberg 2011). It is important to understand these hallmarks, as prevention and treatment can be targeted to stop their acquisition.

9.4 RISK FACTORS FOR CANCER

The factors that increase the chances of a person developing cancer are called "risk factors for cancers." It has been estimated that approximately one-third of cancer deaths are due to five behavioral risk factors: namely, tobacco use, high body mass index (BMI), low consumption of fruits and vegetables, a lack of physical activity, and alcohol consumption (WHO 2015a). Risk factors for cancers are elaborated as follows:

- *Inheritance or family history of cancer*: Genetic mutations can be inherited and are responsible for 5%–10% of all cancer cases. More than 50 hereditary cancer syndromes have been identified that increase the susceptibility of an individual to developing cancer (National Cancer Institute 2015). Some of these include hereditary breast and ovarian cancer syndrome, which increases the risk of breast, ovarian, and fallopian tube cancer in females and prostate cancer in males; familial adenomatous polyposis, which increases the risk of colorectal cancer; hereditary nonpolyposis colon cancer, which increases the risk of colorectal cancer and cancers of the stomach, small bowel, and pancreas; and Li-Fraumeni syndrome, which increases the risk of soft tissue sarcoma, osteosarcoma, leukemia, breast cancer, brain cancer, and adrenocortical cancer (American Society of Clinical Oncology). A meta-analysis of 52 case control studies showed that the risk of breast cancer increases almost twofold in women with at least one relative with breast cancer; the risk was higher in women less than 50 years of age and also for those whose relative was diagnosed with breast cancer before 50 years (Pharoah et al. 1997). In another meta-analysis of 59 studies, the pooled risk estimate for colorectal cancer for those who had a family history of the same in one relative was found to be 2.24

(95% confidence interval [CI] 2.06–2.43), which increased to 3.97 (95% CI 2.60–6.06) for those with a history of cancer in at least two relatives (Butterworth et al. 2006).

- *Tobacco*: Tobacco leads to an estimated 20% of cancer deaths and 70% of lung cancer deaths annually. It is said to be the single greatest preventable risk factor for cancer worldwide (WHO 2015a). Each puff of a cigarette consists of thousands of chemicals and 60 well-established carcinogens (Centers for Disease Control and Prevention 2010). Many types of cancer can be caused by tobacco smoking and these include cancer of the lungs, mouth, esophagus, larynx (voice box), stomach, kidneys, pancreas, cervix, and bladder. Seventy percent of all lung cancers can be attributed to tobacco (WHO 2015b). Secondhand smoke has also been found to be a risk factor for lung cancer in nonsmoking males and females (Oberg et al. 2011). Smokeless tobacco (chewing tobacco) increases the risk of cancers of the mouth, esophagus, and pancreas; 50% of mouth cancers in India and Sudan can be attributed to smokeless tobacco products (Boffetta et al. 2008).

- *Alcohol*: Approximately 2.8% of all cancers can be attributed to alcohol consumption. The highest numbers of cancers due to alcohol have been found to be colon cancer in men and breast cancer in women (Pandeya et al. 2015). Researchers have found causal association between alcohol and cancers of the mouth, larynx, pharynx, esophagus, liver, colon, rectum, and breast (in women) (Boffetta and Hashibe 2006). The relative risk (RR) of pharynx and oral cavity cancer ranges between 3.2 and 9.2 for the consumption of more than four drinks per day (Goldstein et al. 2010).

- *Unhealthy diet*: About 30%–40% of all cancer cases have been associated with poor dietary habits (Divisi et al. 2006; WHO 2011). One in 10 cancers in the United Kingdom is caused by an unhealthy diet (Parkin 2011). In a recent study in Australia, 6.1% of all cancers in the year 2010 could be attributed to inadequate diet (Whiteman et al. 2015b). Unhealthy diet can lead to cancers of the oral cavity, pharynx, esophagus, stomach, intestine, colon, rectum, and lungs (Whiteman et al. 2015a).

- *Lack of physical activity*: It has been estimated that physical inactivity is responsible for 10% of breast cancers and 10% of colon cancers worldwide (Lee et al. 2012). In Australia, more than 1500 cancer cases, including cancers of the colon, postmenopausal breast cancers, and endometrial cancers, could be attributed to insufficient physical activity in 2010. In this study, insufficient physical activity was defined as less than 60 min of physical activity at least 5 days/week. The researchers suggested that if the people who performed less than the required amount of physical activity would have increased their activity levels by 30 min/week, 17% ($n = 314$) of cancers attributable to insufficient physical activity could have been avoided (Olsen et al. 2015). Physical activity can reduce the risk of colon, breast, endometrial, lung, and pancreatic cancer (Lee 2003).

- *Overweight and obesity*: There is growing evidence of a link between obesity and cancers. In the United States, 6% of all incident cases of cancers

(4% in males and 7% in females) can be attributed to obesity (Polednak 2008). BMI and cancer have a dose-responsive relationship. Compared to a BMI of <25 kg/m^2, women with a BMI of 25.0–29.9 kg/m^2 have an 8% increased risk of cancer, which rises to 18%, 32%, and 62% in those with a BMI of 30.0–34.9 kg/m^2, 35.0–39.9 kg/m^2, and ≥40 kg/m^2, respectively. Cancer risk increases for men who have a BMI≥30 kg/m^2. In men with a BMI of 30.0–34.9 kg/m^2, cancer risk increases by 9%, with a BMI of 35.0–39.9 kg/m^2, risk increases by 20%, and for BMI≥40 kg/m^2, risk increases by 52%, compared with men with a BMI of<30 kg/m^2 (Calle et al. 2003). A meta-analysis of 141 observational prospective studies with 282,137 incident cancer cases has shown that a rise in BMI of 5 kg/m^2 is strongly associated (RR>1.5) with esophageal, thyroid, colon, and renal cancers in men and to endometrial, gall bladder, esophageal, and renal cancers in women (Renehan et al. 2008). The World Cancer Research Fund (WRCF) also reported on epidemiological evidence between body fatness and pancreatic, colorectal, and postmenopausal breast cancer (Marmot et al. 2007).

- *Chronic infections*: In 2008, 16.1% of new cancer cases were attributable to infections: 22.9% in less developed countries and 7.4% in more developed countries (De Martel et al. 2012). *Helicobacter pylori*, hepatitis B and C, and the human papilloma viruses have been found to cause gastric, liver, and cervix uteri cancers (De Martel et al. 2012). Epstein–Barr virus (EBV) and human T-cell leukemia virus type 1 (HTLV-1) have also been postulated in cancer causation (Butel 2000). EBV can cause Burkitt's lymphoma, Hodgkin's lymphoma, lymphoproliferative disorder in immunocompromised patients, and nasopharyngeal and gastric carcinoma (Pattle and Farrell 2006). HTLV-1 causes adult T-cell leukemia in 5% of its carriers (Matsuoka 2003).

- *Environmental chemicals*: Many environmental chemicals, including asbestos, vinyl chloride, aristolochic acid, chloromethyl ether, chloromethyl methyl ether, ethylene oxide, formaldehyde, mustard gas, styrene, and sulfuric acid among others, have been linked to cancers of the lungs, nasopharynx, larynx, liver, breast, blood, and kidneys (Blair and Kazerouni 1997; Burcham 2013). Air pollutants, particularly particulate matter (PM$_{10}$ and PM$_{2.5}$), also increase lung cancer risk (Raaschou-Nielsen et al. 2013).

Figure 9.1 shows risk factors for cancers and their plausible mechanisms of action.

9.5 RELATION OF UNHEALTHY DIET TO CANCER

The association of individual food items with cancer risk is challenging to study, as the human diet is composed of a variety of food groups and dietary patterns in which nutrients interact with each other to have an impact on health outcomes. The nutrients in foods or dietary patterns may have synergistic or antagonistic effects. For example, the health benefits of fruits and vegetables in cancer and cardiovascular disease risk reduction can be attributed to the synergistic effect of phytochemicals

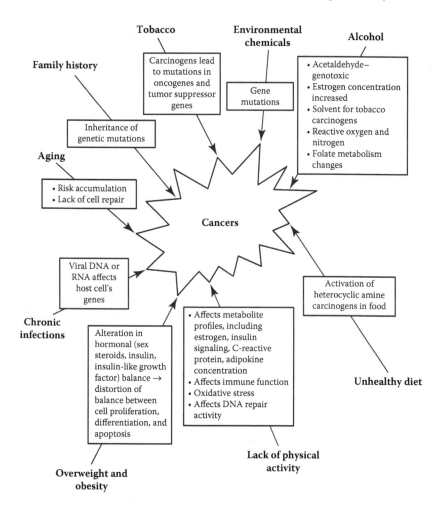

FIGURE 9.1   Risk factors for cancers and their mechanisms of action.

present in whole fruits and vegetables (Liu 2003). On the other hand, vitamin E (α-tocopherol) interacts with selenium or selenomethionine to increase the risk of prostate cancer (Albanes et al. 2014). A high intake of alcohol combined with low methionine and low folate increases the risk of colon cancer in healthy men by three times and distal colon cancer by seven times (Giovannucci et al. 1995).

Many foods, when consumed in excess, have been shown to increase cancer risk. Hence the foods that should be avoided for preventing cancers are:

- *Red meat*: A meta-analysis of 28 prospective studies revealed that high daily consumption of red meat has a linear association with an increased risk of colorectal cancer (Chan et al. 2011). One of the mechanisms for cancer causation by red meat is the production of carcinogens called N-nitroso compounds in the bowel, mediated by the heme present in red meat (Bingham et al. 1996; Cross et al. 2003). Another mechanism is the production of heterocyclic amines when meat is cooked at high temperatures, which are also thought to be carcinogenic (Norat et al. 2002).

- *White bread and starchy foods*: The Oxford Vegetarian Study, composed of 11,140 vegetarians and nonvegetarians, found that people who eat 15 or more slices of white bread per week have a greater risk of colon cancer compared with those who ate less than 15 slices, even after adjusting for alcohol and smoking (Sanjoaquin et al. 2004). Another case control study in Uruguay concluded that rice, white bread, salted meat, stewed meat, potatoes, and tubers increase the risk of gastric cancers (De Stefani et al. 2004). These foods that are rich in starch may contribute to cancer risk by acid-catalyzed nitrosation in the stomach due to the lack of buffering capacity, besides causing physical damage to the gastric mucosa (Kono and Hirohata 1996). Insulin resistance due to energy-rich foods has also been postulated as one of the theories for cancer causation (Arcidiacono et al. 2012; Bruce et al. 2000).
- *High-fat diet*: High-fat intake has been associated with bladder cancer (Steinmaus et al. 2000).
- *Diet sodas and sugar-containing sodas*: The Nurses' Health Study and the Health Professionals Follow-Up Study found that in men diet soda (≥1 serving/day) is associated with a risk of non-Hodgkin lymphoma and multiple myeloma, while the consumption of sugar-sweetened soda is associated with non-Hodgkin lymphoma (Schernhammer et al. 2012). They also reported the association of diet soft drinks with leukemia in both men and women. One of the suggested mechanisms is that the aspartame present in diet sodas breaks down to methanol, aspartic acid, and phenylalanine at or above room temperature; methanol is then converted to formaldehyde in the body, which is carcinogenic (Schernhammer et al. 2012). Body weight gain/obesity due to sugar-containing beverages might contribute to cancer risk.
- *Alcohol*: 3.2%–3.7% of all cancer deaths can be attributed to alcohol in the United States (Nelson et al. 2013). Light-to-moderate alcohol drinking minimally increases the risk of all cancers, while the consumption of ≥30 g/day has been more strongly associated with cancers in smokers and ex-smokers than those never smoked (Cao et al. 2015). For women, an intake of 5.0–14.9 g/day of alcohol has been associated with an increased risk of cancer, especially breast cancer (Cao et al. 2015). A case control study in Spain found that alcohol consumption can increase the risk of breast cancer in women by almost twofold (Gago-Dominguez et al. 2016).

Apart from food composition, the manner in which it is cooked can also have an impact on the risk of developing cancer. In China, women who wait for fumes to be emitted from cooking oil before beginning to cook have been shown to have a higher risk of lung cancer than those who do not (Ko et al. 2000). Pooled analysis from seven studies with 5105 cases and 6535 controls concluded that the risk of lung cancer increases in those using predominantly coal and wood for cooking compared with nonsolid fuels—that is, oil, gas, and electricity (Hosgood et al. 2010). In a case control study, firewood cooking has been associated with a risk of esophageal cancer (Mlombe et al. 2015). In Korea, charcoal-grilled beef in moderate and high amounts has been shown to increase the risk of gastric cancer (Kim et al. 2002). The use of a wood stove and the consumption of charcoal-grilled meat has been associated with oral cancers in Brazil (Franco et al. 1989).

9.6 FOODS THAT PREVENT CANCER

The following foods have been found to prevent cancer:

- *Fiber*: High dietary fiber, particularly from cereals and whole grains, has been shown to decrease the risk of colorectal cancer significantly in a meta-analysis of 25 prospective studies (Aune et al. 2011). An increment of 10 g/day of fiber in the diet can reduce the risk of gastric cancer by 44% (Zhang et al. 2013). Dietary fiber reduces the risk of colorectal cancer by reducing the contact of intestinal content from the gut mucosa. It also may act through stimulating anaerobic fermentation in the large intestine, leading to the production of short-chain fatty acids such as butyrate, which induces apoptosis and reduces cell proliferation (Norat et al. 2015). A high-fiber diet has also been shown to reduce estrogen and androstenedione levels, which has been shown to decrease mammary tumor growth, angiogenesis, and metastasis in animal models (Norat et al. 2015). A high-fiber diet is also a rich source of phytoestrogens, which are estrogen-like compounds and hence can modulate hormone-dependent cancers such as breast cancer (Norat et al. 2015).
- *Fruits and vegetables*: A meta-analysis of 16 observational studies has shown that the intake of fruits and vegetables can decrease the risk of oral cancers by 49% and 50%, respectively (Pavia et al. 2006). Another meta-analysis found that 3 servings of fruit per day can reduce the risk of colorectal cancer by 15% and 5 servings of vegetables per day can reduce this risk by 14% (Johnson et al. 2013). Phytophenols in fruits and vegetables have multiple properties that help in the prevention of cancers, such as being oxidative-agent scavengers, anti-inflammatories, detoxifiers, and inhibitors of platelet aggregation and antimicrobial activity (Norat et al. 2015). Folate, vitamins B_6, C, D and E, carotenoids, selenium, and phytochemicals present in vegetables and fruits reduce cancer risk by their antioxidative mechanisms, inhibiting cell proliferation, maintaining DNA methylation, and inducing cell cycle arrest (Norat et al. 2015).
- *Fish*: The Health Professionals Follow-Up Study, including 47,882 men followed for 12 years, concluded that eating fish three times a week is associated with a reduced risk of prostate cancer compared with those eating fish less than twice a month (Augustsson et al. 2003). A European prospective investigation, including 478,040 males and females followed for an average of 4.8 years, found that the consumption of more than 80 g of fish per day can decrease the risk of colorectal cancer by 31% compared with consuming less than 10 g/day (Norat et al. 2005). A plausible mechanism for

this is the presence of fatty acids in fish such as eicosapentaenoic acid and docosahexaenoic acid, which inhibit carcinogenesis (Larsson et al. 2004). Vitamin D and retinol in the fish may also play a role in cancer prevention. The Health Professionals Study did not find a difference in the results of fish intake even after adjusting for vitamin D and retinol intake. Evidence regarding the use of fish oil supplements for cancer prevention is sparse (Augustsson et al. 2003).

- *Tomatoes*: One serving (200 g) of raw tomatoes per day can decrease the risk of prostate cancer by 22%, as shown by a meta-analysis of 10 cohort studies (Etminan et al. 2004). Lycopene in tomatoes is thought to have anticancer properties as it inhibits cancer cell proliferation, protects cellular lipoprotein and DNA, and is antioxidant in nature (Etminan et al. 2004).

- *Green tea*: The polyphenolic compounds in green tea possess antioxidant and anticarcinogenic properties. Seven observational studies with 77,777 study participants showed an inverse association of green tea with the risk of gastric (stomach) cancer (Liu et al. 2008). A large cohort study in Japan called the Japan Public Health Centre (JPHC) study, including 72,943 participants followed for 8–11 years, concluded that the risk of cancer in the distal third of the stomach reduces by 49% for women consuming 5 cups/day of green tea compared with 1 cup/day; no such association was found for men (Sasazuki et al. 2004). These findings are not consistent for all the gastrointestinal cancers (Liu et al. 2008).

- *Coffee*: The Nurses' Health Study, with 67,470 females between the ages of 34 and 59 years followed up for 26 years, showed that the risk of endometrial cancer reduces by 25% in those consuming 4 cups or more of coffee per day compared with females consuming 1 cup or less per day. No such association was found between tea and endometrial cancer risk (Je et al. 2011). Phenolic and other active compounds in coffee such as chlorogenic acid and caffeine act as antioxidants and also decrease insulin and free estradiol concentrations, which leads to the prevention of endometrial cancers (Je et al. 2011).

- *Nuts*: Nuts have been found to be protective against colorectal, prostate, and endometrial cancers in different countries (Falasca et al. 2014). A large cohort study in Taiwan that recruited 11,917 females and 12,026 males in the age range of 30–65 years concluded that the frequent consumption of peanuts and peanut products can reduce the risk of colorectal cancers in males by 27% and in females by 58% (Yeh et al. 2006). The Nurses' Health Study in the United States also found that women who consumed ≥56 g of nuts per week had a 13% lower risk of colorectal cancers compared with those who rarely consumed them (Yang et al. 2015). In a case control study in Greece, the consumption of pulses, nuts, and seeds was inversely associated with endometrial cancer (Petridou et al. 2002). The phytochemicals in nuts have been shown to inhibit cell proliferation and angiogenesis and potentiate apoptosis, which all have a role in cancer prevention and control (Falasca et al. 2014).

9.7 DIETARY PATTERNS TO PREVENT CANCER

The following dietary patterns have been found to decrease the risk of cancers.

- *Mediterranean diet*: The Mediterranean diet is characterized by a high intake of fruits, vegetables, legumes, unrefined cereals and whole grains, nuts, and olive oil, moderate consumption of wine with meals, fish and seafood, eggs, and dairy products, and a low intake of sweets and red meat. Evidence has shown that this dietary pattern reduces the risk of all cancers both in men and women, but the association of the Mediterranean diet with specific cancers shows varying findings.

  A multicenter prospective cohort study called the European Prospective Investigation into Cancer and Nutrition (EPIC), comprised of 142,605 males and 335,873 females, concluded that greater adherence to the Mediterranean dietary pattern can reduce the risk of all cancers in males by 4.7% and in females by 2.4% (Couto et al. 2011). A study in Cyprus, where people traditionally adhere to the Mediterranean diet, found that there was no association between Mediterranean diet adherence scores and the risk of breast cancer. Nevertheless, a dietary pattern composed of vegetables, fruits, legumes, and olive oil reduced the risk of breast cancer in Greek Cypriot women (Demetriou et al. 2012). Another study in Sweden also found no association of adherence to the Mediterranean diet with breast cancer in women aged 30–49 years (Couto et al. 2013). An Italian subset of the EPIC study including 45,275 participants showed that adherence to the Mediterranean diet, as measured by the Italian Mediterranean index, reduced the risk of colorectal cancers in general in both males and females, but was not affective in decreasing the risk of cancers of the proximal colon (Agnoli et al. 2013). A meta-analysis of 21 cohort studies and 12 case control studies comprised of 1,431,461 participants showed that adherence to the Mediterranean diet reduces the risk of colorectal cancer by 14%, aerodigestive cancer by 56%, and prostate cancer by 4%. This meta-analysis did not find a significant association between the Mediterranean diet and breast cancer, pancreatic cancer, or gastric cancer (Schwingshackl and Hoffmann 2014). A recent update of this meta-analysis, including 56 observational studies and 1,784,404 participants, showed that adherence to the Mediterranean diet reduces the risk of colorectal cancer by 17%, breast cancer by 7%, gastric cancer by 27%, prostate cancer by 4%, liver cancer by 42%, head and neck cancer by 60%, pancreatic cancer by 52%, and respiratory cancer by 90% (Schwingshackl and Hoffmann 2015).

- *Paleolithic diet*: Also called the Paleo diet, Caveman diet, or Stone Age diet, this diet is composed of foods similar to those consumed by humans in prehistoric times. The main composition of the diet is fish, lean meat, fruits, vegetables, root vegetables, eggs, and nuts. It is devoid of refined food such as dairy products, processed oils, grains, salt, alcohol, and coffee.

  A case control study in the United States, showed that the Paleo diet reduces the risk of colorectal adenomas by 16% and 29% when compared with community controls and endoscopy-negative controls, respectively (Whalen et al. 2014). The Paleo diet may contribute to cancer prevention by reducing systemic inflammation and oxidative stress, similar to that of the Mediterranean diet (Whalen et al. 2015). Evidence regarding the role of the Paleo diet in cancer prevention is scarce and more research is needed in this regard.

- *Prudent/healthy diet*: The prudent/healthy dietary pattern is predominantly composed of plant food and less red and processed meat. It can reduce the risk of breast cancer by 11% (Brennan et al. 2010) and the risk of gastric cancer by 25% (Bertuccio et al. 2013). A systematic review of cohort studies from 2000 to 2011 showed an inverse association of the prudent/healthy dietary pattern with the risk of colorectal cancer (Yusof et al. 2012). Dietary patterns composed of fruits, vegetables, and lean protein can also reduce the risk of head and neck squamous cell carcinoma by 47% (Bradshaw et al. 2012). A pooled analysis of 22 case control studies also showed that a dietary pattern consisting of a high intake of fruits and vegetables and a low intake of red meat reduced the risk of head and neck cancers by 10% (Chuang et al. 2012).
- *Vitamin and fiber pattern*: An Italian case control study found that a "vitamin and fiber" dietary pattern can reduce the risk of esophageal cancer by 50% (Bravi et al. 2012). This type of dietary pattern is composed of the frequent consumption of vitamin C, total fiber, soluble carbohydrates, total folate, and beta-carotene equivalents.
- *Polyunsaturated fatty acids and vitamin D*: The Italian case control study by Bravi et al. (2012) found that a dietary pattern consisting of polyunsaturated fatty acids, vitamin D, and niacin can reduce the risk of esophageal cancer by 42%.
- *Dietary Approach to Stop Hypertension (DASH) diet*: The DASH diet is composed of large amounts of fruits and fruit juices, grains, vegetables, and low-fat dairy products, small amounts of fish, poultry, meat, nuts, seeds, and legumes, and very small amounts of snacks and sugar. It has been shown to reduce the risk of colorectal cancer by 33% in Canadian adult men (Jones-McLean et al. 2015). The high fiber content, vitamins, minerals, and antioxidants in the DASH diet are related to the prevention of various types of cancers (Onvani et al. 2015).

Table 9.1 summarizes the foods and dietary patterns that can increase and decrease the risk of cancers.

9.8 FOODS HELPFUL IN THE TREATMENT OF CANCER

The following foods have been found to be beneficial in cancer patients.

- *Fish oil*: 2 g of fish oil supplements per day, providing 0.4 g of docosahexaenoic acid and 0.3 g of eicosapentaenoic acid per day, has been shown to be beneficial in patients receiving cancer chemotherapy. It increases weight by an average of 1.7 kg in 8 weeks, polymorphonuclear cell (mainly neutrophil) numbers by an average of 29%, phagocytosis by an average of 14%,

TABLE 9.1

Foods and Dietary Patterns That Increase and Decrease the Risk of Cancer

Food and Dietary Patterns That Increase Cancer Risk	Food and Dietary Patterns That Decrease Cancer Risk
Foods	**Foods**
• Red meat	• Fiber
• White bread and starchy foods	• Fruits and vegetables
• High-fat diet	• Fish
• Diet sodas and sugar-containing sodas	• Tomato
• Alcohol	• Green tea
	• Coffee
Dietary Patterns	• Nuts
• Animal products and related components	
• High intake of alcohol combined with low methionine and low folate	**Dietary Patterns**
	• Mediterranean diet
	• Paleolithic diet
	• Prudent/healthy diet
	• Vitamin and fiber pattern
	• Polyunsaturated fatty acids and vitamin D
	• DASH diet

and superoxide production by an average of 28%. This implies that fish oil helps in combating reductions in neutrophil numbers and function while the patient is having chemotherapy as cancer treatment (Bonatto et al. 2012).

- *Green tea*: A hospital-based cohort study in Japan showed that breast cancer recurrence can decrease by 31% by consuming 3 or more cups of green tea per day. This was observed in females previously being treated for stages 1 and 2 of breast cancer (Inoue et al. 2001).
- *Ginger*: According to preclinical studies, ginger possesses antineoplastic and chemopreventive properties. *In vitro* studies have shown that ginger has anticancer properties and can be used in the treatments of ovarian cancer (Rhode et al. 2007), cancers of the gastrointestinal tract (Prasad and Tyagi 2015), and prostate cancer (Karna et al. 2012).
- *Curcumin*: Curcumin is an active compound in turmeric, used as a spice in Indian curries. A phase-2 clinical study has shown that 8 g of curcumin per day is effective in the treatment of pancreatic cancer (Dhillon et al. 2008). Curcumin has also been found to be effective in the treatment of colon cancer and multiple myeloma (Shehzad, Wahid, and Lee 2010).
- *Cruciferous vegetables*: Cruciferous vegetables, including broccoli, cauliflower, cabbage, Brussels sprouts, kale, mustard, and chard greens, have been shown to decrease the progression of prostate cancer by 59% in men diagnosed with nonmetastatic prostate cancer in the United States (Richman et al. 2012). The Shanghai Women's Health Study showed that the high prediagnosis intake of cruciferous vegetables by Chinese women with lung cancer improved the cancer survival rate by 31% (Wu et al. 2015).

- *Nuts*: A PREDIMED nutrition intervention trial including 7216 men and women aged 55–80 years old concluded that more than 3 servings of nuts per week, 1 serving equal to 28 g of nuts, can reduce cancer mortality by 40% (Guasch-Ferré et al. 2013). It also showed that more than 3 servings per week of walnuts (1 serving = 28 g of walnuts) can reduce cancer mortality by 54% (Guasch-Ferré et al. 2013).

9.9   DIETARY PATTERNS TO TREAT CANCER

Studies have shown that the following dietary patterns are beneficial to cancer patients in terms of reducing the risk of mortality and cancer recurrence.

- *Mediterranean diet*: A recent meta-analysis of 56 observational studies has shown that the Mediterranean dietary pattern reduces overall cancer mortality by 13% (Schwingshackl and Hoffmann 2015). Researchers have shown that the Mediterranean diet is linked to a 22% lower risk of mortality in men diagnosed with prostate cancer (Kenfield et al. 2014). A European intervention trial reported that a Mediterranean dietary pattern consisting of the high consumption of olive oil, fruits, vegetables, fish, and lean meat reduces the risk of recurrence of colorectal adenomas in women by 50% (Cottet et al. 2005).
- *Prudent/healthy diet*: The Life after Cancer Epidemiology study, including 1091 participants diagnosed with early stage breast cancer, showed that the risk of overall mortality in those adherent to the prudent dietary pattern reduced by 43% (Kwan et al. 2009). In postmenopausal women, a diet composed of high dietary fiber, fruits, and vegetables—that is, a plant-based diet low in dietary fat—increases overall survival after breast cancer diagnosis (Jaiswal McEligot et al. 2006). A randomized controlled trial has shown reduced fat intake in breast cancer patients to decrease the breast cancer relapse rate by 24% (Chlebowski et al. 2006).

9.10   HOME REMEDIES TO PREVENT CANCER

In addition to the foods and dietary patterns mentioned above for the prevention of various types of cancers, many food products used in cooking have been found to possess anticancer properties. Research with regard to its use in population studies is limited; nevertheless, the following natural compounds/spices/herbs can be consumed for cancer prevention. (Caution should be taken for allergies.)

- *Cinnamon*: This spice comes from the inner bark of cinnamon trees, grown in Sri Lanka, southern parts of India, China, Indonesia, and Vietnam. Cinnamon possesses strong antioxidant, anti-inflammatory, and antibacterial properties. The antitumor properties of cinnamon can inhibit breast, ovarian, and lung cancers and leukemia (Hamidpour et al. 2015).
- *Turmeric*: This spice consists of a compound called curcumin, which has been used in Ayurvedic, Indian, and Chinese traditional medicine. Curcumin can modulate the cellular pathways of inflammation, cell proliferation, and invasion, eventually leading to the death of the tumor cells

(Teiten et al. 2010). Researchers have suggested curcumin to be an ideal chemopreventive agent for various cancers due to its low toxicity, easy availability, and affordability, the only limitation being its poor bioavailability for clinical use (Park et al. 2013).

- *Garlic*: Meta-analyses of 18 studies has shown that the consumption of raw and cooked garlic, excluding garlic supplements, can reduce the risk of colorectal cancer by 31% and stomach cancer by 47% (Fleischauer et al. 2000). The consumption of raw and cooked garlic in these studies ranged from 3.5 g/week to more than 28.8 g/week (Fleischauer et al. 2000). The consumption of garlic two or more times per week has been shown to reduce the risk of lung cancer by 44% in Chinese populations, and this association has a dose-responsive pattern (Jin et al. 2013).

- *Rosemary*: This plant is grown in many parts of the world and is used as a herb in cooking. Animal and cell culture studies have shown that rosemary can inhibit tumor cells in many organs, including the breasts, liver, stomach, colon, skin, and blood (Ngo et al. 2011). Further studies are required to evaluate its effectiveness in clinical and population settings.

9.11   NUTRITIONAL COUNSELING FOR CANCER

Nutrition counseling for cancer prevention should be offered to all patients in clinical settings and communities, irrespective of age and gender, as cancer effects them all. This can be done when patients come in for the screening and treatment of cancers and other non-communicable diseases and their risk factors. Nutrition counseling for cancer prevention can also be offered at health camps.

Populations can be made aware of the symptoms of cancer and should be told that if they observe any of the symptoms, they should seek medical attention. According to the American Cancer Society, the general signs and symptoms of cancers include unexplained weight loss, fever, fatigue, pain, and skin changes such as hyperpigmentation, redness, itching, and excessive hair growth. Site-specific signs and symptoms include changes in bowel habits or bladder function, sores that do not heal, white patches or spots in the mouth, bleeding from any orifice of the body, excessive discharge, a thickening or lump in the breast or other body parts, an inability to swallow, recent changes in warts or moles or new skin changes, and continuous coughing or hoarseness (American Cancer Society 2014b). If a patient comes in with any of these symptoms, information regarding cancer screening can be given (Smith et al. 2015).

Nutrition history taking should inquire about the foods and dietary patterns consumed. Diets can be assessed by food frequency questionnaires, 24-hours dietary recalls, and diet histories. Nutrition counseling for cancer prevention and treatment should include advice about foods and dietary patterns that increase and decrease the risk of cancers (Table 9.1). What foods should be added to or avoided in the diet in accordance with the nutrition history and cooking style should also be a part of nutrition counseling for cancer prevention and treatment.

Table 9.2 elaborates on nutrition counseling for cancer prevention and treatment.

TABLE 9.2
Nutritional Counseling for Cancers

Components of Counseling	Description
Symptoms and signs	• *Generalized*: Unexplained weight loss, fatigue, pain (e.g., headache or backache), loss of appetite, fever, skin changes (e.g., hyperpigmentation, jaundice, redness, itching, or excessive growth of hair) • *System specific*: Change in bowel habits or urinary function, bleeding from any orifice of the body (e.g., blood in stools), lumps, recent skin changes (e.g., growth or change in color of moles/warts), difficulty in swallowing, hoarseness of voice, continuous cough, excessive discharge
Nutritional history: Questions to be asked by health expert	Dietary assessment can be done in the form of a *diet history*, *24-hour recall*, *dietary log*, and *food frequency questionnaire*. These should inquire about • Amount of dietary fiber consumed • Intake of fruits and vegetables • Consumption of fish, meat, and poultry • Consumption of legumes, grains, nuts, and seeds • Consumption of alcohol • Intake of sugar-sweetened beverages • Cooking style
Examination and investigations	General physical examination and systematic examination can be done for cancer screening and diagnosis (Jarvis 2015).
Diagnosis	If you make a diagnosis or suspect cancer, refer to the concerned physician.
Nutritional management	Advise patients about Healthful Eating As Lifestyle (HEAL) based on the *foods and dietary patterns for the prevention and treatment of cancers* as explained in this chapter. Give precautionary guidelines and safety concerns when recommending home-based remedies.

9.12 CASE STUDIES

In continuation of the information given in this chapter about Healthful Eating As Lifestyle for cancers, assess the following scenarios and answer the questions about nutrition counseling.

9.12.1 Case Study 1

A 35-year-old female comes to your clinic with a family history of breast cancer. She does not have any of the generalized or local symptoms of breast cancer, but is concerned about her dietary habits. Her BMI is 30 kg/m^2. (*Pointer*: Assess the risk factors and refer to the sections on foods and dietary patterns for the prevention of cancers [Sections 9.6 and 9.7].)

Give responses to the following:

1. How will you assess her dietary pattern/food intake?
2. What are the risk factors in this patient for breast cancer?
3. What dietary advice will you give to your client?

9.12.2 CASE STUDY 2

A 65-year-old male patient recently diagnosed with stage 1 prostate cancer is referred to you for nutrition counseling. He is fond of his high-fat diet and consumes very small amounts of vegetables. (*Pointer*: Refer to the sections on food and dietary patterns for the treatment of cancers [Sections 9.8 and 9.9].)

Give responses to the following:

1. What dietary pattern will you recommend to reduce his risk of mortality due to prostate cancer?
2. What foods will you suggest for the treatment of prostate cancer in this patient?

REFERENCES

Agnoli, Claudia, Sara Grioni, Sabina Sieri, Domenico Palli, Giovanna Masala, Carlotta Sacerdote, Paolo Vineis et al. 2013. Italian Mediterranean index and risk of colorectal cancer in the Italian section of the EPIC cohort. *Int J Cancer* 132 (6):1404–1411.

Albanes, Demetrius, Cathee Till, Eric A. Klein, Phyllis J. Goodman, Alison M. Mondul, Stephanie J. Weinstein, Philip R. Taylor et al. 2014. Plasma tocopherols and risk of prostate cancer in the Selenium and Vitamin E Cancer Prevention Trial (SELECT). *Cancer Prev Res (Phila)* 7 (9):886–895.

American Cancer Society. 2014a. The history of cancer. Accessed November 15, 2015. http://www.cancer.org/acs/groups/cid/documents/webcontent/002048-pdf.pdf.

American Cancer Society. 2014b. Signs and symptoms of cancer. Accessed February 21, 2016. http://www.cancer.org/cancer/cancerbasics/signs-and-symptoms-of-cancer.

American Society of Clinical Oncology. Hereditary cancer-related syndromes. Accessed November 16, 2015. http://www.cancer.net/navigating-cancer-care/cancer-basics/genetics/hereditary-cancer-related-syndromes.

Arcidiacono, Biagio, Stefania Iiritano, Aurora Nocera, Katiuscia Possidente, Maria T. Nevolo, Valeria Ventura, Daniela Foti, Eusebio Chiefari, and Antonio Brunetti. 2012. Insulin resistance and cancer risk: An overview of the pathogenetic mechanisms. *Exp Diabetes Res* 2012:789174.

Augustsson, Katarina, Dominique S. Michaud, Eric B. Rimm, Michael F. Leitzmann, Meir J. Stampfer, Walter C. Willett, and Edward Giovannucci. 2003. A prospective study of intake of fish and marine fatty acids and prostate cancer. *Cancer Epidemiology Biomarkers Prev* 12 (1):64–67.

Aune, Dagfinn, Doris S. M. Chan, Rosa Lau, Rui Vieira, Darren C. Greenwood, Ellen Kampman, and Teresa Norat. 2011. Dietary fibre, whole grains, and risk of colorectal cancer: Systematic review and dose-response meta-analysis of prospective studies. *BMJ* 343:d6617.

Bertuccio, P., V. Rosato, A. Andreano, M. Ferraroni, A. Decarli, V. Edefonti, and C. La Vecchia. 2013. Dietary patterns and gastric cancer risk: A systematic review and meta-analysis. *Ann Oncol* 24 (6):1450–1458.

Bingham, S. A., B. Pignatelli, J. R. A. Pollock, A. Ellul, C. Malaveille, G. Gross, S. Runswick, J. H. Cummings, and I. K. O'Neill. 1996. Does increased endogenous formation of N-nitroso compounds in the human colon explain the association between red meat and colon cancer? *Carcinogenesis* 17 (3):515–523.

Blair, Aaron, and Neely Kazerouni. 1997. Reactive chemicals and cancer. *Cancer Causes Control* 8 (3):473–490.

Boffetta, Paolo, and Mia Hashibe. 2006. Alcohol and cancer. *Lancet Oncol* 7 (2):149–156.

Boffetta, Paolo, Stephen Hecht, Nigel Gray, Prakash Gupta, and Kurt Straif. 2008. Smokeless tobacco and cancer. *Lancet Oncol* 9 (7):667–675.

Bonatto, Sandro J. R., Heloisa H. P. Oliveira, Everson A. Nunes, Daniele Pequito, Fabiola Iagher, Isabela Coelho, Katya Naliwaiko et al. 2012. Fish oil supplementation improves neutrophil function during cancer chemotherapy. *Lipids* 47 (4):383–389.

Bradshaw, Patrick T., Anna Maria Siega-Riz, Marci Campbell, Mark C. Weissler, William K. Funkhouser, and Andrew F. Olshan. 2012. Associations between dietary patterns and head and neck cancer in the Carolina head and neck cancer epidemiology study. *Am J Epidemiol* 175 (12):1225–1233.

Bravi, F., V. Edefonti, G. Randi, W. Garavello, C. La Vecchia, M. Ferraroni, R. Talamini, S. Franceschi, and A. Decarli. 2012. Dietary patterns and the risk of esophageal cancer. *Ann Oncol* 23 (3):765–770.

Brennan, Sarah F., Marie M. Cantwell, Chris R. Cardwell, Louiza S. Velentzis, and Jayne V. Woodside. 2010. Dietary patterns and breast cancer risk: A systematic review and meta-analysis. *Am J Clin Nutr* 91 (5):1294–1302.

Bruce, W. Robert, Thomas M. S. Wolever, and Adria Giacca. 2000. Mechanisms linking diet and colorectal cancer: The possible role of insulin resistance. *Nutr Cancer* 37 (1):19–26.

Burcham, Philip C. 2013. Chemicals and cancer. In *An Introduction to Toxicology*, 221–256. Springer, London.

Butel, Janet S. 2000. Viral carcinogenesis: Revelation of molecular mechanisms and etiology of human disease. *Carcinogenesis* 21 (3):405–426.

Butterworth, Adam S., Julian P. T. Higgins, and Paul Pharoah. 2006. Relative and absolute risk of colorectal cancer for individuals with a family history: A meta-analysis. *Eur J Cancer* 42 (2):216–227.

Calle, Eugenia E., Carmen Rodriguez, Kimberly Walker-Thurmond, and Michael J. Thun. 2003. Overweight, obesity, and mortality from cancer in a prospectively studied cohort of U.S. adults. *N Engl J Med* 348 (17):1625–1638.

Cao, Yin, Walter C. Willett, Eric B. Rimm, Meir J. Stampfer, and Edward L. Giovannucci. 2015. Light to moderate intake of alcohol, drinking patterns, and risk of cancer: Results from two prospective U.S. cohort studies. *BMJ* 351:h4238.

Centers for Disease Control and Prevention. 2010. How tobacco smoke causes disease: The biology and behavioral basis for smoking-attributable disease: A report of the surgeon general. Atlanta, GA: Centers for Disease Control and Prevention.

Chan, D. S., Rosa Lau, Dagfinn Aune, Rui Vieira, Darren C. Greenwood, Ellen Kampman, and Teresa Norat. 2011. Red and processed meat and colorectal cancer incidence: Meta-analysis of prospective studies. *PloS One* 6 (6):e20456.

Chlebowski, Rowan T., George L. Blackburn, Cynthia A. Thomson, Daniel W. Nixon, Alice Shapiro, M. Katherine Hoy, Marc T. Goodman et al. 2006. Dietary fat reduction and breast cancer outcome: Interim efficacy results from the Women's Intervention Nutrition Study. *J Natl Cancer Inst* 98 (24):1767–1776.

Chuang, Shu-Chun, Mazda Jenab, Julia E. Heck, Cristina Bosetti, Renato Talamini, Keitaro Matsuo, Xavier Castellsague et al. 2012. Diet and the risk of head and neck cancer: A pooled analysis in the INHANCE Consortium. *Cancer Causes Control* 23 (1):69–88.

Cottet, V., C. Bonithon-Kopp, O. Kronborg, L. Santos, R. Andreatta, M. C. Boutron-Ruault, J. Faivre, and European Cancer Prevention Organisation Study Group. 2005. Dietary patterns and the risk of colorectal adenoma recurrence in a European intervention trial. *Eur J Cancer Prev* 14 (1):21–29.

Couto, E., P. Boffetta, P. Lagiou, P. Ferrari, G. Buckland, K. Overvad, C. C. Dahm et al. 2011. Mediterranean dietary pattern and cancer risk in the EPIC cohort. *Br J Cancer* 104 (9):1493–1499.

Couto, Elisabeth, Sven Sandin, Marie Lof, Giske Ursin, Hans-Olov Adami, and Elisabete Weiderpass. 2013. Mediterranean dietary pattern and risk of breast cancer. *PloS One* 8 (2):e55374.

Cross, Amanda Jane, Jim R. A. Pollock, and Sheila Anne Bingham. 2003. Haem, not protein or inorganic iron, is responsible for endogenous intestinal N-nitrosation arising from red meat. *Cancer Res* 63 (10):2358–2360.

De Martel, Catherine, Jacques Ferlay, Silvia Franceschi, Jerome Vignat, Freddie Bray, David Forman, and Martyn Plummer. 2012. Global burden of cancers attributable to infections in 2008: A review and synthetic analysis. *Lancet Oncol* 13 (6):607–615.

De Stefani, Eduardo, Pelayo Correa, Paolo Boffetta, Hugo Deneo-Pellegrini, Alvaro L. Ronco, and María Mendilaharsu. 2004. Dietary patterns and risk of gastric cancer: A case-control study in Uruguay. *Gastric Cancer* 7 (4):211–220.

Demetriou, Christiana A., Andreas Hadjisavvas, Maria A. Loizidou, Giorgos Loucaides, Ioanna Neophytou, Sabina Sieri, Eleni Kakouri, Nicos Middleton, Paolo Vineis, and Kyriacos Kyriacou. 2012. The Mediterranean dietary pattern and breast cancer risk in Greek-Cypriot women: A case-control study. *BMC cancer* 12:113.

Dhillon, Navneet, Bharat B. Aggarwal, Robert A. Newman, Robert A. Wolff, Ajaikumar B. Kunnumakkara, James L. Abbruzzese, Chaan S. Ng, Vladimir Badmaev, and Razelle Kurzrock. 2008. Phase II trial of curcumin in patients with advanced pancreatic cancer. *Clin Cancer Res* 14 (14):4491–4499.

Divisi, Duilio, Sergio Di Tommaso, and Salvatore Salvemini. 2006. Diet and cancer. *Acta Biomed* 77 (2):118–123.

Etminan, Mahyar, Bahi Takkouche, and Francisco Caamano-Isorna. 2004. The role of tomato products and lycopene in the prevention of prostate cancer: A meta-analysis of observational studies. *Cancer Epidemiol Biomarkers Prev* 13 (3):340–345.

Falasca, Marco, Ilaria Casari, and Tania Maffucci. 2014. Cancer chemoprevention with nuts. *J Natl Cancer Inst* 106 (9):pii: dju238.

Fleischauer, Aaron T., Charles Poole, and Lenore Arab. 2000. Garlic consumption and cancer prevention: Meta-analyses of colorectal and stomach cancers. *Am J Clin Nutr* 72 (4):1047–1052.

Franco, Eduardo L., Luiz P. Kowalski, Benedito V. Oliveira, M. Paula Curado, Raimunda N. Pereira, M. Estela Silva, Antonio S. Fava, and Humberto Torloni. 1989. Risk factors for oral cancer in Brazil: A case control study. *Int J Cancer* 43 (6):992–1000.

Gago-Dominguez, Manuela, J. Esteban Castelao, Francisco Gude, Maite Pena Fernandez, Miguel E. Aguado-Barrera, Sara Miranda Ponte, Carmen M. Redondo et al. 2016. Alcohol and breast cancer tumor subtypes in a Spanish Cohort. *SpringerPlus* 5 (1):1–9.

Giovannucci, Edward, Eric B. Rimm, Alberto Ascherio, Meir J. Stampfer, Graham A. Colditz, and Walter C. Willett. 1995. Alcohol, low-methionine-low-folate diets, and risk of colon cancer in men. *J Natl Cancer Inst* 87 (4):265–273.

Goldstein, Binh Y., Shen-Chih Chang, Mia Hashibe, Carlo La Vecchia, and Zuo-Feng Zhang. 2010. Alcohol consumption and cancer of the oral cavity and pharynx from 1988 to 2009: An update. *Eur J Cancer Prev* 19 (6):431–465.

Guasch-Ferré, Marta, Mònica Bulló, Miguel Ángel Martínez-González, Emilio Ros, Dolores Corella, Ramon Estruch, Montserrat Fitó et al., and PREDIMED study group. 2013.

Frequency of nut consumption and mortality risk in the PREDIMED nutrition intervention trial. *BMC Med* 11:164.

Hamidpour, Rafie, Mohsen Hamidpour, Soheila Hamidpour, and Mina Shahlari. 2015. Cinnamon from the selection of traditional applications to its novel effects on the inhibition of angiogenesis in cancer cells and prevention of Alzheimer's disease, and a series of functions such as antioxidant, anticholesterol, antidiabetes, antibacterial, antifungal, nematicidal, acaracidal, and repellent activities. *J Tradit Complement Med* 5 (2):66–70.

Hanahan, Douglas, and Robert A. Weinberg. 2011. Hallmarks of cancer: The next generation. *Cell* 144 (5):646–674.

Hosgood, H. Dean, Paolo Boffetta, Sander Greenland, Yuan-Chin Amy Lee, John McLaughlin, Adeline Seow, Eric J. Duell, Angeline S. Andrew, David Zaridze, and Neonila Szeszenia-Dabrowska. 2010. In-home coal and wood use and lung cancer risk: A pooled analysis of the International Lung Cancer Consortium. *Environ Health Perspect* 118 (12):1743–1747.

Inoue, Manami, Kazuo Tajima, Mitsuhiro Mizutani, Hiroji Iwata, Takuji Iwase, Shigeto Miura, Kaoru Hirose, Nobuyuki Hamajima, and Suketami Tominaga. 2001. Regular consumption of green tea and the risk of breast cancer recurrence: Follow-up study from the Hospital-Based Epidemiologic Research Program at Aichi Cancer Center (HERPACC), Japan. *Cancer Lett* 167 (2):175–182.

International Agency for Research on Cancer. 2015. World Cancer Report 2014. WHO. Accessed November 15, 2015. http://www.iarc.fr/en/publications/books/wcr/wcr-order. php.

Jaiswal McEligot, Archana, Joan Largent, Argyrios Ziogas, David Peel, and Hoda Anton-Culver. 2006. Dietary fat, fiber, vegetable, and micronutrients are associated with overall survival in postmenopausal women diagnosed with breast cancer. *Nutr Cancer* 55 (2):132–140.

Jarvis, Carolyn. 2015. *Physical Examination and Health Assessment*. Saint Louis, MO: Elsevier Health Sciences.

Je, Youjin, Susan E. Hankinson, Shelley S. Tworoger, Immaculata DeVivo, and Edward Giovannucci. 2011. A prospective cohort study of coffee consumption and risk of endometrial cancer over a 26-year follow-up. *Cancer Epidemiol Biomarkers Prev* 20 (12):2487–2495.

Jin, Zi-Yi, Ming Wu, Ren-Qiang Han, Xiao-Feng Zhang, Xu-Shan Wang, Ai-Ming Liu, Jin-Yi Zhou, Qing-Yi Lu, Zuo-Feng Zhang, and Jin-Kou Zhao. 2013. Raw Garlic Consumption as a protective factor for lung cancer, a population-based case-control study in a Chinese population. *Cancer Prev Res (Phila)* 6 (7):711–718.

Johnson, Constance M., Caimiao Wei, Joe E. Ensor, Derek J. Smolenski, Christopher I. Amos, Bernard Levin, and Donald A. Berry. 2013. Meta-analyses of colorectal cancer risk factors. *Cancer Causes Control* 24 (6):1207–1222.

Jones-McLean, E., J. Hu, L. S. Greene-Finestone, and M. de Groh. 2015. A DASH dietary pattern and the risk of colorectal cancer in Canadian adults. *Health Promot Chronic Dis Prev Can* 35 (1):12–20.

Karna, Prasanthi, Sharmeen Chagani, Sushma R. Gundala, Padmashree C. G. Rida, Ghazia Asif, Vibhuti Sharma, Meenakshi V. Gupta, and Ritu Aneja. 2012. Benefits of whole ginger extract in prostate cancer. *Br J Nutr* 107 (4):473–484.

Kenfield, Stacey A., Natalie DuPre, Erin L. Richman, Meir J. Stampfer, June M. Chan, and Edward L. Giovannucci. 2014. Mediterranean diet and prostate cancer risk and mortality in the health professionals follow-up study. *Eur Urol* 65 (5):887–894.

Kim, Hyun Ja, Woong Ki Chang, Mi Kyung Kim, Sang Sun Lee, and Bo Youl Choi. 2002. Dietary factors and gastric cancer in Korea: A case control study. *Int J Cancer* 97 (4):531–535.

Ko, Ying-Chin, Li Shu-Chuan Cheng, Chien-Hung Lee, Jhi-Jhu Huang, Ming-Shyan Huang, Eing-Long Kao, Hwei-Zu Wang, and Hsiang-Ju Lin. 2000. Chinese food cooking and lung cancer in women nonsmokers. *Am J Epidemiol* 151 (2):140–147.

Kono, Suminori, and Tomio Hirohata. 1996. Nutrition and stomach cancer. *Cancer Causes Control* 7 (1):41–55.

Kwan, Marilyn L., Erin Weltzien, Lawrence H. Kushi, Adrienne Castillo, Martha L. Slattery, and Bette J. Caan. 2009. Dietary patterns and breast cancer recurrence and survival among women with early-stage breast cancer. *J Clin Oncol* 27 (6):919–926.

Larsson, Susanna C., Maria Kumlin, Magnus Ingelman-Sundberg, and Alicja Wolk. 2004. Dietary long-chain n-3 fatty acids for the prevention of cancer: A review of potential mechanisms. *Am J Clin Nutr* 79 (6):935–945.

Lee, I. Min. 2003. Physical activity and cancer prevention: Data from epidemiologic studies. *Med Sci Sports Exerc* 35 (11):1823–1827.

Lee, I. Min, Eric J. Shiroma, Felipe Lobelo, Pekka Puska, Steven N. Blair, Peter T. Katzmarzyk, and Lancet Physical Activity Series Working Group. 2012. Effect of physical inactivity on major non-communicable diseases worldwide: An analysis of burden of disease and life expectancy. *Lancet* 380 (9838):219–229.

Liu, Jianping, Jianmin Xing, and Yutong Fei. 2008. Green tea (*Camellia sinensis*) and cancer prevention: A systematic review of randomized trials and epidemiological studies. *Chin Med* 3 (1):12.

Liu, Rui Hai. 2003. Health benefits of fruit and vegetables are from additive and synergistic combinations of phytochemicals. *Am J Clin Nutr* 78 (3):517S–520S.

Marmot, Michael, Tola, Atinmo, Tim, Byers, Junshi, Chen, Tomio, Hirohata, Alan, Jackson, Philip, W. James, Laurence, N. Kolonel, Shiriki, Kumanyika, and Claus, Leitzmann. 2007. *Food, Nutrition, Physical Activity, and the Prevention of Cancer: A Global Perspective*. Washington, DC: American Institute for Cancer Research.

Matsuoka, Masao. 2003. Human T-cell leukemia virus type I and adult T-cell leukemia. *Oncogene* 22 (33):5131–5140.

Mlombe, Y. B., N. E. Rosenberg, L. L. Wolf, C. P. Dzamalala, K. Challulu, J. Chisi, N. J. Shaheen, Mina C. Hosseinipour, and C. G. Shores. 2015. Environmental risk factors for oesophageal cancer in Malawi: A case-control study. *Malawi Med J* 27 (3):88–92.

National Cancer Institute. 2015. The genetics of cancer. Accessed November 16, 2015. http://www.cancer.gov/about-cancer/causes-prevention/genetics.

National Library of Medicine. 2015. Carcinogen. Accessed November 16, 2015. http://ghr.nlm.nih.gov/glossary=carcinogen.

Nelson, David E., Dwayne W. Jarman, Jurgen Rehm, Thomas K. Greenfield, Gregoire Rey, William C. Kerr, Paige Miller, Kevin D. Shield, Yu Ye, and Timothy S. Naimi. 2013. Alcohol-attributable cancer deaths and years of potential life lost in the United States. *Am J Public Health* 103 (4):641–648.

Ngo, Suong N. T., Desmond B. Williams, and Richard J. Head. 2011. Rosemary and cancer prevention: Preclinical perspectives. *Crit Rev Food Sci Nutr* 51 (10):946–954.

NIH—National Cancer Institute. 2015. Cancer (malignant neoplasm). Accessed November 15, 2015. http://www.ncbi.nlm.nih.gov/pubmedhealth/PMHT0015630.

Norat, Teresa, Sheila Bingham, Pietro Ferrari, Nadia Slimani, Mazda Jenab, Mathieu Mazuir, Kim Overvad et al. 2005. Meat, fish, and colorectal cancer risk: The European Prospective Investigation into Cancer and Nutrition. *J Natl Cancer Inst* 97 (12):906–916.

Norat, Teresa, Annekatrin Lukanova, Pietro Ferrari, and Elio Riboli. 2002. Meat consumption and colorectal cancer risk: Dose-response meta-analysis of epidemiological studies. *Int J Cancer* 98 (2):241–256.

Norat, Teresa, Chiara Scoccianti, Marie-Christine Boutron-Ruault, Annie Anderson, Franco Berrino, Michele Cecchini, Carolina Espina, Tim Key, Michael Leitzmann, and Hilary

Powers. 2015. European Code against Cancer 4th edition: Diet and cancer. *Cancer Epidemiol* 39 (Suppl 1):S56–S66.

Oberg, Mattias, Maritta S. Jaakkola, Alistair Woodward, Armando Peruga, and Annette Pruss-Ustun. 2011. Worldwide burden of disease from exposure to second-hand smoke: A retrospective analysis of data from 192 countries. *Lancet* 377 (9760):139–146.

Olsen, Catherine M., Louise F. Wilson, Christina M. Nagle, Bradley J. Kendall, Christopher J. Bain, Nirmala Pandeya, Penelope M. Webb, and David C. Whiteman. 2015. Cancers in Australia in 2010 attributable to insufficient physical activity. *Aust N Z J Public Health* 39 (5):458–463.

Onvani, Shokouh, Fahimeh Haghighatdoost, and Leila Azadbakht. 2015. Dietary Approaches to Stop Hypertension (DASH): Diet components may be related to lower prevalence of different kinds of cancer; A review on the related documents. *J Res Med Sci* 20 (7):707–713.

Pandeya, Nirmala, Louise F. Wilson, Penelope M. Webb, Rachel E. Neale, Christopher J. Bain, and David C. Whiteman. 2015. Cancers in Australia in 2010 attributable to the consumption of alcohol. *Aust N Z J Public Health* 39 (5):408–413.

Park, Wungki, A. R. M. Ruhul Amin, Zhuo Georgia Chen, and Dong M. Shin. 2013. New perspectives of curcumin in cancer prevention. *Cancer Prev Res (Phila)* 6 (5):387–400.

Parkin, D. Max. 2011. The fraction of cancer attributable to lifestyle and environmental factors in the UK in 2010. *Br J Cancer* 105:S2–S5.

Pattle, Samuel B., and Paul J. Farrell. 2006. The role of Epstein–Barr virus in cancer. *Expert Opin Biol Ther* 6 (11):1193–1205.

Pavia, Maria, Claudia Pileggi, Carmelo G. A. Nobile, and Italo F. Angelillo. 2006. Association between fruit and vegetable consumption and oral cancer: A meta-analysis of observational studies. *Am J Clin Nutr* 83 (5):1126–1134.

Petridou, Eleni, Simon Kedikoglou, Panagiotis Koukoulomatis, Nick Dessypris, and Dimitrios Trichopoulos. 2002. Diet in relation to endometrial cancer risk: A case-control study in Greece. *Nutr Cancer* 44 (1):16–22.

Pharoah, Paul D. P., Nicholas E. Day, Stephen Duffy, Douglas F. Easton, and Bruce A. J. Ponder. 1997. Family history and the risk of breast cancer: A systematic review and meta-analysis. *Int J Cancer* 71 (5):800–809.

Polednak, Anthony P. 2008. Estimating the number of U.S. incident cancers attributable to obesity and the impact on temporal trends in incidence rates for obesity-related cancers. *Cancer Detect Prev* 32 (3):190–199.

Prasad, Sahdeo, and Amit K. Tyagi. 2015. Ginger and its constituents: Role in prevention and treatment of gastrointestinal cancer. *Gastroenterol Res Pract* 2015:142979.

Raaschou-Nielsen, Ole, Zorana J. Andersen, Rob Beelen, Evangelia Samoli, Massimo Stafoggia, Gudrun Weinmayr, Barbara Hoffmann, Paul Fischer, Mark J. Nieuwenhuijsen, and Bert Brunekreef. 2013. Air pollution and lung cancer incidence in 17 European cohorts: Prospective analyses from the European Study of Cohorts for Air Pollution Effects (ESCAPE). *Lancet Oncol* 14 (9):813–822.

Renehan, Andrew G., Margaret Tyson, Matthias Egger, Richard F. Heller, and Marcel Zwahlen. 2008. Body-mass index and incidence of cancer: A systematic review and meta-analysis of prospective observational studies. *Lancet* 371 (9612):569–578.

Rhode, Jennifer, Sarah Fogoros, Suzanna Zick, Heather Wahl, Kent A. Griffith, Jennifer Huang, and J. Rebecca Liu. 2007. Ginger inhibits cell growth and modulates angiogenic factors in ovarian cancer cells. *BMC Complement Altern Med* 7:44.

Richman, Erin L., Peter R. Carroll, and June M. Chan. 2012. Vegetable and fruit intake after diagnosis and risk of prostate cancer progression. *Int J Cancer* 131 (1):201–210.

Sanjoaquin, M. A., P. N. Appleby, M. Thorogood, J. I. Mann, and T. J. Key. 2004. Nutrition, lifestyle and colorectal cancer incidence: A prospective investigation of 10,998 vegetarians and non-vegetarians in the United Kingdom. *Br J Cancer* 90 (1):118–121.

Sasazuki, Shizuka, Manami Inoue, Tomoyuki Hanaoka, Seiichiro Yamamoto, Tomotaka Sobue, and Shoichiro Tsugane. 2004. Green tea consumption and subsequent risk of gastric cancer by subsite: The JPHC Study. *Cancer Causes Control* 15 (5):483–491.

Schernhammer, Eva S., Kimberly A. Bertrand, Brenda M. Birmann, Laura Sampson, Walter C. Willett, and Diane Feskanich. 2012. Consumption of artificial sweetener- and sugar-containing soda and risk of lymphoma and leukemia in men and women. *Am J Clin Nutr* 96 (6):1419–1428.

Schwingshackl, Lukas, and Georg Hoffmann. 2014. Adherence to Mediterranean diet and risk of cancer: A systematic review and meta-analysis of observational studies. *Int J Cancer* 135 (8):1884–1897.

Schwingshackl, Lukas, and Georg Hoffmann. 2015. Adherence to Mediterranean diet and risk of cancer: An updated systematic review and meta-analysis of observational studies. *Cancer Med* 4 (12):1933–1947.¡

Shehzad, Adeeb, Fazli Wahid, and Young Sup Lee. 2010. Curcumin in cancer chemoprevention: Molecular targets, pharmacokinetics, bioavailability, and clinical trials. *Arch Pharm (Weinheim)* 343 (9):489–499.

Smith, Robert A., Deana Manassaram-Baptiste, Durado Brooks, Mary Doroshenk, Stacey Fedewa, Debbie Saslow, Otis W. Brawley, and Richard Wender. 2015. Cancer screening in the United States, 2015: A review of current American Cancer Society guidelines and current issues in cancer screening. *CA Cancer J Clin* 65 (1):30–54.

Steinmaus, Craig M., Sandra Nunez, and Allan H. Smith. 2000. Diet and bladder cancer: A meta-analysis of six dietary variables. *Am J Epidemiol* 151 (7):693–702.

Teiten, Marie-Hélène, Serge Eifes, Mario Dicato, and Marc Diederich. 2010. Curcumin: The paradigm of a multi-target natural compound with applications in cancer prevention and treatment. *Toxins (Basel)* 2 (1):128–162.

Trichopoulos, Dimitrios, Frederick P. Li, and David J. Hunter. 1996. What causes cancer? *Sci Am* 275 (3):80–84.

Weinberg, Robert A. 1996. How cancer arises. *Sci Am* 275 (3):62–71.

Whalen, Kristine A., Marji McCullough, W. Dana Flanders, Terryl J. Hartman, Suzanne Judd, and Roberd M. Bostick. 2014. Paleolithic and Mediterranean diet pattern scores and risk of incident, sporadic colorectal adenomas. *Am J Epidemiol* 180 (11):1088–1097.

Whalen, Kristine, Marji McCullough, W. Dana Flanders, Terryl J. Hartman, Suzanne Judd, and Roberd M. Bostick. 2015. Paleolithic and Mediterranean diet pattern scores and their associations with biomarkers of inflammation and oxidative balance. *Cancer Res* 75 (15 Suppl):1889–1889.

Whiteman, David C., Penelope M. Webb, Adele C. Green, Rachel E. Neale, Lin Fritschi, Christopher J. Bain, D. Max Parkin, Louise F. Wilson, Catherine M. Olsen, and Christina M. Nagle. 2015a. Cancers in Australia in 2010 attributable to modifiable factors: Introduction and overview. *Aust N Z J Public Health* 39 (5):403–407.

Whiteman, David C., Penelope M. Webb, Adele C. Green, Rachel E. Neale, Lin Fritschi, Christopher J. Bain, D. Max Parkin, Louise F. Wilson, Catherine M. Olsen, and Christina M. Nagle. 2015b. Cancers in Australia in 2010 attributable to modifiable factors: Summary and conclusions. *Aust N Z J Public Health* 39 (5):477–484.

World Health Organization. 2011. Cancer linked with poor nutrition. Accessed November 23, 2015. http://www.euro.who.int/en/health-topics/noncommunicable-diseases/cancer/news/news/2011/02/cancer-linked-with-poor-nutrition.

WHO. 2015a. Cancer. Accessed November 15, 2015. http://www.who.int/mediacentre/factsheets/fs297/en.

WHO. 2015b. Cancer prevention. Accessed November 20, 2015. http://www.who.int/cancer/prevention/en.

Wu, Qi-Jun, Gong Yang, Wei Zheng, Hong-Lan Li, Jing Gao, Jing Wang, Yu-Tang Gao, Xiao-Ou Shu, and Yong-Bing Xiang. 2015. Pre-diagnostic cruciferous vegetables intake and lung cancer survival among Chinese women. *Sci Rep* 5:10306.

Yang, M., F. B. Hu, E. L. Giovannucci, M. J. Stampfer, W. C. Willett, C. S. Fuchs, K. Wu, and Y. Bao. 2015. Nut consumption and risk of colorectal cancer in women. *Eur J Cancer*. doi:10.1038/ejcn.2015.66. (Epub ahead of print).

Yeh, Chih-Ching, San-Lin You, Chien-Jen Chen, and Fung-Chang Sung. 2006. Peanut consumption and reduced risk of colorectal cancer in women: A prospective study in Taiwan. *World J Gastroenterol* 12 (2):222–227.

Yusof, Afzaninawati Suria, Zaleha Md Isa, and Shamsul Azhar Shah. 2012. Dietary patterns and risk of colorectal cancer: A systematic review of cohort studies (2000–2011). *Asian Pac J Cancer Prev* 13 (9):4713–4717.

Zhang, Zhizhong, Gelin Xu, Minmin Ma, Jie Yang, and Xinfeng Liu. 2013. Dietary fiber intake reduces risk for gastric cancer: A meta-analysis. *Gastroenterology* 145 (1):113–120. e3.

10 HEAL for Mental Health Issues

Karen M. Davison, Ann S. Hatcher, and David Benton

CONTENTS

10.1 WHAT IS MENTAL HEALTH?

In 1999, U.S. Surgeon General David Satcher issued a report on mental health and mental illness and stated, "There is no health without mental health," a saying that is often reiterated by recognized health authorities globally. The World Health Organization (WHO) defines mental health as "a state of well-being in which every individual realizes his or her own potential, can cope with the normal stresses of life, can work productively and fruitfully, and is able to make a contribution to her or his community" (WHO 2011). Based on the WHO's definition, someone who is mentally healthy is not simply a person who does not have any psychopathologies such as depression and anxiety. Rather, mental health and illness are considered related dimensions of a two-continua model (Figure 10.1), viewed as subjective evaluations with respect to the core components of the WHO's definition of positive mental health (Westerhof and Keyes 2008) that include emotional, psychological, and social well-being. "Flourishing" is a state where individuals combine a high level of subjective well-being with an optimal level of psychological and social functioning. Similarly, "languishing" refers to a state where low levels of subjective well-being are combined with low levels of psychological and social well-being. Those who are not languishing or flourishing are considered to be in moderate mental health. This definition parallels the definition of depression in the fifth edition of the American Psychiatric Association's *Diagnostic and Statistical Manual of Mental Disorders* (DSM-5) (American Psychiatric Association 2013), which includes both feelings of

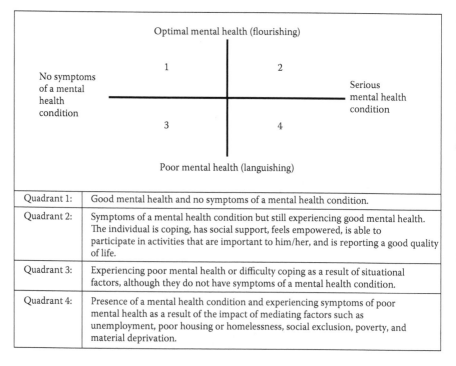

Quadrant 1:	Good mental health and no symptoms of a mental health condition.
Quadrant 2:	Symptoms of a mental health condition but still experiencing good mental health. The individual is coping, has social support, feels empowered, is able to participate in activities that are important to him/her, and is reporting a good quality of life.
Quadrant 3:	Experiencing poor mental health or difficulty coping as a result of situational factors, although they do not have symptoms of a mental health condition.
Quadrant 4:	Presence of a mental health condition and experiencing symptoms of poor mental health as a result of the impact of mediating factors such as unemployment, poor housing or homelessness, social exclusion, poverty, and material deprivation.

FIGURE 10.1 Two-continua model for mental health assessment. (From Canadian Mental Health Association, *Mental Health Promotion*, Canadian Mental Health Association, Toronto, 2006; CLM Keyes, *J Health Soc Behav*, 43(2), 207–222, 2002.)

anhedonia (feeling sadness or a loss of interest and pleasure) and reported problems in functioning (such as problems in appetite, sleeping, or fatigue). The two-continua model of mental illness and health has been validated across a number of international samples across the life span (Keyes 2005, 2006; Suldo and Shaffer 2008; Westerhof and Keyes 2008). Figure 10.1 shows the two-continua model for mental health assessment.

10.2 WHAT ARE MENTAL HEALTH CONDITIONS?

Each quadrant of the two-continua model (Figure 10.1) highlights one of the four possible experiences people may have with respect to their mental health (Canadian Mental Health Association 2006; Keyes 2002). Included in the model are serious mental health conditions. For the purposes of this chapter, reference will be made to mental health conditions rather than mental disorders or illnesses, the latter of which suggest that individuals who have them are always symptomatic and do not have periods of remission or good mental health. Mental health conditions comprise a broad range of problems and symptoms due to an alteration in brain or nervous system function. They are generally characterized by some combination of abnormal thoughts, emotions, behavior, and relationships with others. Examples are schizophrenia, depression, and substance use disorders (WHO 2015). Mental health conditions, therefore, are conditions that are formally diagnosed using either of the internationally recognized criteria that include the fifth edition of the American Psychiatric Association's *Diagnostic and Statistical Manual of Mental Disorders* (DSM-5) (American Psychiatric Association 2013) or those outlined in the mental and behavioral disorders section of the WHO's International Statistical Classification of Diseases and Related Health Problems, 10th revision. In reference to the two-continua model, languishing individuals function as poorly on most outcomes as those with a mental health condition who have symptoms. Individuals who are flourishing but have periods mental symptoms (e.g., fewer missed days of work) function better than those with moderate mental health, who in turn function better than individuals who are languishing and have episodes of mental illness.

10.3 FOOD GROUPS AND DIETARY PATTERNS TO PREVENT MENTAL ILL HEALTH

10.3.1 THE INTERSECTIONS OF NUTRITION AND MENTAL ILL HEALTH

Social and biological sciences have provided insight into the role of risk and protective factors in the development of poor mental health and diet as a modifiable target for prevention and mental health promotion (Figure 10.2). Research suggests that mental health conditions are associated with neurotransmitter imbalances, hypothalamic–pituitary–adrenal axis (HPA) disturbances, dysregulated inflammatory pathways, microbiome imbalance, increased oxidative and nitrosative damage, neuroprogression, and mitochondrial disruptions (Berk et al. 2013; Lopresti et al. 2012; Maes

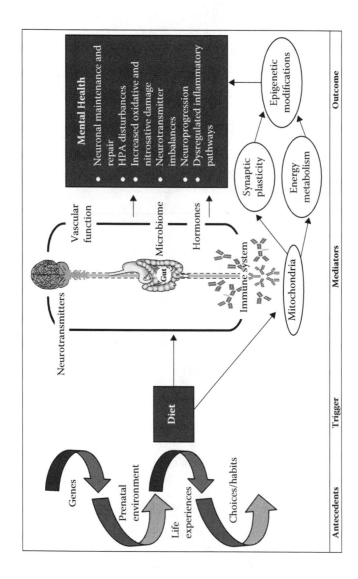

FIGURE 10.2 Schematic relationships between diet and mental health. (From J.S. Grigoleit et al., *PLoS One*, 6(12):e28330, 2011; S. Romero et al., *J Clin Psychiatry*, 70(10), 1452–1460, 2009; M. Berk et al., *BMC Med*, 12, 200, 2013.)

et al. 2013), and all of these pathways require enzymes and coenzymes that are derived from nutrients. Nutrients commonly associated with mental health include polyunsaturated fatty acids (particularly the omega-3 types), minerals such as zinc, magnesium, selenium, copper, and iron, B vitamins such as folate, vitamin B_6, and vitamin B_{12}, antioxidants such as vitamins C and E, and vitamin D (Kaplan et al. 2007; Maddock et al. 2013). Researchers have also explored the relationship between intakes of specific food groups (e.g., fruits, vegetables, fish, milk, and red meat) and dietary patterns (e.g., vegetarian and traditional diets) that may impact on mental health. While most of the evidence draws on the use of heterogeneous measures of diet and mental health from observational studies and does not always control for confounders such as education, general health consciousness, activity, and affluence, the findings seem relatively consistent and compelling. Figure 10.2 shows the relationship between diet and mental health.

10.3.2 DIETARY PATTERNS AND MENTAL HEALTH

Several investigations have connected "healthy" dietary patterns to a lower risk of depression, anxiety, bipolar disorder, and suicide in adults. Cross-sectional and longitudinal studies that compared "healthy" (e.g., focused on whole foods, Mediterranean-style diets) and "unhealthy" diets based on food frequency questionnaires have shown that decreased adherence to low-quality diets (e.g., more processed foods, nutrient poor) are associated with new diagnoses of depression (Chrysohoou et al. 2004), dysthymia, or anxiety disorders (Jacka et al. 2011) or high depression scores (Sarandol et al. 2007). Various population studies have linked traditional diet patterns such as Mediterranean, Japanese, and Norwegian dietary practices to a lowered risk of anxiety or depression (Jacka et al. 2010; Jacka et al. 2011; Rienks et al. 2013; Sanchez-Villegas et al. 2009). A 2013 study found that among nearly 90,000 Japanese men and women, a prudent diet characterized by more vegetables, fruit, potatoes, soy products, mushrooms, seaweed, and fish correlated with a lower risk of suicide (Nanri et al. 2013).

10.3.3 FOODS, FOOD GROUPS, AND MENTAL HEALTH

Two recent reviews drawing on observational and randomized clinical trials (RCTs) suggested that a high intake of fruits, vegetables, fish, and whole grains and modest amounts of dairy and lean meats may be protective against depression (Lai et al. 2014; Opie et al. 2015); a high intake of fish may also be protective against Alzheimer's disease (AD) (Xu et al. 2015). However, a more recent longitudinal investigation of the relationship between fruit and vegetable intake and mental health suggests that health behaviors such as smoking and physical activity have a larger impact on depression than diet (Kingsbury et al. 2015). In recent years, some research specific to milk and milk product intake and its relationship to cognitive function and psychological well-being have indicated that higher-fat products that contain primarily saturated fat are associated with poor psychological functioning (Crichton et al. 2010) and that higher milk and milk product intake in postmenopausal women is associated with new diagnoses of depression (Pasco et al. 2015).

10.3.4 Diet across the Life Span and Mental Health

Links between nutrition and mental health have also been shown in different developmental periods across the life span. Several studies have indicated that mothers with low-quality diets during the perinatal period and up to the first 5 years of their child's life increase the risk of attention problems and aggressive behavior as well as anxious and depressive symptoms in their children (Jacka et al. 2013). Similar findings have been found in childhood and adolescence. For example, a review of seven studies revealed a consistent trend between a higher intake of nutrient-dense foods, including vegetables, salads, fruits, and fish, and lower rates of depression, low mood, emotional problems, and anxiety (O'Neil et al. 2014). Conversely, a consistent and positive relationship between an "unhealthy" dietary pattern (i.e., a higher intake of saturated fat, sugar, refined starches, and processed foods) and poorer mental health in youth was found. However, it is important to note that many studies included in this review did not take socioeconomic status into account, which may explain the observed relationship rather than diet or mental health alone.

In early-to-late adulthood, the nutrition and mental health research has largely focused on factors associated with cognitive decline, forms of dementia, and depression. High intakes of saturated and polyunsaturated fat (excluding the omega-3s), processed sugar, and excess calories contribute to body-wide oxidative stress, weight gain and obesity, dyslipidemia, hyperglycemia, and atherosclerosis, which are risk factors that have been linked to cognitive decline (Arvanitakis et al. 2004; Gustafson et al. 2003; Kalmijn 2000; Kivipelto et al. 2006). Observational studies suggest that energy-dense diets containing excess fat (particularly saturated and trans fat) are associated with an increased risk of mental health conditions (Gougeon et al. 2015; Whitmer et al. 2005). Conversely, Mediterranean-style diets that emphasize vegetables, fruits, whole grains, fish, legumes, and nuts may protect against the development of depressive symptoms in older age (Skarupski et al. 2013). In a recent study of disadvantaged elderly Brazilians, fruit and vegetable intakes that exceeded the WHO's recommendations (>400 g) were significantly associated with reduced cognitive impairment (Pastor-Valero et al. 2014). Much scientific attention has been focused on antioxidants, particularly vitamins C and E, in the prevention of Alzheimer's disease. Shrinkage of the brain begins in young adulthood, suggesting that dietary influences will take place from that time onward over a period of many decades. In a meta-analysis, high vitamin C and/or E intake showed a trend of attenuating risk by about 26%. However, no significant association was indicated with a concurrent intake of these antioxidants (Xu et al. 2015).

10.4 FOOD GROUPS AND DIETARY PATTERNS TO TREAT MENTAL HEALTH CONDITIONS

Medical nutrition therapy is recognized as a cornerstone of treatment for mental health conditions that can help optimize the structure and function of neurons and brain centers, as well as contribute to self-reliance and healthy body image. Lifestyle interventions, including diet and exercise, are viable and effective adjunct strategies in the treatment of mental health conditions (Bauer et al. 2016). In this section, dietary interventions are discussed for different mental health conditions.

10.4.1 ANXIETY DISORDERS

Anxiety disorders are a group of conditions in which anxiety and avoidance behavior are prominent, including separation anxiety disorder, selective mutism, specific phobia, social phobia, panic disorder, agoraphobia, and generalized anxiety disorder (American Psychiatric Association 2013). Several epidemiological studies have found associations between poor diet quality and anxiety; however, the underlying mechanisms to explain these links are largely based on animal studies. Current recommendations are that individuals with anxiety disorders should consume a high-quality diet with low levels of caffeine (Tenore et al. 2015) to minimize symptoms.

10.4.2 ATTENTION DEFICIT HYPERACTIVITY DISORDER

Attention deficit hyperactivity disorder (ADHD) includes inattention (e.g., distractibility), hyperactivity, and/or impulsivity (e.g., fidgeting, excessive running, interrupting others). Individuals with ADHD tend to have deficiencies of polyunsaturated fatty acids, zinc, magnesium, and iron. Serum ferritin and zinc levels may be low; supplementation of iron and zinc helps symptoms if there is deficiency (Kiddie et al. 2010; Konofal et al. 2008). If the child is food sensitive, an additive-free diet (no food colors or preservatives) might improve symptoms (Schab and Trinh 2004) but must be monitored by a registered dietitian to ensure adequacy. Though sugar is thought to cause hyperactivity, a meta-analysis of well-designed studies assessing the impact of sucrose on the behavior of children produced no evidence that it has an adverse influence (Benton 2008). Individuals with ADHD should be checked for celiac disease and, if present, a gluten-free diet can improve behavior (Niederhofer and Pittschieler 2006).

10.4.3 AUTISM

Based on the DSM-5 criteria, individuals with autism spectrum disorder (ASD) show symptoms from early childhood that can occur along a spectrum and can include communication deficits, dependence on routines, high sensitivity to changes in the environment, or intense focus on inappropriate items (American Psychiatric Association 2013). Studies appear to suggest that the diets of children with ASD tend to lack in milk and milk products, fiber, calcium, iron, and vitamins D and E (Herndon et al. 2009). Some may respond to an increased intake of omega-3 fats, especially docosahexaenoic acid (DHA), ranging from 1 to 3 g/day. Gluten-free and casein-free diets are only recommended if there has been a diagnosis of an intolerance or allergy to foods containing the allergens (Marí-Bauset et al. 2014).

10.4.4 BIPOLAR AND RELATED DISORDERS

Bipolar disorders include a history of manic, mixed, or hypomanic episodes, usually with a concurrent or previous history of one or more major depressive episodes

(Brenner 2014). Up to 65% of individuals with bipolar disorder meet the criteria for at least one comorbid mental health condition (McElroy et al. 2001); the most common include anxiety, substance use, ADHD, and personality disorders. The cyclical nature of bipolar disorder presents unique challenges for nutritional interventions. During mania, large amounts of sugar, caffeine, and food may be consumed or there may be periods of not eating (American Dietetic Association and Dietitians of Canada 2000). If the individual is in a controlled environment, measures can be put into place to ensure healthy foods are available in order to prevent weight gain from overeating. If they are not eating, providing nutritious foods and beverages that are easy to consume while someone is on the go (e.g., energy bars, fruit smoothies) will help ensure adequate nutrition is provided. Selenium, folic acid (folate), omega-3 fatty acids, and tryptophan are substances that have all been implicated in keeping moods stable and good food sources of these should be emphasized in the diet (Mahan and Escott-Stump 2007).

10.4.5 DEPRESSIVE DISORDERS

Depressive disorders include chronic depression (dysthymia), disruptive mood dysregulation, and major depressive and premenstrual dysphoric disorders. Most of the criteria for major depressive disorder are identical in DSM-IV and DSM-5; the disorder is defined by one or more major depressive episodes (MDE) and the lifetime absence of mania and hypomania (Uher et al. 2014). Depression often leads to weight changes as appetite may increase or decrease. The tendency to carry excess weight in this population may be exacerbated by a preference for higher-calorie liquids and/or convenience foods and a sedentary lifestyle (American Dietetic Association and Dietitians of Canada 2000). Others may undereat due to feelings such as not being worthy enough to eat, lacking motivation or energy to prepare foods, or somatic delusions of not being able to eat. A well-balanced diet with protein/calorie supplementation may help as well as structuring eating for mood stability throughout the day; enteral feedings may be needed for those who refuse food. Similar to other mental health conditions, celiac disease is common in this population and testing to rule out this condition is recommended. Depressive disorders often coexist with eating disturbances (Davison et al. 2014), thereby requiring behavioral interventions to normalize eating.

10.4.6 TRAUMA- AND STRESSOR-RELATED DISORDERS

Trauma- and stressor-related disorders include conditions such as reactive attachment disorder, disinhibited social engagement disorder, post-traumatic stress disorder (PTSD), acute stress disorder, or adjustment disorders. Approximately 40%–60% of people with PTSD have symptoms that become chronic, and comorbidities such as major depression, anxiety, or substance abuse are common and may require therapeutic diet interventions. Recent studies have described an association of PTSD symptoms with fast food and soda consumption and unhealthy dieting behaviors (i.e., purging and food avoidance) in young women (Hirth et al. 2011). Individuals with adverse childhood experiences are at increased risk of developing maladaptive coping strategies, including stress-induced emotional eating (Evers et al. 2010). Emerging research suggests that targeting emotional dysregulation may provide benefits for those exposed to childhood trauma. For example, focusing on controlling caloric intake in those exposed to trauma may reduce the risk of obesity, which is associated with emotional dysregulation (Michopoulos et al. 2015). Nutritional guidelines that include a focus on antioxidants (e.g., beta-carotene, vitamin C, vitamin E, and selenium) may help counteract the effects of stress (American Dietetic Association and Dietitians of Canada 2000).

10.4.7 DISRUPTIVE, IMPULSE CONTROL, AND CONDUCT DISORDERS

Disruptive, impulse control, and conduct disorders include oppositional defiant disorder, pyromania, kleptomania, intermittent explosive disorder, conduct disorder, and dyssocial personality disorder (American Psychiatric Association 2013). Clinical trial data that included baseline dietary (dietary survey) and behavioral (i.e., overt aggression scale, life history of aggression, conflict tactics scale, self-rated impatience and irritability) assessments of 945 adult men and women indicated that dietary trans fatty acids (dTFA) were associated with greater aggression (Golomb et al. 2012). However, the roles of natural versus manufactured dTFA were not separated. Based on an assessment of relationships between biochemical indicators of diet and aggression in forensic psychiatric patients, the consumption of ample sources of omega-3 fats and supplementation with vitamin D is recommended (Zaalberg et al. 2015). The role of diet in antisocial behavior in children has been the subject of some studies. A meta-analysis of five well-designed studies found that elimination diets reduced hyperactivity-related symptoms (Benton 2007). Supplementation with polyunsaturated fatty acids decreased violence, but there was no indication of influence on hyperactivity. Three studies reported that vitamin/mineral supplementation reduced antisocial behavior.

10.4.8 EATING DISORDERS

This group of conditions includes anorexia nervosa (AN), bulimia nervosa (BN), and binge eating disorder (BED) (American Psychiatric Association 2013). AN involves the refusal by the individual to maintain a minimal normal body weight (e.g., less than 85% of expected), intense fear of gaining weight, and significant body image disturbances. AN usually begins in females during the teen years or young adulthood. The goals for AN treatment are to restore normal body weight and eating habits. A weight gain of 0.5–1.5 kg/week is considered a safe goal and may be achieved by increasing social activity, reducing physical activity, and using schedules for eating. Many start with a short hospital stay and then are followed through a day treatment program. For severe and life-threatening malnutrition, the person may need enteral or parenteral feedings.

BN is a condition in which a person binges on food or has regular episodes of overeating and feels a loss of control. The affected person then uses various purging methods, such as vomiting, laxatives, enemas, diuretics, or excessive exercise to prevent weight gain (American Psychiatric Association 2000). Most often, a stepped nutrition intervention approach is used. Support groups may be helpful for patients with mild conditions who do not have any health problems. Cognitive behavioral therapy and nutritional therapy are the preferred treatments for BN that does not respond to support groups.

BED is characterized by the consumption of large amounts of food in a 2 h time period, accompanied by a perceived loss of control (American Psychiatric Association 2000). BED, or compulsive eating, is often triggered by chronic dieting and involves periods of overeating, often in secret and often carried out as a means of deriving comfort. Because BED involves both weight and eating disorder concerns, researchers and professionals in both the obesity and eating disorder fields perceive treatment goals differently. Eating disorder experts suggest binge eating is best approached by treating underlying psychological problems, whereas obesity experts think that excess weight should be addressed first. BED often presents itself in those seeking weight loss surgery; these individuals should be screened for disordered eating and treated as needed (American Dietetic Association 2011).

Nutritional care as part of a multidisciplinary team approach is important in the treatment of eating disorders. A variety of counseling techniques are utilized that include cognitive behavioral therapy, dialectical behavioral therapy, motivational interviewing, and mindfulness. In the counseling of those with eating disturbances, a history of trauma and antecedents of food behaviors are explored. Nutrition intervention supports experimentation with new behaviors and the adoption of healthy eating patterns (American Dietetic Association 2011; Wanden-Berghe et al. 2011). Eating disorders are often found with conditions such as depression, anxiety, body dysmorphic disorder, chemical dependency, or personality disorders, which require additional counseling skills (Wilson and Syako 2009).

Eating disorder not otherwise specified (EDNOS) refers to eating disturbances of clinical severity that fall outside the diagnostic criteria of eating disorders (Fairburn et al. 2007). Night eating syndrome (NES), one example of EDNOS, is a syndrome consisting of morning anorexia, evening hyperphagia, and insomnia. People with NES typically have more frequent eating episodes (9.3 vs. 4.2 in 24 hours), more daily caloric intake between 8:00 p.m. and 6:00 a.m., and frequent nighttime awakenings (Birketvedt et al. 1999). They tend toward carbohydrate-rich nighttime snacks with a high carbohydrate-to-protein ratio (7:1) (Birketvedt et al. 1999). The aims of treatment are regular meal consumption earlier in the daytime, shifting the timing of caloric intake, and increased protein intake.

10.4.9 NEUROCOGNITIVE DISORDERS

Those with mild neurocognitive disorder have mild cognitive deficits in one or more of the same domains but can function independently (i.e., have intact instrumental activities of daily living), often through increased effort or compensatory strategies. Major neurocognitive disorders have the same characteristics as the mild classifications; however, the cognitive decline is significant. Dementia is described as a clinical syndrome with impairment in multiple neuropsychological and behavioral domains, including memory, cognition, visuospatial skills, and language (Franczak and Maganti 2004). Alzheimer's disease (AD) is the most common form of dementia. Unintentional weight loss is one of the main hallmarks of AD and the loss of weight can continue as the condition progresses (Gillette Guyonnet et al. 2007). Interventions such as a high-energy, high-protein diet, facilitating the ability to self-feed with adaptive equipment such as lip plates, specialized cups, and weighted utensils, guided feeding techniques, or food texture modification can help prevent the loss of weight.

10.4.10 Schizophrenia Spectrum Disorders

Schizophrenia spectrum disorders include a range of unusual behaviors such as delusions, hallucinations, disorganized speech, or disorganized or catatonic behavior that cause profound disruption in the lives of people with the condition. Schizophrenia spectrum disorders are considered the most severe of the DSM-5 conditions and are often complicated by physical and psychiatric comorbidities, including metabolic syndrome, cardiovascular disease, chronic obstructive pulmonary disease, type 2 diabetes, tuberculosis, HIV, hepatitis B and C, periodontal disease (Casey et al. 2011; Cournos et al. 2005; Friedlander and Marder 2002), anxiety, depression, PTSD, obsessive-compulsive disorder, and substance use issues (Hermle et al. 2013), all having nutritional implications. Individuals with schizophrenia tend to have diets that are high in energy and fat, and low in fruits and vegetables, fiber, vitamin C, and beta-carotene (McCreadie and Scottish 2003). Nutritional interventions are usually related to symptoms (e.g., catatonia) or the side effects of medications. Second-generation antipsychotic treatment is associated with metabolic side effects that include various degrees of weight gain, dyslipidemia, susceptibility to type 2 diabetes, and metabolic syndrome (McEvoy et al. 2005; Newcomer 2005). Nutritional interventions should be focused to prevent and treat these conditions as outlined in the earlier chapters.

For individuals that have hallucinations related to smell and taste, a loss of pleasure from eating and food safety risks may occur (Gaines 2010). Flavor enhancement of food with appropriate seasonings might help make the food more enjoyable, and taking precautions with measuring devices, thermometers, and timers will help to avoid relying on aroma and taste to determine meal quality and readiness (Green et al. 2008). Celiac disease in schizophrenia has double the prevalence of general populations. Testing for this condition is advised and if confirmed a gluten-free diet should be implemented (Cascella et al. 2011).

10.4.11 Substance Use Disorders

Substance use disorders include conditions usually defined by the type of substance used (e.g., alcohol, illicit drugs, prescription or over-the-counter medications, tobacco) and include a maladaptive pattern of use leading to significant impairment or distress, tolerance (e.g., increased need for the substance to achieve effects), and withdrawal (Hasin et al. 2013). The consumption of different substances can have profound effects on health and nutritional status. These effects occur as a result of the decreased inclusion of foods that provide essential nutrients and calories and alterations in the functioning of body organs (Thompson and Manore 2012). Recovery occurs in different stages and certain nutritional modifications can be beneficial according to the stage.

- *Stage 1: Early recovery*—Emotional and cognitive processing of the fact that the substance use is destroying one's life occurs (Gorski and Miller 1982). Nutritional interventions can include ensuring food intake at regular intervals and encouraging the use of a wider variety of foods than when the individual was consuming the substance. The use of nutritional supplements that provide one to three times the recommended levels of vitamins B and C, magnesium, and zinc aids recovery.
- *Stage 2: Middle recovery (aftercare)*—A commitment to long-term treatment and the lifestyle changes essential to maintaining sobriety are made (Gorski and Miller 1982). For most, the consumption of foods from the recommended food groups is the primary goal of nutritional therapy. For highly motivated clients, experimentation with new food patterns is possible. Clients interested in taking care of the problems resulting from poor nutrition will seek out information and explore the use of nutritional supplements and herbs. The clinician needs to be aware of this pattern and provide education about credible sources of information.
- *Stage 3: Late recovery*—As the client becomes more comfortable with the new lifestyle essential to staying substance-free, an assessment of the life problems that occurred as a result of alcohol and drug abuse becomes possible (Gorski and Miller 1982). The modification of fat and sugar intake, appropriate weight control measures, and addressing the nutritional health problems resulting from substance use are likely to occur at this point of recovery.
- *Maintenance*—Recovery from substance abuse is a life-long process resulting in a continued increase in knowledge and making appropriate changes in lifestyle (Gorski and Miller 1982). As recovery becomes more stable and the body changes with age, appropriate nutritional changes are needed.

Generally speaking, a varied diet rich in healthy carbohydrates, good-quality proteins (lean meat, fish, and vegetable proteins), fresh fruit and vegetables, essential fats (oily fish, nuts), and lots of water (Grotzkyj-Giorgi 2009) help with the recovery process.

10.5 HOME REMEDIES TO PREVENT AND TREAT MENTAL HEALTH CONDITIONS

There has been little study of home remedies to prevent mental health conditions. Investigations that have been conducted tended to be on small sample groups, using varying doses and diverse measures of mental health condition outcomes. In recent years, there have been several studies examining the use of vitamins and minerals in general populations and their effects on mental health. In a meta-analysis of eight randomized and placebo-controlled studies (Long and Benton 2013) that evaluated stress, mild psychiatric symptoms, or mood in the general population and multiple vitamin/mineral supplement use for at least 28 days, the results indicated that supplementation reduced the levels of perceived stress, mild psychiatric symptoms, anxiety, fatigue, and confusion. No improvements were found for depression.

Therapeutic options for those with mental health conditions contain agents that include constituents such as vitamins and minerals, herbs, homeopathic medicines, traditional medicines, probiotics, and other products such as amino acids and essential fatty acids. The use of some of these products (e.g., St. John's wort, dehydroepiandrosterone [DHEA], ginseng, melatonin) may produce negative side effects when combined with conventional management (Lam 2006; Ulbricht et al. 2008). However, other studies have shown that some home remedies result in the requirement of lower doses of medications (Sarris et al. 2011). The following highlights home remedies that have been used for mental health conditions and the evidence that supports them.

- *Ginkgo biloba*: G. biloba (Gb) may increase vasodilation, peripheral blood flow, antioxidant action, and cholinergic transmission by inhibiting acetylcholinesterase. This product may elevate gamma-aminobutyric acid (GABA) and inhibit the neuronal uptake of serotonin, potentiating serotonergic activity. A systematic review of RCTs with meta-analysis (Chen et al. 2015) in the treatment of schizophrenia indicated that the extract of Gb as an adjuvant therapy to antipsychotics in chronic schizophrenia treatment showed differences in ameliorating total and negative symptoms. However, the safety of Gb therapy in chronic schizophrenia treatment needs more evidence as all trials examined were based on Chinese populations. For Alzheimer's disease (AD), Gb may be beneficial. In a systematic review of RCTs (von Gunten et al. 2015), the effects of Gb were assessed for behavioral and psychological symptoms of dementia (BPSD) in confirmed AD and treated for at least 22 weeks. Outcome measures covered BPSD and at least two domains of assessment (i.e., cognition, activities of daily living, clinical global assessment). Four trials ($n = 1628$ outpatients) with mild-to-moderate dementia were included. From baseline in cognition, BPSD, activities of daily living, clinical global impression, and quality of life favored Gb. The pooled analyses provided evidence for Gb (240 mg/d) in the treatment of outpatients suffering from AD or vascular or mixed dementia with BPSD.
- *Kava kava*: A Cochrane review and meta-analysis of seven RCTs using kava preparations (60–280 mg kavalactones) for the treatment of generalized anxiety symptoms found a reduction in the Hamilton Anxiety Rating Scale (HAM-A) scores for kava compared with placebo (p value $= .01$) (Pittler and Ernst 2000).
- *Omega-3 fatty acid*: In a Cochrane review of the efficacy of omega-3 fatty acids as either an alternative or adjunct treatment for bipolar disorder (Montgomery and Richardson 2008), five studies of variable methodological quality were included. Only one study involving 75 participants could be analyzed, and the results indicated a reduction in depression symptoms and clinical global impression scores but not for mania. A 12-week RCT conducted in individuals at high clinical risk of schizophrenia provided

preliminary evidence that an intervention composed of 1.2 g of PUFA (i.e., EPA and DHA) could prevent transition to first-episode psychosis. A recent study notes that PUFA metabolism disturbances are present relatively early in the course of schizophrenia and diminish over time as the disease progresses, and that treatment with antipsychotic medications (e.g., aripiprazole, risperidone) was able to correct aberrant PUFA levels in first episodes, but not in chronic schizophrenia (McEvoy et al. 2013). This suggests that intervention with n-3 PUFA can be more effective when administered early in the course of the disease.

- *S-adenosyl methionine (SAMe)*: SAMe is distributed in body tissues and fluids and plays a role in the immune system, preserves cell membranes, and helps produce and metabolize several brain substances, such as acetylcholine, melatonin, and dopamine. Being deficient in either vitamin B_{12} or vitamin B_6 may reduce body levels of SAMe, leading to the development of depressive symptoms (De Berardis et al. 2013). Several studies have indicated that SAMe monotherapy reduces depression symptoms (Papakostas et al. 2012). When SAMe (800 mg/twice daily) is used as an adjunct to standard therapy in people who are non- or partial responders to selective serotonin reuptake inhibitors or serotonin norepinephrine reuptake inhibitors, positive results are observed (Papakostas et al. 2010).

- *St. John's Wort (Hypericum perforatum)*: St. John's Wort might inhibit the reuptake of serotonin, norepinephrine, dopamine, GABA, and L-glutamate and is often advocated for use in depression. A recent systematic review that investigated whether antidepressants are more effective than placebo in the primary care setting (Linde et al. 2015) found that *H. perforatum* extracts were superior to placebo, with estimated odds ratios between 1.69 and 2.03. While *H. perforatum* extracts have shown some positive results, the limitations of the available evidence make a clear recommendation on their place in clinical practice difficult.

- *Vitamins*: Vitamins B_6, B_9 (folate), and B_{12} have been provided as treatment options for depression and Alzheimer's disease. These vitamins share common pathways in the synthesis of many neurotransmitters (e.g., dopamine, serotonin, norepinephrine, epinephrine, histamine, GABA) (McCarty 2000). A systematic review of 11 RCTs of vitamin B_9 (folate or folic acid) or vitamin B_{12} (cobalamin or cyanocobalamin) and measures of depression (condition or symptoms) found that the short-term use of these vitamins (a few days to a few weeks) does not improve depressive symptoms in adults with major depression treated with antidepressants. However, based on one study, consumption over several weeks to years may decrease the risk of relapse. In two studies, the use of these vitamins showed decreases in the onset of clinically significant symptoms in people at risk (Almeida et al. 2015).

Vitamin D's role in depression is biologically plausible based on mechanisms that include its role in modulating the hypothalamic–pituitary–adrenal axis, regulating adrenalin, noradrenaline, and dopamine production through receptors in the adrenal cortex (Puchacz et al. 1996), and protecting against the depletion of dopamine and serotonin centrally (Cass et al. 2006). Two meta-analyses showed contradictory results for the use of vitamin D supplements in depression (Gowda et al. 2015; Spedding 2014), the limitations of these studies being that most had low levels of depression and sufficient serum vitamin D at baseline, and the vitamin D doses and duration of interventions varied.

- *Multinutrient formulas*: In the past decade, a few studies have examined the use of multinutrient formulas (i.e., vitamins, minerals) in the treatment of mental health symptoms. In a systematic review that examined at least four vitamins and/or minerals (Rucklidge and Kaplan 2015), there was some evidence of efficacy for the use of micronutrients in the treatment of stress, antisocial behavior, and depressed mood in nonclinical and elderly populations. The same review also suggested that the evidence to support micronutrient supplementation in the treatment of autism spectrum disorders, bipolar disorder, ADHD, and substance abuse/dependence is insufficient at this time. Finally, there was no clinical trial evidence for the use of these supplements in clinically depressed or anxious samples, psychosis, or eating disorders.

10.6 NUTRITIONAL COUNSELING FOR MENTAL HEALTH CONDITIONS

Nutritional care in the prevention and management of mental health conditions may help improve or stabilize nutritional status (e.g., identify, prevent, or minimize drug nutrition side effects), identify and correct eating disturbances, optimize medication effectiveness (e.g., prevent or correct nutritional deficiencies), and enable the individual to function at the highest level of independent living.

Figure 10.3 outlines an algorithm that may be used in the assessment and management of nutritional status for those with mental health issues.

Table 10.1 outlines selected condition-specific factors and their impact on nutritional intake.

Considerations for the initial screening of an individual for mental health concerns include

- *Presence of health conditions and/or following a special diet*: Special or therapeutic diets include modifications made to the amount, types, or textures of foods or fluids. These diets may be implemented if a person has a health condition such as cardiovascular disease, ulcers, Crohn's disease, ulcerative colitis, celiac disease, cancer, cerebral palsy, or pancreatitis or any other conditions known to benefit from diet therapy. The individual would benefit from a review by a registered dietitian to ensure the nutritional adequacy of their food intake for optimal mental health.
- *Biochemical measures and genomic markers*: Abnormal lab results for measures such as blood glucose (random, fasting), albumin, cholesterol (total, HDL, LDL), hemoglobin, hematocrit, ferritin, serum creatinine, hemoglobin A_{1C}, prealbumin, total lymphocyte count, liver enzymes, triglycerides, potassium, sodium, folate, vitamin B_{12}, homocysteine, or

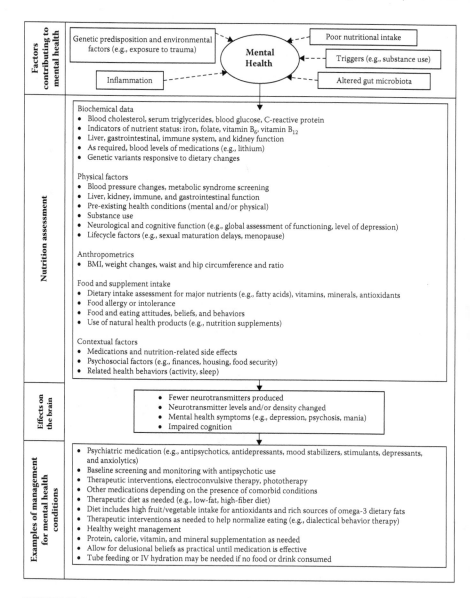

FIGURE 10.3 Nutritional counseling for Healthful Eating As Lifestyle (HEAL) for the prevention and management of mental health conditions. (Adapted from Dietitians of Canada, *Promoting Mental Health through Healthy Eating and Nutritional Care,* © Dietitians of Canada 2012. With permission.)

TABLE 10.1

Selected Condition-Specific Factors and Their Effects on Nutritional Intake

Factors	Description of Effect on Nutritional Intake
Altered circadian rhythm	Altered sleep can lead to increased eating and weight gain
Anxiety, overactivity	Unable to sit long enough to eat or eat "on the go"; increased energy output
Avoidance or social isolation	PTSD-related dissociation; isolation may induce overeating and access to health support; avoiding mealtimes, embarrassed to eat with others, and not shopping for food
Delirium	Delirium associated with poor nutrition
Dementia	Increased or decreased food intake; altered food choices; consumption of inedible substances; disturbances in eating processes and behavior
Depression	Overeating, undereating, comfort eating; feel unworthy of eating, lack of motivation, or poor energy levels; severe lack of appetite; no desire to shop or prepare food; poor food hygiene presenting food safety risks; exacerbated sedentary lifestyle associated with subsequent weight gain; somatic delusions of not being able to eat or being physically too ill to eat; preferences for liquid and/or convenience foods; require less energy to prepare and eat
Disordered eating, body image	Anorexia, bulimia, binge eating; may be prone to food fads, use of herbs or steroids, or eating disorder
Mania	Associated with treatment nonadherence; elevated or irritable mood, rapid speech, and hyperactivity; poor intake may result from distractibility; patients with bipolar disorder are less likely to report that their provider discussed diet habits with them
Megaphagia	Eating large amounts of food; common feature of Kleine–Levin syndrome
Memory or cognitive impairment	Forgetting to eat; forgetting a meal has been taken and overeating; impaired ability to retain new information
Obsessive compulsiveness	May avoid certain foods or food groups
Panic attacks	May use food to soothe anxiety leading to weight gain; may isolate themselves to prevent panic attacks, which may limit diet; may use sedating medication to ease symptoms, which may decrease motivation to eat and/or promote sleep/drowsiness
Pica	Consuming non-nutritive substances
Psychotic symptoms	Delusions about food or hallucinations, causing refusal to eat
Sensory issues	Some (especially children) may have problems with texture and consistency of foods
Sleep problems, insomnia	Can alter intake (usually increased); leads to night eating syndrome and weight gain; fatigue can lead to excess caffeine intake and dehydration
Substance use	Reduced food intake; organ damage alters the utilization of nutrients; malnutrition
Withdrawal	Undereating; delusions regarding fluid and food; lack of interest in eating; ravenous appetite

Source: Adapted from Dietitians of Canada, *Promoting Mental Health through Healthy Eating and Nutritional Care*, © Dietitians of Canada 2012. With permission.

microalbumin should be followed by a dietary assessment to determine where changes may be made to benefit both physical and mental health. In recent years, there has been much work done on the assessment of specific gene variants and their relationship to dietary response to enable the use of nutrition to its fullest potential to address various health issues. Caution must be exercised in recommending nutrigenomics tests to clients as the credibility of the various companies offering these products is variable. In general, it is recommended that clients can be referred to companies that provide tests with sound scientific evidence and that provide consultation with a regulated health professional with appropriate expertise (e.g., a registered dietitian) to review the results and provide a personalized nutrition care plan.

- *Medications*: Consider all types, including those sold over the counter (e.g., laxatives, antacids, enemas), vitamin and mineral supplements, and herbal remedies. Also consider if any of the following are taken: isoniazid (INH), antipsychotics, antiseizure medications, lithium, statins, or monoamine oxidase inhibitors (MAOI). Careful assessment of food intake as well as home remedies and medications will minimize the potential for adverse events. Furthermore, many medications used in the treatment of mental health conditions have nutrition-related side effects (Table 10.2) that must be considered in treatment. For those taking second-generation antipsychotics, metabolic monitoring is needed (Table 10.3).

Table 10.2 shows the nutrition-related side effects of selected medications. Table 10.3 shows the recommended schedule for monitoring patients taking second-generation antipsychotic medications.

- *Behavioral eating assessment*: Careful assessment of behaviors that can impact nutrition and mental health status should be undertaken. Examples may include eating nonfood or unsafe food items, regurgitating or self-inducing, taking excess fluids, eating a limited range of foods, using laxatives, diuretics, or diet pills, and chronic dieting.
- *Body measures*: Anthropometric measures of height, weight, waist circumference, and hip circumference should be undertaken for the calculations of BMI and waist-to-hip ratio, and compared with appropriate age/ethnic-specific standards. In addition, assessment for any significant weight changes (defined as 5% in 1 month, 7.5% in 2 months, or 10% in 6 months) should be made. Where required, review and adjust food intake or activity level to help achieve a healthy body weight.

Nutritional treatment for mental health conditions will require the use of therapeutic interventions. Table 10.4 highlights common therapeutic approaches in nutrition and mental health care.

TABLE 10.2
Selected Medications and Their Nutrition-Related Side Effects

Medication Group	Some Possible Nutrition-Related Side Effects
Analgesics/substance use treatment drugs	Anorexia, nausea, vomiting, constipation, decreased appetite, weight changes, menstrual irregularities with long-term use, sleep disturbances
Antianxiety (anxiolytic)/ sedative hypnotics	Constipation, sweating, nausea, vomiting, diarrhea, weight changes, edema
Anticonvulsants/ anti-epileptic	Nausea, vomiting, decreased appetite, weight increase, vitamin D deficiency, GI complaints, can alter blood glucose and lipids, trembling of hands
Antidepressants: SSRIs, SNRIs, and MAOIs	Nausea, vomiting, diarrhea, abdominal discomfort, dry mouth, constipation, sweating, anorexia, dyspepsia, insomnia

SSRIs: Interact with diabetes medications; weight loss occurs with acute treatment but not sustained with chronic treatment; tends to be more pronounced in those with excess weight; weight gain reported; up to 18% of people gain more than 7% body weight with chronic use. Rate of bone loss higher in SSRI users; increased risk of fractures in women and older adults

SNRIs: Increase blood cholesterol; reduce growth in children; sedation or insomnia; cases of elevated liver enzymes, hepatitis, bilirubinemia, and jaundice with venlafaxine

MAOIs: Hypertension; requires low-tyramine diet |
Antinarcolepsy/drugs for ADHD/stimulants	Anorexia, weight loss, HT, anemia
Antipsychotics typical ("first generation")	Dry mouth, constipation, weight gain; abdominal pain, water intoxication, mouth ulcerations; can alter blood glucose and lipids; hyperprolactinemia (can alter menstrual cycle); bone mineral density loss
Antipsychotics atypical/ novel ("second-generation" or "SGA")	Dry mouth, constipation, diarrhea, sweating, weight gain (primarily adipose tissue); dysphagia; requires metabolic monitoring (Table 10.3)
Antipsychotics ("third generation")	Appear to have less metabolic effect than SGAs; constipation, dysphagia, nausea, and vomiting (usually dissipates quickly)
Drugs for treatment of dementia	Nausea, vomiting, diarrhea, constipation, anorexia (occurs early in treatment); elevated liver transaminases in about 50% in first 12 weeks of treatment
Hypnotics/sedatives	Altered appetite; weight loss
Mood stabilizers/ antimanics	GI upset (initial), thirst, polyuria (may persist), dry mouth, metallic taste (composition of saliva altered), edema, weight changes (gain in 60%), hyperglycemia, hyperammonemia, acute pancreatitis, hypothyroidism, blood/serum calcium, phosphorous, and magnesium; weight gain (usually >4 kg) may be related to increased appetite, fluid retention, altered carbohydrate and fat metabolism, hypothyroidism

Source: Adapted from Dietitians of Canada, *Promoting Mental Health through Healthy Eating and Nutritional Care*, © Dietitians of Canada 2012. With permission.

TABLE 10.3
Recommended Schedule for Monitoring Individuals Taking Second-Generation Antipsychotics

Factor	Baseline	4 Weeks	8 Weeks	12 Weeks	Quarterly	Annually	Every 5 Years
Personal/family history	√					√	
Weight (BMI)	√	√	√	√	√		
Waist circumference	√					√	
Blood pressure	√			√		√	
Fasting plasma glucose	√			√		√	
Fasting lipid profile	√			√			√

Note: Second-generation antipsychotics include clozapine, olanzapine, ziprasidone, risperidone, and olanzapine-fluoxetine (combination).

Schedule based on
- National Cholesterol Education Program, Executive Summary of the Third Report of the National Cholesterol Education Program (NCEP) Expert Panel on the Detection, Evaluation, and Treatment of High Blood Cholesterol in Adults (ATP III), *JAMA* 285:2486–97, 2001.
- JW Newcomer and D Haupt, The metabolic effects of antipsychotic medication, *Can J Psychiatry* 51:480–491, 2006.
- American Diabetes Association, Consensus development conference on antipsychotic drugs and obesity and diabetes, *Diabetes Care* 27:596–601, 2004.
- Center for Quality Assessment and Improvement in Mental Health, Metabolic monitoring toolkit. Available at: http://www.cqaimh.org/pdf/tool_metabolic.pdf. Accessed February 1, 2016.

10.7   CASE STUDIES

10.7.1   CASE STUDY 1

Ashley is a 20-year-old white female who is in her second year of university. Her grades were previously all As but they have fallen substantially. She has come to you with complaints of headaches, difficulty concentrating, irritability, bloating, early satiety, constipation, and amenorrhea for 6 months. She has been a lacto-ovo-vegetarian for 1 year and restricts her intake to two meals/day (lunch and dinner). She limits the calories she consumes to a maximum 800 kcal/day and has a BMI of 18.5. You also discover that she self-harms by cutting on occasion. Give responses to the following questions:

1. What additional information will you need to assess Ashley more thoroughly?
2. What immediate nutrition interventions would you suggest?
3. You have ordered blood work and find the following: low potassium, low ferritin, and high creatine phosphokinase (an enzyme found mainly in the heart, brain, and skeletal muscle). What do these results suggest?
4. What long-term nutrition care will she need?

TABLE 10.4

Therapeutic Approaches in Nutrition and Mental Health Care

Therapeutic Approach	Description	Targeted Mental Health Conditions
Cognitive behavioral therapy (CBT)	Focus on how thoughts affects actions.	Eating disorders (BN, BED)
Mindfulness; mindfulness-based stress reduction (MBSR); mindfulness-based eating awareness training (MB-EAT)	Nonjudgmental awareness of the present moment; using all the senses to increase pleasure and connection to hunger/satiety cures.	Eating disorders; concurrent disorders; weight management
Dialectical behavior therapy (DBT)	A form of CBT, combined with mindfulness and validation strategies; core strategies blend a focus of both acceptances and change (dialectic).	Chronic suicidality; eating disorders; personality disorders
Solution-focused brief therapy (SFBT)	Goal-oriented; focuses on solutions versus problems; competency-based (the client is the expert).	Eating disorders; weight management
Acceptance and commitment therapy (ACT)	Based on experiential avoidance models: disordered behavior is often due to efforts to avoid/escape aversive internal experiences; uses nonjudgmental, mindful acceptance; commitment toward clarified goals and values.	Eating disorders

Source: Adapted from Dietitians of Canada, *Promoting Mental Health through Healthy Eating and Nutritional Care*, © Dietitians of Canada 2012. With permission.

10.7.2 CASE STUDY 2

Allen is a 52-year-old married male with two sons. He has come to see you as he has racing thoughts, irritability, variable appetite, and weight loss. Based on questions you have asked you have also discovered that he likes to drink two to three beers on weeknights and five to six beers per day on the weekends. His high- and low-density lipoproteins are normal; however, his triglycerides are high. He also has low folate levels and his thyroid levels are normal. His BMI is 26 kg/m². Give responses to the following questions:

1. What additional information will you need to assess Allen more thoroughly?
2. What immediate nutrition interventions would you suggest?
3. What ongoing monitoring would you recommend to ensure Allen's nutrition status is optimal?

REFERENCES

Almeida OP, Ford AH, and Flicker L. 2015. Systematic review and meta-analysis of randomized placebo-controlled trials of folate and vitamin B_{12} for depression. *Int Psychogeriatr* 27(5):727–737.

American Dietetic Association. 2011. Position of the American Dietetic Association: Nutrition intervention in the treatment of eating disorders. *J Am Diet Assoc* 111:1236–1241.

American Dietetic Association and Dietitians of Canada. 2000. *Manual of Clinical Dietetics*, 6th edn. Chicago: American Dietetics Association.

American Psychiatric Association. 2000. *Diagnostic and Statistical Manual of Mental Disorders* (DSM-IV-TR). Washington, DC: American Psychiatric Association.

American Psychiatric Association. 2013. *Diagnostic and Statistical Manual of Mental Disorders*, 5th edn. Arlington, VA: American Psychiatric Publishing.

Arvanitakis Z, Wilson RS, Bienias JL, Evans DA, and Bennett DA. 2004. Diabetes mellitus and risk of Alzheimer disease and decline in cognitive function. *Arch Neurol* 61:661–666.

Bauer IE, Gálvez JF, Hamilton JE, Balanzá-Martínez V, Zunta-Soares GB, Soares JC, and Meyer TD. 2016. Lifestyle interventions targeting dietary habits and exercise in bipolar disorder: A systematic review. *J Psychiatr Res* 74:1–7.

Benton D. 2007. The impact of diet on anti-social, violent and criminal behaviour. *Neurosci Biobehav Rev* 31(5):752–774.

Benton D. 2008. Sucrose and behavioral problems. *Crit Rev Food Sci Nutr* 48(5):385–401.

Berk M, Williams LJ, Jacka FN, O'Neil A, Pasco JA, Moylan S, Allen NB et al. 2013. So depression is an inflammatory disease, but where does the inflammation come from? *BMC Med* 12:200.

Birketvedt GS, Florholmen J, Sundsfjord J, Osterud B, Dinges D, Bilker W, and Stunkard A. 1999. Behavioral and neuroendocrine characteristics of the night-eating syndrome. *JAMA* 282(7):657–663.

Brenner CJ, Shyn SI. 2014. Diagnosis and management of bipolar disorder in primary care: A DSM-5 update. *Med Clin North Am* 98(5):1025–1048.

Canadian Mental Health Association. 2006. *Mental Health Promotion*. Toronto: Canadian Mental Health Association.

Cascella NG, Kryszak D, Bhatti B, Gregory P, Kelly DL, McEvoy JP, Fasano A, and Eaton WW. 2011. Prevalence of celiac disease and gluten sensitivity in the United States clinical antipsychotic trials of intervention effectiveness study population. *Schizophr Bull* 37(1):94–100.

Casey DA, Rodriguez M, Northcott C, Vickar G, and Shihabuddin L. 2011. Schizophrenia: Medical illness, mortality, and aging. *Int J Psychiatry Med* 41(3):245–251.

Cass WA, Smith MP, and Peters LE. 2006. Calcitriol protects against the dopamine- and serotonin-depleting effects of neurotoxic doses of methamphetamine. *Ann NY Acad Sci* 1074:261–271.

Chen X, Hong Y, and Zheng P. 2015. Efficacy and safety of extract of *Ginkgo biloba* as an adjunct therapy in chronic schizophrenia: A systematic review of randomized, double-blind, placebo-controlled studies with meta-analysis. *Psychiatry Res* 228(1):121–127.

Chrysohoou C, Panagiotakos DB, Pitsavos C, Das UN, and Stefanadis C. 2004. Adherence to the Mediterranean diet attenuates inflammation and coagulation process in healthy adults: The ATTICA Study. *J Am Coll Cardiol* 44(1):152–158.

Cournos F, McKinnon K, and Sullivan G. 2005. Schizophrenia and comorbid human immunodeficiency virus or hepatitis C virus. *J Clin Psychiatry* 66 (Suppl 6):27–33.

Crichton GE, Murphy KJ, and Bryan J. 2010. Dairy intake and cognitive health in middle-aged South Australians. *Asia Pac J Clin Nutr* 19(2):161–171.

Davison KM, Marshall-Fabien GL, and Gondara L. 2014. Sex differences and eating disorder risk among psychiatric conditions, compulsive behaviors and substance use in a screened Canadian national sample. *Gen Hosp Psychiatry* 36(4): 411–414.

De Berardis D, Marini S, Serroni N, Rapini G, Iasevoli F, Valchera A, Signorelli M et al. 2013. S-adenosyl-L-methionine augmentation in patients with stage II treatment-resistant major depressive disorder: An open label, fixed dose, single-blind study. *Scientific World Journal* 2013:204649.

Evers C, Marijn Stok F, and de Ridder DT. 2010. Feeding your feelings: Emotion regulation strategies and emotional eating. *Pers Soc Psychol Bull* 36(6):792–804.

Fairburn CG, Cooper Z, Bohn K, O'Connor ME, Doll HA, and Palmer RL. 2007. The severity and status of eating disorder NOS: Implications for DSM-V. *Behav Res Ther* 45(8):1705–1715.

Franczak MB and Maganti R. 2004. Neurodegenerative disorders: Dementias. *Neurology* 8(4):2.

Friedlander AH and Marder SR. 2002. The psychopathology, medical management, and dental implications of schizophrenia. *J Am Dental Assoc* 133(5):603–610.

Gaines AD. 2010. Anosmia and hyposmia. *Allergy Asthma Proc* 31(3):185–189.

Gillette Guyonnet S, Abellan Van Kan G, Alix E, Andrieu S, Belmin J, Berrut G et al. 2007. International academy on nutrition and aging expert group: Weight loss and Alzheimer's disease. *J Nutr Health Aging* 11(1):38–48.

Golomb BA, Evans MA, White HL, and Dimsdale JE. 2012. Trans fat consumption and aggression. *PLoS One* 7(3):e32175.

Gorski TT and Miller M. 1982. *Counseling for Relapse Prevention*. Independence, MO: Herald House.

Gougeon L, Payette H, Morais J, Gaudreau P, Shatenstein B, and Gray-Donald K. 2015. Dietary patterns and incidence of depression in a cohort of community-dwelling older Canadians. *J Nutr Health Aging* 19(4):431–436.

Gowda U, Mutowo MP, Smith BJ, Wluka AE, and Renzaho AM. 2015. Vitamin D supplementation to reduce depression in adults: Meta-analysis of randomized controlled trials. *Nutrition* 31(3):421–429.

Green TL, McGregor LD, and King KM. 2008. Smell and taste dysfunction following minor stroke: A case report. *Can J Neurosci Nurs* 30(2):10–13.

Grigoleit JS, Kullmann JS, Wolf OT, Hammes F, Wegner A, Jablonowski S, Engler H, Gizewski E, Oberbeck R, and Schedlowski M. 2011. Dose-dependent effects of endotoxin on neurobehavioral functions in humans. *PLoS One* 6(12):e28330.

Grotzkyj-Giorgi M. 2009. Nutrition and addiction: Can dietary changes assist with recovery? *Drugs and Alcohol Today* 9(2):24–28.

Gustafson D, Rothenberg E, Blennow K, Steen B, and Skoog I. 2003. An 18-year follow-up of overweight and risk of Alzheimer disease. *Arch Intern Med* 163:1524–1528.

Hasin DS, O'Brien CP, Auriacombe M, Borges G, Bucholz K, Budney A, Compton WM et al. 2013. DSM-5 criteria for substance use disorders: Recommendations and rationale. *Am J Psychiatry* 170(8):834–851.

Hermle L, Szlak-Rubin R, Täschner KL, Peukert P, and Batra A. 2013. Substance use associated disorders: Frequency in patients with schizophrenic and affective psychoses. *Nervenarzt* 84(3):315–325.

Herndon AC, DiGuiseppi C, Johnson SL, Leiferman J, and Reynolds A. 2009. Does nutritional intake differ between children with autism spectrum disorders and children with typical development? *Journal of Autism and Developmental Disorders* 39:212–222.

Hirth JM, Rahman M, and Berenson AB. 2011. The association of posttraumatic stress disorder with fast food and soda consumption and unhealthy weight loss behaviors among young women. *J Womens Health (Larchmt)* 20(8):1141–1149.

Jacka FN, Mykletun A, Berk M, Bjelland I, and Tell GS. 2011. The association between habitual diet quality and the common mental disorders in community-dwelling adults: The
Hordaland Health study. *Psychosom Med* 73(6):483–490.

Jacka FN, Pasco JA, Mykletun A, Williams LF, Hodge AM, O'Reilly SL, Nicholson GC,
Kotowicx MA, and Berk M. 2010. Association of Western and traditional diets with
depression and anxiety in women. *Am J Psychiatry* 167:305–311.

Jacka FN, Ystrom E, Brantsaeter AL, Karevold E, Roth C, Haugen M, Meltzer HM, Schjolberg
S, and Berk M. 2013. Maternal and early postnatal nutrition and mental health of offspring by age 5 years: A prospective cohort study. *J Am Acad Child Adolesc Psychiatry*
52(10):1038–1047.

Kalmijn S. 2000. Fatty acid intake and the risk of dementia and cognitive decline: A review of
clinical and epidemiological studies. *J Nutr Health Aging* 4:202–207.

Kaplan BJ, Crawford SG, Field CJ, and Simpson JSA. 2007. Vitamins, minerals, and mood.
Psychol Bull 133(5):747–760.

Keyes CLM. 2002. The mental health continuum: From languishing to flourishing. *J Health
Soc Behav* 43(2):207–222.

Keyes CLM. 2005. Mental illness and/or mental health? Investigating axioms of the complete
state model of health. *J Consult Clin Psychol* 73(3):539–548.

Keyes CLM. 2006. Mental health in adolescence: Is America's youth flourishing? *Am J
Orthopsychiatry* 76(3):395–402.

Kiddie JY, Weiss MD, Kitts DD, Ley-Milne R, and Wasdell MB. 2010. Nutritional status of
children with attention deficit hyperactivity disorder: A pilot study. *Int J Pediatr* 2010:
767318.

Kingsbury M, Dupuis G, Jacka F, Roy-Gagnon MH, McMartin SE, and Colman I. 2015.
Associations between fruit and vegetable consumption and depressive symptoms:
Evidence from a national Canadian longitudinal survey. *J Epidemiol Community Health*
70(2):155–161.

Kivipelto M, Ngandu T, Laatikainen T, Winblad B, Soininen H, and Tuomilehto J. 2006. Risk
score for the prediction of dementia risk in 20 years among middle aged people: A longitudinal, population-based study. *Lancet Neurol* 5:735–741.

Konofal E, Lecendreux M, Deron J, Marchand M, Cortese S, Zaim M, Mouren MC, and
Arnulf I. 2008. Effects of iron supplementation on attention deficit hyperactivity disorder in children. *Pediatr Neurol* 38(1):20–26.

Lai JS, Hiles S, Bisquera A, Hure AJ, McEvoy M, and Attia J. 2014. A systematic review and
meta-analysis of dietary patterns and depression in community-dwelling adults. *Am J
Clin Nutr* 99(1):181–197.

Lam RW. 2006. Sleep disturbances and depression: A challenge for antidepressants. *Int Clin
Psychopharmacol* 21:S25–S29.

Linde K, Kriston L, Rücker G, Jamil S, Schumann I, Meissner K, Sigterman K, and Schneider
A. 2015. Efficacy and acceptability of pharmacological treatments for depressive disorders in primary care: Systematic review and network meta-analysis. *Ann Fam Med*
13(1):69–79.

Long SJ and Benton D. 2013. Effects of vitamin and mineral supplementation on stress, mild
psychiatric symptoms, and mood in nonclinical samples: A meta-analysis. *Psychosom
Med* 75(2):144–153.

Lopresti AL, Hood SD, and Drummond PD. 2012. Multiple antidepressant potential modes
of action of curcumin: A review of its anti-inflammatory, monoaminergic, antioxidant,
immune-modulating and neuroprotective effects. *J Psychopharmacol* 26(12):1512–1524.

Maddock J, Berry DJ, Geoffroy MC, Power C, and Hyppönen E. 2013. Vitamin D and common mental disorders in mid-life: Cross-sectional and prospective findings. *Clin Nutr*
32(5):758–764.

Maes M, Kubera M, Leunis JC, Berk M, Geffard M, and Bosmans E. 2013. In depression, bacterial translocation may drive inflammatory responses, oxidative and nitrosative stress (O&NS), and autoimmune responses directed against O&NS-damaged neoepitopes. *Acta Psychiatr Scand* 127:344–354.

Mahan KL and Escott-Stump S. 2007. *Krause's Food and Nutrition Therapy*, 12th edn. Philadelphia, PA: Elsevier/Saunders.

Marí-Bauset S, Zazpe I, Mari-Sanchis A, Llopis-González A, and Morales-Suárez-Varela M. 2014. Evidence of the gluten-free and casein-free diet in autism spectrum disorders: A systematic review. *J Child Neurol* 29(12):1718–1727.

McCarty MF. 2000. High-dose pyridoxine as an "anti-stress" strategy. *Med Hypotheses* 54:803–807.

McCreadie R and Scottish Schizophrenia Lifestyle Group. 2003. Diet, smoking, and cardiovascular risk in people with schizophrenia: Descriptive study. *Br J Psychiatry* 183:534–539.

McElroy SL, Altshuler LL, Suppes T, Keck PE Jr, Frye MA, Denicoff KD, Nolen WA et al. 2001. Axis I psychiatric comorbidity and its relationship to historical illness variables in 288 patients with bipolar disorder. *Am J Psychiatry* 158:420–426.

McEvoy J, Baillie RA, Zhu H, Buckley P, Keshavan MS, Nasrallah HA, Dougherty GG, Yao JK, and Kaddurah-Daouk R. 2013. Lipidomics reveals early metabolic changes in subjects with schizophrenia: Effects of atypical antipsychotics. *PLoS One* 8(7):e68717.

McEvoy JP, Meyer JM, Goff DC, Nasrallah HA, Davis SM, Sullivan L, Meltzer HY, Hsiao J, Scott Stroup T, and Lieberman JA. 2005. Prevalence of the metabolic syndrome in patients with schizophrenia: Baseline results from the Clinical Antipsychotic Trials of Intervention Effectiveness (CATIE) schizophrenia trial and comparison with national estimates from NHANES III. *Schizophr Res* 80(1):19–32.

Michopoulos V, Powers A, Moore C, Villarreal S, Ressler KJ, and Bradley B. 2015. The mediating role of emotion dysregulation and depression on the relationship between childhood trauma exposure and emotional eating. *Appetite* 91:129–136.

Montgomery P and Richardson AJ. 2008. Omega-3 fatty acids for bipolar disorder. *Cochrane Database Syst Rev* 2:CD005169.

Nanri A, Mizoue T, Poudel-Tandukar K, Noda M, Kato M, Kurotani K, Goto A, Oba S, Inoue M, Tsugane S, and Japan Public Health Center–Based Prospective Study Group. 2013. Dietary patterns and suicide in Japanese adults: The Japan Public Health Center–Based Prospective Study. *Br J Psychiatry* 203(6):422–427.

Newcomer JW. 2005. Second-generation (atypical) antipsychotics and metabolic effects: A comprehensive literature review. *CNS Drugs* 19(Suppl 1): 1–93.

Niederhofer H and Pittschieler K. 2006. A preliminary investigation of ADHD symptoms in persons with celiac disease. *J Atten Disord* 10(2):200–204.

O'Neil A, Quirk SE, Housden S, Brennan SL, Williams LJ, Pasco JA, Berk M, and Jacka FN. 2014. Relationship between diet and mental health in children and adolescents: A systematic review. *Am J Public Health* 104(10):e31–e42.

Opie RS, O'Neil A, Itsiopoulos C, and Jacka FN. 2015. The impact of whole-of-diet interventions on depression and anxiety: A systematic review of randomised controlled trials. *Public Health Nutr* 18(11):2074–2093.

Papakostas GI, Cassiello CF, and Iovieno N. 2012. Folates and S-adenosylmethionine for major depressive disorder. *Can J Psychiatry* 57(7):406–413.

Papakostas GI, Mischoulon D, Shyu I, Alpert JE, and Fava M. 2010. S-adenosyl methionine (SAMe) augmentation of serotonin reuptake inhibitors for antidepressant nonresponders with major depressive disorder: A double-blind, randomized clinical trial. *Am J Psychiatry* 167(8):942–948.

Pasco JA, Williams LJ, Brennan-Olsen SL, Berk M, and Jacka FN. 2015. Milk consumption and the risk for incident major depressive disorder. *Psychother Psychosom* 84(6):384–386.

Pastor-Valero M, Furlan-Viebig R, Menezes PR, da Silva SA, Vallada H, and Scazufca M. 2014. Education and WHO recommendations for fruit and vegetable intake are associated with better cognitive function in a disadvantaged Brazilian elderly population: A population-based cross-sectional study. *PLoS One* 9(4):e94042.

Pittler MH and Ernst EE. 2000. Efficacy of kava extract for treating anxiety: Systematic review and meta-analysis. *J Clin Psychopharm* 20(1):84–89.

Puchacz E, Stumpf W, Stachowiak EK, and Stachowiak MK. 1996. Vitamin D increases expression of the tyrosine hydroxylase gene in adrenal medullary cells. *Mol Brain Res* 36:193–196.

Rienks J, Dobson AJ, and Mishra GD. 2013. Mediterranean dietary pattern and prevalence and incidence of depressive symptoms in mid-aged women: Results from a large community-based prospective study. *Eur J Clin Nutr* 67(1):75–82.

Romero S, Birmaher B, Axelson DA, Iosif AM, Williamson DE, Gill MK, Goldstein BI et al. 2009. Negative life events in children and adolescents with bipolar disorder. *J Clin Psychiatry* 70(10):1452–1460.

Rucklidge JJ and Kaplan BJ. 2015. Broad-spectrum micronutrient formulas for the treatment of psychiatric symptoms: A systematic review. *Expert Rev Neurother* 13(1):49–73.

Sanchez-Villegas A, Delgado-Rodriguez M, Alonso A, Schlatter J, Lahortiga F, Majem LS, and Martinez-Bonzalez MA. 2009. Association of the Mediterranean dietary pattern with the incidence of depression: The Seguimiento Universidad de Navarra/University of Navarra follow-up (SUN) cohort. *Arch Gen Psychiatry* 66:1090–1098.

Sarandol A, Sarandol E, Eker SS, Erdinc S, Vatansever E, and Kirli S. 2007. Major depressive disorder is accompanied with oxidative stress: Short-term antidepressant treatment does not alter oxidative-antioxidative systems. *Hum Psychopharmacol* 22:67–73.

Sarris J, Mischoulon D, and Schweitzer I. 2011. Adjunctive nutraceuticals with standard pharmacotherapies in bipolar disorder: A systematic review of clinical trials. *Bipolar Disord* 13:454–465.

Schab DW and Trinh NH. 2004. Do artificial colors promote hyperactivity in children with hyperactive syndromes? A meta-analysis of double-blind placebo-controlled trials. *J Dev Behav Pediatr* 25(6):423–434.

Skarupski KA, Tangney CC, Li H, Evans DA, and Morris MC. 2013. Mediterranean diet and depressive symptoms among older adults over time. *J Nutr Health Aging* 17(5):441–445.

Spedding S. 2014. Vitamin D and depression: A systematic review and meta-analysis comparing studies with and without biological flaws. *Nutrients* 6(4):1501–1518.

Suldo SM and Shaffer EJ. 2008. Looking beyond psychopathology: The dual-factor model of mental health in youth. *School Psych Rev* 37:52–68.

Tenore GC, Daglia M, Orlando V, D'Urso E, Saadat SH, Novellino E, Nabavi SF, and Nabavi SM. 2015. Coffee and depression: A short review of literature. *Curr Pharm Des* 21(34):5034–5040.

Thompson J and Manore M. 2012. *Nutrition: An Applied Approach*. New York: Benjamin Cummings.

Uher R, Payne JL, Pavlova B, and Perlis RH. 2014. Major depressive disorder in DSM-5: Implications for clinical practice and research of changes from DSM-IV. *Depress Anxiety* 31(6):459–471.

Ulbricht C, Chao W, Costa D, Rusie-Seamon E, Weissner W, and Woods J. 2008. Clinical evidence of herb-drug interactions: A systematic review by the natural standard research collaboration. *Curr Drug Metab* 9:1063–1120.

von Gunten A, Schlaefke S, and Überla K. 2015. Efficacy of *Ginkgo biloba* extract EGb 761® in dementia with behavioural and psychological symptoms: A systematic review. *World J Biol Psychiatry* Aug 27:1–12.

Wanden-Berghe RG, Sanz-Valero J, and Wanden-Berghe C. 2011. The application of mindfulness to eating disorders treatment: A systematic review. *Eat Disord* 19(1):34–48.

Westerhof GJ and Keyes CLM. 2008. Mental health is more than the absence of mental illness. *Maandblad geestelijke volksgezondheid* 63:808–820.

Wilson GT and Syako R. 2009. Frequency of binge eating episodes in bulimia nervosa and binge ED: Diagnostic considerations. *Int J Eat Disord* 42:603–610.

World Health Organization. 2010. *International Statistical Classification of Diseases and Related Health Problems* 10th Revision. Geneva, CHE: World Health Organization.

WHO. 2011 *Mental Health: A State of Well-Being.* Geneva, Switzerland: World Health Organization.

WHO. 2015. *Mental Disorders.* Geneva, Switzerland: World Health Organization.

Xu W, Tan L, Wang HF, Jiang T, Tan MS, Tan L, Zhao QF, Li JQ, Wang J, and Yu JT. 2015. Meta-analysis of modifiable risk factors for Alzheimer's disease. *J Neurol Neurosurg Psychiatry* 86(12):1299–1306.

Zaalberg A, Wielders J, Bulten E, van der Staak C, Wouters A, and Nijman H. 2015. Relationships of diet-related blood parameters and blood lead levels with psychopathology and aggression in forensic psychiatric inpatients. *Crim Behav Ment Health* 2016 Jul;26(3):196–211. doi: 10.1002/cbm.1954.

11 HEAL and Physical Activity

Ranjit Mohan Anjana, Vaidya Ruchi,
Vasudevan Sudha, Unnikrishnan
Ranjit, and Rajendra Pradeepa

CONTENTS

11.1 INTRODUCTION

Non-communicable diseases (NCDs), which include diabetes, cardiovascular disease (heart disease and stroke), cancers, chronic respiratory diseases, hypertension, obesity, and mental illness, have emerged as pandemics in recent years, with disproportionately higher rates in developing countries (Terzic and Waldman 2011). The World Health Organization (WHO) estimates that NCDs account for 80% of the global burden of disease, causing 7 out of every 10 deaths in the low- and middle-income countries (LMICs) of the world (WHO 2013). According to the WHO, it is estimated that the global NCD burden will increase by 17% in the next 10 years (WHO 2013).

The majority of NCDs occur due to the synergistic effects of behavioral risk factors such as physical inactivity, unhealthy diets, tobacco consumption, and the harmful use of alcohol. The greatest effects of these risk factors are observed increasingly in LMICs and in poorer people within all countries, mirroring the underlying socioeconomic determinants (poverty, illiteracy, social inequality, and poor health infrastructure). Physical inactivity is increasingly becoming prevalent in LMICs and already constitutes one of the leading causes of mortality (WHO 2009). There is concern about unhealthy diets in LMICs, although large regional differences are observed (Popkin 2006). Thus, promoting a balance between healthy food choices (energy input) and regular physical activity (PA) (energy output) is imperative in preventing NCDs.

11.1.1 BURDEN DUE TO PHYSICAL INACTIVITY

Physical inactivity is now identified as the fourth leading risk factor for global mortality (WHO 2010). According to Beaglehole et al. (2011), approximately 3.2 million deaths each year are attributable to physical inactivity and both physical inactivity and unhealthy diets are considered priority areas for international action. Globally, it is estimated that physical inactivity is responsible for between 6% and 10% of the major NCDs, including coronary heart disease (6.0%), type 2 diabetes (7.0%), breast cancer (10.0%), and colon cancer (10.0%). By eliminating physical inactivity, the life expectancy of the world's population may be expected to increase by 0.68 years (Lee et al. 2012). Evidence shows that adequate levels of PA are associated with a 30% reduction in the risk of ischemic heart disease, a 27% reduction in the risk of diabetes, and 21%–25% reduction in the risk of breast and colon cancer (Paffenbarger et al. 1994; Lee et al. 1995).

Physical inactivity levels are rising in many countries, with major implications for increases in the prevalence of NCDs worldwide (WHO 2010). A global report from 2000, comprised of 14 subregions, reported that 17.7% of the global population aged ≥15 years were not engaged in any kind of PA (WHO 2002), and that nearly 58% were not achieving the recommended amount of activity (USDHHS 2008). The World Health Survey, a large cross-sectional study, was done in 70 countries in 2002 and 2003 by the WHO (Guthold et al. 2008). This showed that the prevalence of physical inactivity for Indian men was 9.3%, whereas for women it was 15.2%. The International Prevalence Study on Physical Activity was a 20-country study done from 2002 to 2004 on 52,746 adults aged 18–65 years (Bauman et al. 2009). The prevalence of high PA varied from 21% to 63%. Low PA varied from 9% to 43%. A review conducted by Ng and Popkin (2012) looked at patterns of PA across time among adults in the United States, the United Kingdom, China, Brazil, and India. The review showed that across all countries studied, PA levels are on a downward trend and sedentary time is increasing across the globe. A more recent report from the WHO states that the prevalence of physical inactivity is highest in the Americas and the Eastern Mediterranean region (WHO Global Health Observatory 2012). In all regions, physical inactivity is higher in women than men, with the greatest disparity in

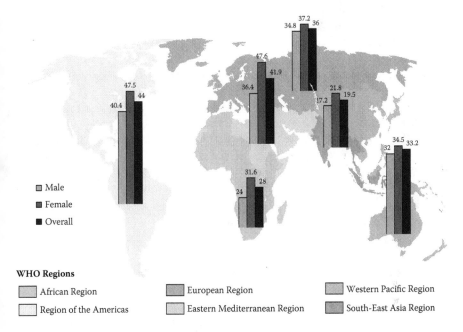

FIGURE 11.1 World map showing gender-wise prevalence of physical inactivity (age standardized). *Note*: 30 min of moderate activity less than five times per week or 20 min of vigorous activity less than three times of per week, or equivalent. (From WHO, Global Health Observatory, 2012).

the Eastern Mediterranean region. Although physical inactivity is more prevalent in high-income countries, the poorer countries are fast catching up. The *Lancet* released a PA series on the various aspects of physical activity. In this series, a study by Hallal et al. (2012) looked at physical inactivity levels across the globe. They obtained estimates for physical inactivity in adults aged 15 years or older from 122 countries, representing 88.9% of the world's population. The results showed that 31.1% of adults worldwide were physically inactive.

Figure 11.1 summarizes the gender-wise prevalence of physical inactivity worldwide.

11.1.2 Adverse Health Outcomes Due to Physical Inactivity

Low levels of PA are a major risk factor for ill health and mortality from all causes. A wide spectrum of adverse effects can occur with decreased PA, ranging from those that cause minimal inconvenience to those that are life threatening. Physical inactivity is a primary cause of the initiation of 35 separate pathological and clinical conditions (Booth et al. 2012). Strong evidence shows that physical inactivity increases the risk of many adverse health conditions, including the major NCDs (type 2 diabetes, CHD, stroke, cancer), and shortens life expectancy, which presents a major public health problem globally. Too much sitting and other sedentary activities can increase the risk of NCDs.

Globally, Lee et al. (2012) estimated that the elimination of physical inactivity would prevent between 6% and 10% of the major NCDs (coronary heart disease, type 2 diabetes, and breast and colon cancers) and increase life expectancy. The study also reported that inactivity is responsible for 9% of premature mortality. Physical inactivity is responsible for 5.8% of the burden of coronary heart disease worldwide, ranging from 3.2% in Southeast Asia to 7.8% in the Eastern Mediterranean. Similarly, the burden of diabetes attributable to physical inactivity is 7.2% worldwide, ranging from 3.9% in Southeast Asia to 9.6% in the Eastern Mediterranean. Worldwide, 10.1% of breast cancers and 10.4% of colon cancers are attributable to decreased PA.

11.2 PHYSICAL ACTIVITY AND HEALTH

11.2.1 WHAT IS PHYSICAL ACTIVITY?

According to the WHO, physical activity (PA) is defined as any bodily movement produced by muscles that requires energy expenditure, including activities undertaken while working, playing, carrying out household chores, traveling, and engaging in recreational pursuits (WHO 2015). From time immemorial, PA has been an essential component of human life and inextricably linked to survival. However, in this modern era of industrialization and mechanization, PA has taken a backseat. Physical inactivity has become a global problem not just in developed nations but in developing nations as well. Regular PA decreases the risk of non-communicable diseases by small-to-moderate degrees (Vuori 2014).

The term "physical activity" should not be mistaken with "exercise." Caspersen et al. (1985) have defined exercise as a subcategory of physical activity that is planned, structured, and repetitive, done to maintain or improve one or more components of physical fitness. Researchers sometimes use the terms "leisure time physical activity" or "recreational physical activity" as synonyms for exercise. Studies have shown that in rapidly growing large cities of the developing world, physical inactivity is an even greater problem, with more than half of the population of adults being insufficiently active. Urbanization has resulted in several environmental factors that discourage participation in physical activity, particularly in the transport and occupational domains. In developing countries, less than a quarter of the population exercises regularly (Anjana et al. 2015). Even in rural areas, sedentary activities (e.g., watching television, sleeping, sitting) are increasing. More than 90% of individuals in both urban and rural areas of India do no recreational physical activity at all (Anjana et al. 2015a).

11.2.2 TYPES OF EXERCISES

Exercise is generally grouped into two types depending on the overall effect they have on the human body. These are

- *Aerobic exercise* can be defined as those activities that use oxygen to adequately meet energy demands during exercise via aerobic metabolism (Anjana 2014). Aerobic activity usually involves using large muscle groups repetitively and rhythmically and can be performed for extended periods of time. This helps to improve cardiorespiratory fitness. Aerobic exercises including cycling, walking, running, hiking, and playing tennis focus on increasing cardiovascular endurance (Wilmore and Knuttgen 2003). Regular aerobic exercise has significant cardiovascular benefits (Mersy 1991).

- *Resistance or strength training* involves the physical training of a muscle or group of muscles to improve muscle strength and endurance—for example, weight lifting. When properly performed, strength training can provide significant health benefits as well as improvement in overall health and well-being. This type of exercise can also help maintain lean body mass, decrease the risk of osteoporosis, and develop coordination and balance. In contrast to aerobic exercise, resistance training mainly has long-term physiological effects. The effects of regular resistance training include increased muscle strength (up to 30%), muscle mass (10%–12%), and stamina, increased ability to sustain high-intensity exercise for longer periods of time, increased glucose utilization even in the resting state, and better postural stability in older individuals (Sigal et al. 2004).

11.2.3   How Much Physical Activity Is Recommended?

International guidelines regarding PA have been mostly developed from studies done in the West. The WHO has developed the Global Recommendations on Physical Activity for Health for the prevention of NCDs (WHO 2010). These recommendations are relevant for the following health outcomes: cardiorespiratory health (coronary heart disease, cardiovascular disease, stroke, and hypertension), metabolic health (diabetes and obesity), musculoskeletal health (bone health, osteoporosis), cancers (breast and colon cancer), functional health, the prevention of falls, and depression. The recommendations emphasize the need for at least 150 min of moderate-intensity aerobic physical activity throughout the week or at least 75 min of vigorous-intensity aerobic physical activity throughout the week, or an equivalent combination of moderate- and vigorous-intensity activity. Aerobic activity should be performed in bouts at least 10 min in duration. For additional health benefits, adults should increase their moderate-intensity aerobic physical activity to 300 min per week or engage in 150 min of vigorous-intensity aerobic physical activity per week, or an equivalent combination of moderate- and vigorous-intensity activity. In addition, muscle-strengthening activities involving major muscle groups should be done on 2 or more days a week. These recommendations are relevant to all healthy adults aged 18–64 years unless specific medical conditions indicate to the contrary. Pregnant and postpartum women and persons with cardiac events may need to take extra precautions and seek medical advice before striving to achieve the recommended levels of PA. Adults aged 65 years or older with poor mobility should perform PA on 3 or more days per week so as to enhance their balance and prevent falls as well as to improve cardiorespiratory and muscular fitness, maintain bone and functional health, and reduce the risk of NCDs, depression, and cognitive decline. When adults aged 65 years or older cannot do the recommended amounts of PA due to health conditions, they should be as physically active as their abilities and conditions allow.

11.2.4 Mechanisms and Benefits of Physical Activity

Understanding the mechanisms that link physical activity with NCDs is useful in designing prevention and treatment modalities. PA may decrease the risk of various cancers by several mechanisms. PA might work through reducing the amount of adipose tissue, which lowers the production of sex hormones (estrogens and androgens), insulin, leptin, and inflammatory markers, and improves immune function, thereby decreasing exposure to these potentially carcinogenic hormones and peptides and reducing cancer risk (McTiernan 2008).

Bowles and Laughlin (2011), after critical analysis of the literature, have put forth several potential mechanisms for the decreased morbidity and mortality from coronary heart disease in physically active individuals. They include attenuated plaque progression, the enhancement of regression and outward remodeling, the stabilization of vulnerable plaques (preventing plaque rupture), infarct sparing due to myocardial preconditioning, the correction of autonomic imbalance, improved endothelial function and collateralization, and a reduction in myocardial oxygen demand, thrombosis, and inflammatory mediator release from skeletal muscle and adipose tissue.

In individuals with type 2 diabetes, exercise improves glucose tolerance and insulin sensitivity (Albright et al. 2000). Aerobic exercise and resistance training improve glucose disposal in type 2 diabetes. In individuals with type 2 diabetes, both hepatic and peripheral insulin resistance respond positively to regular moderate-intensity aerobic activity. Resistance training improves muscle strength and endurance and body composition.

There is evidence to suggest that exercise can improve mental health by reducing anxiety, depression, and cognitive decline. It has also been found to alleviate symptoms such as low self-esteem and social withdrawal (Callaghan 2004; Guszkowska 2004). The potential mechanisms of exercise in individuals with mental disorders include psychological factors such as increased self-efficacy, a sense of mastery, distraction, and changes in self-concept, as well as physiological factors such as increased central norepinephrine transmission, changes in the hypothalamic adrenocortical system, serotonin synthesis and metabolism, and endorphins (Craft and Perna 2004).

Being physically active plays a vital role in ensuring health and well-being. The benefits of exercise extend far beyond weight management. Physical activity benefits many parts of the body—the heart, skeletal muscles, bones, blood (e.g., cholesterol levels), the immune system, the nervous system—reduces many of the risk factors for NCDs, and improves overall quality of life.

Regular PA reduces the risk of NCDs and premature death by several biological mechanisms. Regular PA has been shown to improve body composition (reduced abdominal adiposity and improved weight control) (Tremblay et al. 1990), lipid profiles (reduced triglyceride levels, increased high-density lipoprotein [HDL] cholesterol levels and decreased low-density lipoprotein [LDL]-to-HDL ratios) (Berg

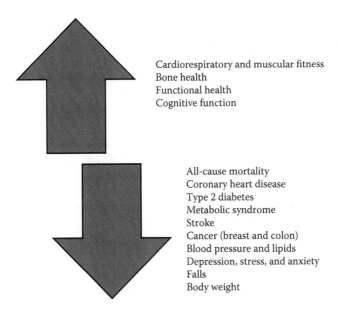

Cardiorespiratory and muscular fitness
Bone health
Functional health
Cognitive function

All-cause mortality
Coronary heart disease
Type 2 diabetes
Metabolic syndrome
Stroke
Cancer (breast and colon)
Blood pressure and lipids
Depression, stress, and anxiety
Falls
Body weight

FIGURE 11.2 Benefits of physical activity.

et al. 1997; Enkhmaa et al. 2015), glucose homeostasis and insulin sensitivity (Hawley 2004; Hawley and Lessard 2008), and psychological well-being (reduced stress, anxiety, and depression) (Nabkasorn et al. 2006). Studies have also shown that PA reduces blood pressure (Paffenbarger et al. 1991) and systemic inflammation (Adamopoulos et al. 2001), and enhances endothelial function (Kobayashi et al. 2003). Figure 11.2 summarizes the various benefits of physical activity.

11.3 HEALTHFUL EATING AND PHYSICAL ACTIVITY FOR PREVENTION AND CONTROL OF NON-COMMUNICABLE DISEASES

Large RCTs provide evidence as to the effectiveness of diet and PA in the prevention of diabetes and other NCDs. The Da Qing IGT and Diabetes Study conducted among 577 adults with impaired glucose tolerance (IGT) in the city of Da Qing, China, aimed to observe the effects of diet, exercise, and a combination of both on the incidence of non-insulin-dependent diabetes mellitus (NIDDM) (Pan et al. 1997). In the *dietary arm*, individual goals were framed for total calories and quantities of cereals, vegetables, milk, and oil consumed. Participants were encouraged to consume more vegetables, control the intake of alcohol, and reduce the intake of simple sugars. In the *exercise arm*, activities were defined based on intensity as mild, moderate, strenuous, or very strenuous. Participants were taught and encouraged to increase their leisure time exercise by at least 1 U/day. After 6 years of follow-up, the cumulative incidence of NIDDM was 43.8% in the diet group, 41.1% in the exercise group, and 46% in the combined group ($p = <.05$).

The Finnish Diabetes Prevention Study (DPS) was carried out to observe the short- and long-term effects of diet and exercise among 522 middle-aged adults with IGT (Lindstrom et al. 2003). Supervised, individually tailored, circuit-type, moderate-intensity resistance training sessions were offered free of charge. Exercise competitions and voluntary group walking and hiking were also organized. Significantly greater improvements were observed in fasting plasma glucose, 2 h plasma glucose, HbA_{1C}, total cholesterol-to-HDL ratio, and triglyceride levels in the intervention group compared with the control group ($p = <.01$) after 1 and 3 years of follow-up.

The Diabetes Prevention Program (DPP) Research Group carried out a large randomized clinical trial on 3234 nondiabetic U.S. adults with elevated fasting and postload plasma glucose. The study was designed to see the effectiveness of lifestyle intervention inclusive of diet, exercise, and behavioral modification over treatment with metformin. After 3 years of follow-up, the lifestyle intervention reduced the incidence of type 2 diabetes by 58%, whereas the group intervened with metformin showed only 31% reduction (Diabetes Prevention Program Research Group 2002).

Our experience with the recently completed Diabetes Community Lifestyle Improvement Program (D-CLIP), an RCT that aimed at the prevention of diabetes in adults with any form of prediabetes, showed a 32% relative risk reduction for diabetes in the intervention arm compared with the control group even after 3 years of follow-up. The study compared the standard of care (control group) with a culturally tailored lifestyle education curriculum (healthy diet and physical activity) based on the U.S. DPP (intervention group) (Weber et al. 2015).

A randomized trial of 492 sedentary adults was conducted in Florida to study the effect of moderate-to-high-intensity walking on cardiorespiratory fitness. The study showed that 30 min walking at a high intensity (65%–75% of heart rate reserve) for 5–7 days/week produced long-term improvements not only on cardiorespiratory fitness but also on HDL-C and the total cholesterol-to-HDL-C ratio (Duncan et al. 2005).

The HERITAGE family study carried out on 675 healthy, normolipidemic adults in the United States to study the effect of a 20-week exercise intervention on plasma lipids showed a significant decrease in VLDL triglycerides ($p = <.01$) and apolipoprotein A ($p = .002$) 24 hours after the intervention. There was a significant increase ($p = <.001$) in HDL-C levels in the intervention group (3.6%) and an inverse correlation ($r = -.241$) was observed between the increase in HDL-C and a change in body fat only in men. There was no significant change in total cholesterol, LDL-C, and apolipoprotein B in the study participants (Leon et al. 2000).

The population attributable risk for excess cases of type 2 diabetes due to lack of moderate-to-vigorous physical activity can range from 3% in Finland to 40% in Canada (Laaksonen et al. 2010; Lee et al. 2012; USDHHS 2008). A 10-year follow up study of the Chennai Urban Rural Epidemiological Study (CURES) on Asian Indians has shown that around 50% of diabetes could be eliminated if physical activity and diet patterns improved in this population (Anjana et al. 2015). A large international study involving 52 countries has shown that about 12% of myocardial infarctions could be eliminated if these populations had regular physical activity (Yusuf et al. 2004).

Thus, increases in PA and healthful eating can improve health substantially. Moderate-to-vigorous-intensity physical activity along with healthful eating has an established preventive role in cardiovascular disease, type 2 diabetes, obesity, and some cancers.

11.4 BARRIERS TO PHYSICAL ACTIVITY

Traditionally, populations in developing countries were mostly engaged in physically active occupations, and the concept of leisure time PA was relatively unknown to these countries. The current levels of physical inactivity are to an extent due to insufficient involvement in PA during leisure time. Similarly, an increase in the use of "passive" modes of transport has been associated with decreased PA levels, and with occupations becoming less labor-intensive with the advent of urbanization and mechanization, most PA has to be derived from leisure time. There are several barriers, both internal and external, to exercise. Internal barriers include factors that are influenced by the individual's own decision-making—for example, lack of time, emotions, laziness, and fear of exercise—while external barriers include factors that are outside of the individual's own control—such as weather, cultural barriers, lack of exercise facilities, and lack of social support (Korkiakangas et al. 2009).

According to Sallis and Hovell (1990), the various barriers to PA include high-density traffic (fear of being injured), pollution, a lack of parks, sidewalks, sports/recreation facilities, and time, low self-motivation and encouragement, inconvenience, finding exercise boring, low self-efficacy, and a lack of self-management skills, such as the ability to set personal goals, monitor progress, or reward progress toward such goals. In the Diabetes Community Lifestyle Improvement Program (D-CLIP), conducted with 1281 participants, the most frequently cited barriers to exercise were not having enough time and space to exercise (Anjana et al. 2015). In another study (Vaz and Bharathi 2000), a lack of time and motivation were the most cited reasons for being unable to achieve exercise goals.

11.5 WAYS TO INCREASE PHYSICAL ACTIVITY

Efforts to increase physical activity need to take place at the individual, family, community, and population levels to be maximally effective. Individuals should be made aware of the importance and benefits of PA, the implications and health penalties of inactivity, and the ways and means to improve PA in daily life. Individuals should also be provided information on what types of exercise to do, how much to do, and what precautions to take. Involving the family in physically active pursuits such as cleaning, gardening, and so on, is a simple and inexpensive way of promoting activity. Limiting screen time (TV and computers) is essential to reducing sedentary time and needs to be inculcated from childhood.

At the community and government levels, efforts should focus on modifying the built environment so as to make offices, neighborhoods, and cities more "exercise friendly." Studies have shown a clear link between health, physical activity, and the built environment (Mohan and Pradeepa 2007). The provision of well-lit and spacious stairways and walkways, the construction of dedicated pedestrian footpaths and bicycle lanes, and safe and spacious parks and gardens will go a long way to encouraging people to engage in more PA (Foster and Hillsdon 2004). An earlier study by our group showed a 277% increase in the exercise levels of the residents of a middle-income colony in Chennai after the construction of a park with a walking track by the residents themselves (Deepa et al. 2011; Mohan et al. 2006). Similar government-funded as well as community-driven efforts are needed so as to improve levels of leisure time PA.

Table 11.1 shows various strategies to increase physical activity.

TABLE 11.1
Strategies to Increase Physical Activity at Various Levels

Levels	Strategies
Individual	• Set aside time for exercise every day. • Motivation is key; if self-motivation is not possible, then peer groups can be tried. • Awareness of what exercises to do is essential, so ask a health professional before starting an exercise program. • In addition to exercises, moving around to accumulate 10,000 steps/day will improve health. • Limit TV watching and sedentary time.
Family	• Schedule time for physical activity. • Get the whole family involved in household chores such as cleaning, gardening, and so on. • Encourage children to join a sports team or try a new physical activity. • Play actively with children or grandchildren. • Limit TV time and keep the TV out of children's bedrooms. • Encourage and engage the family in more outdoor activities together.
Community (workplace)	• Provide wide, well-lit stairs in multistoried buildings. • Provide spaces for outdoor and indoor games. • Construct gyms. • Encourage employers to adopt policies that support physical activity such as offering flex-time at work sites.
Government	• Construct parks and provide provisions for sports, fitness, and recreational facilities. • Improve lighting and security in public exercise areas such as walking paths and cycling lanes. • Maintaining facilities that promote activity, usable public transport systems, and cycling and walking infrastructure, especially in cities. • Ensure that the public health benefits of both leisure time and transportation-related physical activity are conveyed to state transportation agencies and urban planners. • Put in place legislation to promote the provision of safe open spaces and widespread dedicated walking and cycling facilities throughout built and external environments. • Invest in systems to monitor physical activity patterns in the population.

11.6 PHYSICAL ACTIVITY PROMOTES HEALTHFUL EATING

Those who habitually exercise tend to have a healthier diet. A national longitudinal survey of youths with 6244 respondents in the United States showed that the participants who moved from inadequate exercise to adequate exercise tended to increase their intake of fruits and vegetables, with exercise frequency and fruit and vegetable intake having a linear association (Jayawardene et al. 2015). Choi and Ainsworth (2016) studied the association of food consumption, serum vitamin levels, and markers of metabolic syndrome with the frequency of physical activity in middle-aged adults who completed the National Health and Nutrition Examination Survey (NHANES) 2005–2006. Physical activity was measured by accelerometer-determined steps in men and women. This study found that men who were in the highest tertile of physical activity tended to consume more grains, fruits, and vegetables, whereas the most active women consumed more legumes and vegetables when compared with the sedentary men and women, respectively. Serum vitamin C, vitamin D, α-carotene, trans-β-carotene, cis-β-carotene, lycopene, and γ-tocopherol were significantly positively associated with the daily step count. This implies that people who are physically active tend to have healthful eating behaviors compared with those who are physically inactive/sedentary. Moreover, the odds of having metabolic syndrome risk markers (low HDL cholesterol, hypertriglyceridemia, abdominal obesity, hypertension, hyperglycemia) were significantly higher in the sedentary group compared with the participants who were active.

This clustering of health behavior could have a synergistic effect on various NCDs. Therefore, adhering to a healthy diet along with increased physical activity will reduce the burden due to lifestyle disorders such as obesity, heart diseases, cancer, and diabetes.

11.7 CASE STUDIES

11.7.1 CASE STUDY 1

A 24-year-old male comes to you with a complaint of obesity (BMI 40 kg/m^2). He has tried various weight loss programs but does not adhere to physical activity regimen. Give responses to the following:

- How will you explore the barriers to physical activity in this patient? (*Hint*: Refer to Section 11.4.)
- How will you assist this patient in overcoming the barriers to physical activity? (*Hint*: Refer to Section 11.5.)
- How will you explain the benefits of physical activity for healthful eating to this patient? (*Hint*: Refer to Section 11.6.)

11.7.2 CASE STUDY 2

Mrs. D. S. is a 60-year-old female. She has had type 2 diabetes for 7 years. Her fasting blood sugar levels are not controlled by diet or medication. Her physician has started insulin in this patient, but has sent her to you for nutritional consultation and physical activity recommendations. Give responses to the following:

- What dietary patterns will you recommend for managing diabetes in this patient? (*Hint*: Refer to Chapter 5.)
- What recommendations will you give to this patient about the type and frequency of physical activity? (*Hint*: Refer to Section 11.2.3.)

REFERENCES

Adamopoulos, Stamatis, John Parissis, Christos Kroupis, Michael Georgiadis, Dimitrios Karatzas, George Karavolias, Katerina Koniavitou, Andrew J.S Coats, and Dimitrios Th. Kremastinos. 2001. Physical training reduces peripheral markers of inflammation in patients with chronic heart failure. *Eur Heart J* 22(9): 791–797.

Albright, Ann, Marion Franz, Guyton Hornsby, Andrea Kriska, David Marrero, Irma Ullrich, and Larry S. Verity. 2000. American College of Sports Medicine position stand: Exercise and type 2 diabetes. *Med Sci Sports Exerc* 32(7): 1345–1360.

Anjana Ranjit Mohan. 2014. Physical activity and Type 2 diabetes. *World Clinics Diabetology: Type 2 Diabetes Mellitus*. Mohan V, Ranjit Unnikrishnan (Eds). Jaypee Brothers Medical Publishers. New Delhi. India. 1:74–86.

Anjana, R. M., H. Ranjani, R. Unnikrishnan, M. B. Weber, V. Mohan, and K. M. Venkat Narayan. 2015. Exercise patterns and behaviour in Asian Indians: Data from the baseline survey of the Diabetes Community Lifestyle Improvement Program (D-CLIP). *Diabetes Res Clin Pract* 107(1): 77–84.

Anjana, Ranjit Mohan, Vasudevan Sudha, Divya H. Nair, Nagarajan Lakshmipriya, Mohan Deepa, Rajendra Pradeepa, Coimbatore S. Shanthirani et al. 2015. Diabetes in Asian Indians: How much is preventable? Ten-year follow-up of the Chennai Urban Rural Epidemiology Study (CURES-142). *Diabetes Res Clin Pract* 109(2): 253–261.

Bauman, Adrian, Fiona Bull, Tien Chey, Cora L. Craig, Barbara E. Ainsworth, James F. Sallis, Heather R. Bowles, Maria Hagstromer, Michael Sjostrom, and Michael Pratt. 2009. The international prevalence study on physical activity: Results from 20 countries. *Int J Behav Nutr Phys* Act 6(1): 21.

Beaglehole, Robert, Ruth Bonita, Richard Horton, Cary Adams, George Alleyne, Perviz Asaria, Vanessa Baugh et al. 2011. Priority actions for the non-communicable disease crisis. *Lancet* 377(9775): 1438–1447.

Berg, Aloys, Martin Halle, I. Franz, and Joseph Keul. 1997. Physical activity and lipoprotein metabolism: Epidemiological evidence and clinical trials. *Eur J Med Res* 2 (6): 259–264.

Booth, Frank W., Christian K. Roberts, and Matthew J. Laye. 2012. Lack of exercise is a major cause of chronic diseases. *Compr Physiol* 2(2):1143–1211.

Bowles, Douglas K., and M. Harold Laughlin. 2011. Mechanism of beneficial effects of physical activity on atherosclerosis and coronary heart disease. *J Appl Physiol* 111(1): 308–310.

Callaghan, Patrick. 2004. Exercise: A neglected intervention in mental health care? *J Psychiatr Ment Health Nurs* 11(4): 476–483.

Caspersen, Carl J., Kenneth E. Powell, and Gregory M. Christenson. 1985. Physical activity, exercise, and physical fitness: Definitions and distinctions for health-related research. *Pub Health Rep* 100(2): 126.

Choi, Jihyun E., and Barbara E. Ainsworth. 2016. Associations of food consumption, serum vitamins and metabolic syndrome risk with physical activity level in middle-aged adults: The National Health and Nutrition Examination Survey (NHANES) 2005–2006. *Public Health Nutr* 19(9): 1674–83.

Craft, Lynette L., and Frank M. Perna.2004. The benefits of exercise for the clinically depressed. *Prim Care Companion J Clin Psychiatry* 6(3): 104–111.

Deepa, Mohan, Ranjit Mohan Anjana, Datta Manjula, KM Venkat Narayan, and Viswanathan Mohan. 2011. Convergence of prevalence rates of diabetes and cardiometabolic risk factors in middle and low income groups in urban India: 10-year follow-up of the Chennai Urban Population Study. *J Diabetes Sci Technol* 5(4): 918–927.

Diabetes Prevention Program Research Group. 2002. Reduction in the incidence of type 2 diabetes with lifestyle intervention or metformin. *New Engl J Med* 346(6): 393–403.

Duncan, Glen E., Stephen D. Anton, Sumner J. Sydeman, Robert L. Newton, Joyce A. Corsica, Patricia E. Durning, Timothy U. Ketterson, A. Daniel Martin, Marian C. Limacher, and Michael G. Perri. 2005. Prescribing exercise at varied levels of intensity and frequency: A randomized trial. *Arch Intern Med* 165(20): 2362–2369.

Enkhmaa, Byambaa, Prasanth Surampudi, Erdembileg Anuurad, and Lars Berglund. 2015. Lifestyle changes: Effect of diet, exercise, functional food, and obesity treatment, on lipids and lipoproteins. In L. J. De Groot, P. Beck-Peccoz, G. Chrousos et al., eds., *Endotext* (Internet). South Dartmouth, MA: MDText.com, 2000. Accessed April 20, 2016. Available from: https://www.ncbi.nlm.nih.gov/books/NBK326737.

Foster, Charles, and Melvyn Hillsdon. 2004. Changing the environment to promote health-enhancing physical activity. *J Sports Sci* 22(8): 755–769.

Guszkowska, M. 2003. Effects of exercise on anxiety, depression and mood. *Psychiatria polska* 38(4): 611–620.

Guthold, Regina, Tomoko Ono, Kathleen L. Strong, Somnath Chatterji, and Alfredo Morabia. 2008. Worldwide variability in physical inactivity: A 51-country survey. *Am J Prev Med* 34(6): 486–494.

Hallal, Pedro C., Lars Bo Andersen, Fiona C. Bull, Regina Guthold, William Haskell, Ulf Ekelund, and Lancet Physical Activity Series Working Group. 2012. Global physical activity levels: Surveillance progress, pitfalls, and prospects. *Lancet* 380(9838): 247–257.

Hawley J.A. 2004. Exercise as a therapeutic intervention for the prevention and treatment of insulin resistance. *Diabetes Metab Res Rev* 20:383–93.

Hawley, J.A. and Lessard, S.J. 2008. Exercise training-induced improvements in insulin action. *Acta Physiol (Oxf)* 192:127–35.

Jayawardene, Wasantha P., Mohammad R. Torabi, and David K. Lohrmann. 2016. Exercise in young adulthood with simultaneous and future changes in fruit and vegetable intake. *J Am Coll Nutr* 35(1): 59–67.

Kobayashi, Nobuhiko, Yoshio Tsuruya, Takamasa Iwasawa, Nahoko Ikeda, Shigemasa Hashimoto, Takanori Yasu, Hiroto Ueba et al. 2003. Exercise training in patients with chronic heart failure improves endothelial function predominantly in the trained extremities. *Circ J* 67(6): 505–510.

Korkiakangas, Eveliina E., Maija A. Alahuhta, and Jaana H. Laitinen. 2009. Barriers to regular exercise among adults at high risk or diagnosed with type 2 diabetes: A systematic review. *Health Promot Int* 24(4):416–427.

Laaksonen, Maarit A., Paul Knekt, Tommi Härkänen, Esa Virtala, and Hannu Oja. 2010. Estimation of the population attributable fraction for mortality in a cohort study using a piecewise constant hazards model. *Am J Epidemiol* 171(7): 837–847.

Lee, I-Min, and Ralph S. Paffenbarger Jr. 1994. Physical activity and its relation to cancer risk: A prospective study of college alumni. *Med Sci Sports Exerc* 26(7): 831–837.

Lee, I-Min, Eric J. Shiroma, Felipe Lobelo, Pekka Puska, Steven N. Blair, Peter T. Katzmarzyk, and Lancet Physical Activity Series Working Group. 2012. Effect of physical inactivity on major non-communicable diseases worldwide: An analysis of burden of disease and life expectancy. *Lancet* 380(9838): 219–229.

Leon, Arthur S., Treva Rice, Stephen Mandel, Jean-Pierre Despres, Jean Bergeron, Jacques Gagnon, D. C. Rao, James S. Skinner, Jack H. Wilmore, and Claude Bouchard. 2000. Blood lipid response to 20 weeks of supervised exercise in a large biracial population: The HERITAGE Family Study. *Metabolism* 49(4): 513–520.

Lindström, Jaana, Anne Louheranta, Marjo Mannelin, Merja Rastas, Virpi Salminen, Johan Eriksson, Matti Uusitupa, and Jaakko Tuomilehto. 2003. The Finnish Diabetes Prevention Study (DPS) lifestyle intervention and 3-year results on diet and physical activity. *Diabetes Care* 26(12): 3230–3236.

McTiernan, Anne. 2008. Mechanisms linking physical activity with cancer. *Nat Rev Cancer* 8(3): 205–211.

Mersy, David J. 1991. Health benefits of aerobic exercise. *Postgrad Med* 90(1): 103–107.

Mohan, Viswananthan, Coimbatore Subramaniyam Shanthirani, Mohan Deepa, Manjula Datta, O. Dale Williams, and Raj Deepa. 2006. Community empowerment: A successful model for prevention of non-communicable diseases in India; The Chennai urban population study (CUPS-17). *J Assoc Physicians India* 54: 858–862.

Mohan, V. and Pradeepa R. 2007. Redesigning the urban environment to promote physical activity in southern India. *Diabetes Voice* 52:33–35.

Nabkasorn, Chanudda, Nobuyuki Miyai, Anek Sootmongkol, Suwanna Junprasert, Hiroichi Yamamoto, Mikio Arita, and Kazuhisa Miyashita. 2006. Effects of physical exercise on depression, neuroendocrine stress hormones and physiological fitness in adolescent females with depressive symptoms. *Eur J Pub Health* 16(2): 179–184.

Ng S.W., Popkin B.M. 2012. Time use and physical activity: A shift away from movement across the globe. *Obes Rev* 13:659–680.

Paffenbarger, Ralph S., Dexter L. Jung, Rita W. Leung, and Robert T. Hyde. 1991. Physical activity and hypertension: An epidemiological view. *Ann Med* 23(3): 319–327.

Paffenbarger Jr., Ralph S., James B. Kampert, I. Min Lee, Robert T. Hyde, Rita W. Leung, and Alvin L. Wing. 1994. Changes in physical activity and other lifeway patterns influencing longevity. *Med Sci Sports Exerc* 26(7): 857–865.

Pan, Xiao-Ren, Guang-Wei Li, Ying-Hua Hu, Ji-Xing Wang, Wen-Ying Yang, Zuo-Xin An, Ze-Xi Hu et al. 1997. Effects of diet and exercise in preventing NIDDM in people with impaired glucose tolerance: The Da Qing IGT and Diabetes Study. *Diabetes Care* 20(4): 537–544.

Popkin, Barry M. 2006. Global nutrition dynamics: The world is shifting rapidly toward a diet linked with noncommunicable diseases. *Am J Clin Nutr* 84(2): 289–298.

Popkin, Barry M., Linda S. Adair, and Shu Wen Ng. 2012. Global nutrition transition and the pandemic of obesity in developing countries. *Nutr Rev* 70(1): 3–21.

Sallis, James F., and Melbourne F. Hovell. 1990. Determinants of exercise behavior. *Exerc Sport Sci Rev* 18(1): 307–330.

Sigal, Ronald J., Glen P. Kenny, David H. Wasserman, and Carmen Castaneda-Sceppa. 2004. Physical activity/exercise and type 2 diabetes. *Diabetes Care* 27(10): 2518–2539.

Terzic, Andre, and Scott A. Waldman. 2011. Chronic diseases: The emerging pandemic. Thomas Jefferson University, Department of Pharmacology and Experimental Therapeutics Faculty Papers. Paper 12. Accessed April 10, 2016. Available from: http://jdc.jefferson.edu/petfp/12.

Tremblay, A., Despres, J.P, and Leblanc, C. et al. 1990. Effect of intensity of physical activity on body fatness and fat distribution. *Am J Clin Nutr* 51:153–7.

U.S. Department of Health and Human Services. 2008. *Physical Activity Guidelines for Americans*. Washington, DC: U.S. Department of Health and Human Services.

Vaz, Mario, and Ankalmadagu Venkatasubbareddy Bharathi. 1999. Practices and perceptions of physical activity in urban, employed, middle-class Indians. *Indian Heart J* 52(3): 301–306.

Vuori, Ilkka. 2014. Health effects of living habits. *Duodecim: Laaketieteellinen aikakauskirja* 131(8): 729–736.

Weber, Mary Beth, Rekha Harish, Lisa R. Staimez, Ranjit Mohan Anjana, Mohammed K. Ali, K. M. Venkat Narayan et al. 2015. 180-LB reduction in diabetes incidence differs by prediabetes type in a randomized translational trial of prevention. *Diabetes* 64(Suppl 1A): LB46.

Wilmore, Jack H., and Howard G. Knuttgen. 2003. Aerobic exercise and endurance: Improving fitness for health benefits. *Phys Sportsmed* 31(5): 45–51.

World Health Organization. 2002. *The World Health Report 2002: Reducing Risks, Promoting Healthy Life*. Geneva, Switzerland: World Health Organization.

WHO. 2009. *Global Health Risks: Mortality and Burden of Disease Attributable to Selected Major Risks*. Geneva, Switzerland: World Health Organization.

WHO. 2010. *Global Recommendations on Physical Activity for Health*. Geneva, Switzerland: World Health Organization. Accessed January 21, 2016. Available from: http://apps.who.int/iris/bitstream/10665/44399/1/9789241599979_eng.pdf.

WHO. 2012. Global Health Observatory Data Repository. Accessed January 22, 2016. Available from: http://apps.who.int/gho/data/node.home.

WHO. 2013. *Global Action Plan for The Prevention and Control of Noncommunicable Diseases 2013–2020*. Geneva, Switzerland: World Health Organization.

Yusuf, Salim, Steven Hawken, Stephanie Ôunpuu, Tony Dans, Alvaro Avezum, Fernando Lanas, Matthew McQueen et al. 2004. Effect of potentially modifiable risk factors associated with myocardial infarction in 52 countries (the INTERHEART study): Case-control study. *Lancet* 364(9438): 937–952.

12 HEAL and Smoking Cessation

Shirin Anil and Redhwan Al Naggar

CONTENTS

12.1 SMOKING-RELATED MORTALITY AND MORBIDITY

12.1.1 SMOKING KILLS

Tobacco smoking is a preventable risk factor of undue death and illness. Smoking-related deaths as well as illnesses are on the rise, based on the estimates of the World Health Organization (WHO). Tobacco kills approximately 6 million people every year, five million as a result of direct tobacco smoking and 600,000 nonsmokers who are exposed to second-hand smoke (WHO 2015). In 2012, one-fifth of the global population aged 15 years and above smoked tobacco, the tobacco smoking rate being

36% in men and 7% in women (WHO 2016b). This was the case despite widespread knowledge of the aftereffects of cigarette smoking on health.

In addition to cigarettes, many tobacco products have gained popularity in previous years. These include *snus* (smokeless tobacco products), dissolvable tobacco products, e-cigarettes or electronic nicotine delivery systems (ENDS), and water pipes (also referred to as *hookah, hubble bubble*, or *sheesha*) (McMillen et al. 2012). Other tobacco products include cigars, *bidis* (hand-rolled tobacco products common in India), *midwakh* (smoking pipes of Arabian origin), and *kreteks* (O'Connor 2012). All these products are considered less hazardous than cigarettes, whereas they are equally hazardous or even more so, and their health burden is similar (O'Connor 2012).

12.1.2 TOBACCO SMOKING AND CARDIOVASCULAR DISEASE

Smoking is an independent risk factor for cardiovascular disease (CVD). One-third of all CVD deaths can be attributed to cigarette smoking in Western populations (Chen and Boreham 2002). CVD is responsible for 35% of all smoking-related deaths (Ezzati and Lopez 2004). Young smokers who smoke 20 cigarettes per day are 5.6 times more at risk of acute myocardial infarction (AMI) compared with nonsmokers of a similar age (Teo et al. 2006). Smokers are three times more likely to suffer from nonfatal AMI and twice more likely to have sudden cardiac death compared with nonsmokers (Burns 2003; Wannamethee et al. 1995). Cigarette smoking has a role in all phases of atherosclerosis from endothelial dysfunction to acute thrombotic events. Oxidative stress is the potential mechanism by which cigarette smoking results in CVD; it causes inflammation, thrombosis, and oxidation of low-density lipoprotein cholesterol (Ambrose and Barua 2004). Nonsmokers exposed to secondhand smoking are 25% more at risk of developing coronary heart disease (CHD) compared with nonsmokers not exposed to secondhand smoking (He et al. 1999). The toxins present in secondhand smoke affect platelet and endothelial function, oxidative stress, inflammation, atherosclerosis, and heart rate variability in nonsmokers in a similar way to smokers, the effects being as large as 80%–90% of those in smokers, after only minutes or hours of exposure to cigarette smoke (Barnoya and Glantz 2005). Long-term, heavy smoking is associated with hypertension (Hu et al. 2014), which may further increase the risk of CVD.

Cigarette smoking can cause ischemic as well as hemorrhagic stroke (Kurth et al. 2003; Uddin et al. 2008). The risk of stroke in active smokers is four times that of those who never smoke. Passive smokers are 82% more likely to develop stroke and long-term ex-smokers 34% more likely than nonsmokers (Bonita et al. 1999). Nicotine in tobacco is an acute vasoactive and mitogenic substance and has a role in altering the blood–brain barrier and endothelial function, and hence may play a role in the development of stroke (Hawkins et al. 2002). Smoking also exacerbates the effects of high systolic blood pressure on hemorrhagic stroke (Nakamura et al. 2008).

12.1.3 TOBACCO SMOKING AND HYPERTENSION

Cigarette smoke has been postulated to raise blood pressure acutely due to the activation of the sympathetic nervous system (Virdis et al. 2010). The causal relationship of smoking to hypertension is not clear. It is known that smoking leads to endo-thelial dysfunction, which is strongly associated with hypertension (Leone 2011). Hypertensive smokers are more at risk of developing severe forms of hypertension, including malignant and renovascular hypertension, which may be due to the accel-erated atherosclerotic process in smokers (Virdis et al. 2010). Passive smoking is related to endothelial dysfunction in a similar way to active smokers (Holay et al. 2004).

12.1.4 Tobacco Smoking and Type 2 Diabetes

Smoking has also been linked to type 2 diabetes. A meta-analysis of 25 cohort stud-ies including 1.2 million participants showed a dose-responsive relationship between cigarette smoking and the risk of type 2 diabetes. Heavy smokers (who smoke 20 or more cigarettes per day) are 61% more at risk of developing type 2 diabetes and light smokers 29% more at risk than nonsmokers. Former smokers are also 23% more likely to develop type 2 diabetes than active smokers (Willi et al. 2007).

12.1.5 Tobacco Smoking and Chronic Respiratory Disease

Tobacco smoking is one of the major risk factors for the development of chronic obstructive pulmonary disease (COPD). A meta-analysis of 133 COPD studies showed that the risk of COPD in ever-smokers is 2.89 times higher, in current smok-ers 3.51 times higher, and in ex-smokers 2.35 times higher compared with nonsmok-ers (Forey et al. 2011). Tobacco smoking also increases the risk of chronic bronchitis and emphysema (Forey et al. 2011). Current smoking increases asthma severity com-pared with never-smokers and ex-smokers (Siroux et al. 2000). Passive smoking is an independent risk factor for COPD and asthma. The U.S. Black Women's Health Study, which followed 46,182 participants for 16 years, concluded that passive smok-ing increases the risk of asthma by 21% compared with those not exposed to pas-sive smoking (Coogan et al. 2015). Environmental tobacco smoke (ETS) or passive smoking increases the likelihood of COPD by almost fourfold compared with those not exposed to ETS (Hagstad et al. 2014).

12.1.6 Tobacco Smoking and Cancers

Tobacco is responsible for 22% of cancer deaths globally (WHO 2016a). In 2004, 1.6 million out of 7.4 million cancer deaths were attributed to tobacco smoking (WHO 2016a). Smoking increases the risk of cancers of the lungs, larynx, oral cav-ity, pharynx, esophagus, kidneys, bladder, pancreas, and colon in both men and women (Freedman et al. 2015). About 70% of the lung cancer burden can be attrib-uted to tobacco smoking (WHO 2016a). Active smoking has also been associated with breast cancer (Reynolds et al. 2004). The European Prospective Investigation into Cancer and Nutrition (EPIC) study has reported tobacco smoking to be a major risk factor for cervical cancer (Roura et al. 2014). People exposed to secondhand smoke are also at increased risk of developing cancers. A study in Japan of 91,540 nonsmoking wives of smoking and nonsmoking husbands concluded that the risk of lung cancer in the wives of smoking husbands was much higher compared with the wives of nonsmoking husbands, depicting a dose-responsive relationship (Hirayama 2000). Passive smoking has been found to increase the risk of breast cancer among Chinese women (Gao et al. 2013).

12.1.7 TOBACCO SMOKING AND MENTAL HEALTH ISSUES

Smoking has been linked to depression in both cross-sectional and prospective studies. Current smokers are 50% more likely to be depressed than never-smokers and 76% more likely than former smokers (Luger et al. 2014). The risk of depression in current smokers is 62% higher than in never-smokers (Luger et al. 2014). Smoking cessation reduces anxiety, depression and stress, and improves mood as compared to those who continue to smoke (Taylor et al. 2014).

12.2 INTERVENTIONS FOR SMOKING CESSATION

Many smoking cessation interventions have been implemented in developed and developing countries to counteract the adverse health effects, such as non-communicable diseases (NCDs), attributed to a major extent to tobacco smoking. Some of these interventions along with their impacts are as follows:

- *Smoke-free laws*: One year after their implementation, smoke-free laws were shown to reduce hospital admissions due to acute myocardial infarction by an average of 17% in Argentina, Canada, England, France, Ireland, Italy, Scotland, and the United States (Glantz and Gonzalez 2012; Lightwood and Glantz 2009). In Arizona, hospital admissions due to asthma reduced by 22% after smoke-free laws were implemented in workplaces, restaurants, and bars (Herman and Walsh 2011). In Canada, hospital admissions for chronic respiratory disease dropped by 33% 2 years after the enforcement of smoke-free laws in restaurants (Naiman et al. 2010).
- *Advice and assistance from physicians*: The National Health Interview Survey (NHIS) in the United States showed a positive correlation between a health-care provider's advice to quit smoking and the smoker's wish to quit smoking (Kruger et al. 2012). A meta-analysis of 13 studies showed that physicians offering assistance results in more quit attempts, 69% more for offering behavioral support and 39% more for offering medication, compared with advice to quit smoking on medical grounds (Aveyard et al. 2012).
- *Culturally appropriate quit smoking face-to-face interventions*: A systematic review of 17 studies showed that interventions incorporating a package of cultural adaptations that imply high-intensity and embedded family values are more likely to be effective for smoking cessation (Nierkens et al. 2013). Smoking cessation interventions tailored to cultural contexts have been shown to increase quit rates by 2.4 times in a face-to-face intervention group compared with a control group among Indigenous Australians (Marley et al. 2014). In Pakistan, behavioral support intervention and

behavioral support combined with bupropion therapy achieved effective smoking cessation among suspected tuberculosis patients (Siddiqi et al. 2013).

- *Nicotine replacement therapy (NRT)*: A meta-analysis of 53 trials measuring the effectiveness of various forms of NRT (gum, patches, intranasal spray, and inhalers) showed that the odds of abstinence are 71% higher in NRT users compared with the control interventions (Silagy et al. 1994). Another meta-analysis of 12 trials on the long-term efficacy of a single-treatment episode of NRT showed that smoking cessation is enhanced by 99% in NRT users compared with placebo over many years (Etter and Stapleton 2006). The relapse rate for NRT users from 12 months to 2–8 years of follow-up is 30% (Etter and Stapleton 2006).

- *E-cigarettes*: Though e-cigarettes have been used as a strategy for quitting cigarette smoking, it is associated with significantly less quitting among smokers. A meta-analysis of 38 studies showed that the odds of quitting cigarette smoking are 28% lower in smokers who use e-cigarettes compared with those who do not use them (Kalkhoran and Glantz 2016).

- *Text messaging–based smoking cessation*: Text messages are now being used to help smokers to quit smoking. A pilot study in the United States found that the quit rate at 4 weeks after text-messaging intervention was 3.3 times higher compared with the control group (Ybarra et al. 2013). A systematic Cochrane review of five studies reported that long-term quit rates increase by 71% in cell phone intervention for smoking cessation (Whittaker et al. 2012).

- *Smartphone apps for smoking cessation*: Many smartphone applications (apps), both Android- and Apple-based, are available for smoking cessation (Patel et al. 2015). A content analysis of 225 Android smoking cessation apps showed that these apps addressed 2.1 ± 0.9 of the "5As" framework (ask, advise, assess, assist, and arrange follow-up) (Hoeppner et al. 2015), suggested as an effective tobacco cessation counseling tool by the U.S. Public Health Service's clinical practice guidelines (Fiore et al. 2008). A feasibility study of a smoking cessation app called Quit Advisor showed that it was downloaded the most in the United States, followed by the United Kingdom and Australia. The majority of users of this app had never sought professional help to quit smoking and 77.2% were ready to quit within 30 days (BinDhim et al. 2014). A randomized controlled trial in the United States measured the effectiveness of an acceptance and commitment therapy app for smoking cessation called SmartQuit against the National Cancer Institute's app for smoking cessation called QuitGuide. It showed that the quit rate was 13% for SmartQuit and 8% for QuitGuide (Bricker et al. 2014).

- *Physical activity*: For women, supervised exercise three times per week for 12 months along with a cognitive behavioral smoking cessation program has been shown to lead to smoking abstinence in 19.4% of participants at the end of treatment, 16.4% after 3 months, and 11.9% after 12 months (Marcus et al. 1999). Short bouts of exercise such as 10 min moderate-intensity exercise on a stationary cycle have been shown to reduce the desire to smoke as well as withdrawal symptoms in abstaining smokers (Ussher et al. 2001).

- *Nicotine gum, behavioral therapy, and a very low-calorie diet*: An intervention for female smokers consisting of nicotine gum with a behavioral weight control program combined with a very low-calorie diet led to smoking cessation in 50% of the participants after 16 weeks of therapy, and the success rate after 1 year of intervention remained at 28% (Danielsson et al. 1999).

12.3   ADVERSE EFFECTS OF SMOKING ON NUTRITION INTAKE

Tobacco smoking adversely effects eating behavior. National surveys from 15 countries including 47,250 nonsmokers and 35,870 smokers showed that smokers have a higher intake of energy, total fat, saturated fat, cholesterol, and alcohol and lower intakes of fiber, polyunsaturated fat, vitamin C, vitamin E, and beta-carotene compared with nonsmokers (Dallongeville et al. 1998). A population-based survey of a Swiss urban population showed that current heavy smokers both male and female consume less vegetable proteins, carbohydrates, fiber saccharose, fruits, vegetables, and beta-carotene and consume more coffee and alcohol compared with never-smokers. This study also showed that current female smokers eat less complex carbohydrates, cereals, vegetables, and iron (Morabia et al. 1999). A Korean study found that smokers tended to skip breakfast and other meals and drink more coffee compared with nonsmokers (Kim et al. 2003).

Women smokers have a significantly lower consumption of fruits and vegetables and higher consumption of eggs, sugar, coffee, carbonated soft drinks, and alcoholic beverages than nonsmoking females (Larkin et al. 1990). The French E3N-EPIC cohort study including 64,252 women confirmed that current and former smokers tended to consume more on the "alcohol/meat product" pattern (consisting of meat and meat products, alcohol, and coffee; few fruits and soup) and had an inverse relationship with the "processed meat/starchy food" pattern (including fast foods, processed meat, rice/pasta/semolina, and cakes; few vegetables). It also showed an inverse association of current smokers with the "fruit/vegetables" pattern (consisting of vegetables, fruits, seafood, vegetable oil, and yogurt) compared with never-smokers, and former smokers showed a positive association with the "fruit/vegetables" pattern (Touvier et al. 2009). A study on Australian women showed that current smokers consumed 4.1 g less fiber in their diet compared with nonsmokers (Midgette et al. 1993). Figure 12.1 shows a typical smoker's diet.

12.4   ALCOHOL AND SMOKING

Alcohol has been linked to many non-communicable diseases and their risk factors such as hemorrhagic stroke, diabetes, hypertension, atrial fibrillation, and cancer. Of the global burden of deaths due to non-communicable diseases, 3.4% can be attributed to alcohol (Parry et al. 2011).

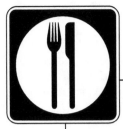

Smoker

⬆ **Intake of**
- Energy
- Total fat, saturated fat, cholesterol
- Alcohol
- Meat and meat products
- Coffee
- Carbonated drinks
- Sugar

⬇ **Intake of**
- Fruits
- Vegetables
- Fiber/complex carbohydrate
- Polyunsaturated fat
- Vitamin C
- Vitamin E
- Beta-carotene
- Iron

FIGURE 12.1   The effects of smoking on diet.

The Dutch National Food Consumption Survey found a strong association between alcohol drinking and tobacco smoking (Veenstra et al. 1993). The same was found by the U.S. Department of Agriculture's Continuing Survey of Food Intakes by Individuals (Ma et al. 2000). Alcohol consumption has an influence on the initiation of smoking, as found in college students in the United States (Reed et al. 2007). Moreover, heavy alcohol drinkers are less likely to attempt to quit smoking and are less likely to succeed even if they attempt to do so. Less alcohol consumption is an independent predictor for smoking cessation, as found in a cohort of cigarette smokers followed for 5 years (Hymowitz et al. 1997). Those who quit alcohol are more likely to succeed in quitting smoking (Zimmerman et al. 1990), and smoking cessation has been associated with a 25% greater likelihood of abstaining from alcohol and other drugs (Prochaska et al. 2004).

The pattern of poor food choices and lower nutrient intake increases with increased consumption of alcohol and smoking (Ma et al. 2000). Due to the clustering of smoking and alcohol consumption and its adverse impact on food choices, interventions and nutritional counseling for healthy dietary patterns should be multifaceted, embedding motivational strategies to quit smoking and alcohol consumption for health promotion.

12.5   HEALTHFUL EATING REDUCES THE CHANCE OF SMOKING

A healthy diet can not only prevent smoking, but can also reduce the frequency of smoking. A cohort study of 1000 smokers showed that the participants who consumed more fruits and vegetables had a significantly longer time to their first cigarette, smoked fewer cigarettes, and had a lower score on the nicotine-dependent syndrome scale compared with those who consumed less fruits and vegetables (Haibach et al. 2013). Another cross-sectional study on youth showed that those who consumed fruits two or more times per day were 53% less likely to be in the higher smoking frequency category compared with those who did not consume fruits, though no association of fruits or vegetables was seen with the frequency of smoking in a longitudinal analysis (Haibach et al. 2015).

12.6   HEALTHFUL EATING HELPS TO QUIT SMOKING

Healthful eating helps smokers to quit smoking and abstain from smoking for longer. A longitudinal study in France and Northern Ireland showed that those who consume more fruits and vegetables are 73% more likely to quit smoking. This association between fruits and vegetables and smoking cessation remained significant even after adjustment for sociodemographic factors, body mass index, and medical diet (Poisson et al. 2012). A study in the United States, found that those who consume higher amounts of fruits and vegetables (being in the highest quartile) and have quit smoking are three times more likely to be abstinent at 30 days, compared with those who consume less or no fruits and vegetables (Haibach et al. 2013).

Certain foods have been linked to the palatability of cigarettes. Fruits/vegetables, dairy products, and noncaffeinated beverages worsen the taste of nonmenthol cigarettes (McClernon et al. 2007). Hence, they help smokers to quit cigarettes.

A pilot study in Japan found that the consumption of oat extract (900 mg of Neuravena for 28 months) can reduce the number of cigarettes smoked per day (from an average of 19.5 cigarettes per day to an average of 8.5 cigarettes per day) (Fuji et al. 2008). This study had a very small sample size and larger studies are needed to give conclusive evidence about the association between oat extract and smoking cessation.

Smoking is associated with lower body weight. Weight increases after smoking cessation due to increased energy intake, reduced exercise, and decreased resting metabolic rate (Pistelli et al. 2009). A meta-analysis of 62 studies showed that 84% of untreated quitters gain an average of 4–5 kg after 12 months of quitting smoking, mostly in the first 3 months of quitting (Aubin et al. 2012). This weight gain can persist up to 8 years after smoking cessation. This hinders smoking abstinence in smokers (Pistelli et al. 2009). To avoid weight gain, many smokers might stay food deprived for long periods while trying to quit smoking. Food deprivation when combined with nicotine deprivation reduces the ability of the smoker to resist smoking (Leeman et al. 2010). Hence, smokers should have frequent healthy meals while trying to quit, as it will increase their ability to resist smoking.

12.7   FOODS AND DIETARY PATTERNS THAT HELP REPAIR DAMAGE CAUSED BY SMOKING

The pathogenesis of diseases caused by tobacco smoking involves oxidative damage due to free radicals. This has been confirmed by a study that showed that the levels of free and esterified F_2-isoprostanes (a novel product of lipid peroxidation) in plasma are significantly higher in smokers compared with nonsmokers (Morrow et al. 1995). Several other biomarkers of oxidative stress, such as hydroxyeicosatetraenoic acid products and 8-hydroxy-2′-deoxyguanosine, are elevated in smokers and some of these still remain high even after a period of abstinence from smoking (Seet et al. 2011). Smoking has a similar effect in passive smokers. Children exposed to passive smoking have significantly lower total antioxidant response compared with children not exposed to passive smoking (Kosecik et al. 2005). Mothers and infants exposed to passive smoking also have a higher oxidative stress index compared with mothers and infants not exposed to passive smoking (Aycicek et al. 2005).

Many foods and nutrients help combat oxidative damage caused by smoking. These include

- *Tualang honey*: Honey is a natural product containing antioxidants. A randomized trial in Malaysia tested the effect of honey supplementation (20 g/day for 12 weeks) on antioxidant status in 64 chronic smokers. Before the intervention, the levels of biomarkers for oxidative stress including F_2-isoprostanes were higher, while glutathione peroxidase was significantly lower in smokers compared with nonsmokers. After the intervention, smokers who were supplemented with Tualang honey had lower levels of F_2-isoprostanes and higher levels of glutathione peroxidase and total antioxidant status compared with the pre-intervention levels (Wan Ghazali et al. 2015). Another study in the same cohort of chronic smokers found that the group supplemented with honey had lower levels of total cholesterol and low-density lipoproteins (LDL) compared with the pre-intervention levels (Wan Ghazali and Mohamed 2015). These findings suggest that honey supplementation in smokers can protect against oxidative damage caused by smoking. This may reduce the risk of cardiovascular disease in smokers.
- *Tomatoes*: Tomatoes contain antioxidants such as vitamin C that help combat free radicals in the blood, protecting against oxidative damage caused by smoking. Coumaric acid and chlorogenic acid in tomatoes are beneficial against the carcinogenic effect of cigarettes. Lycopene is an antioxidant in tomatoes that slows the growth of cancer cells, and cooked tomatoes produce even more lycopene. Vitamin B and potassium in tomatoes help reduce blood pressure and cholesterol levels (Bhowmik et al. 2012).
- *Oranges*: Blood orange juice contains high amounts of vitamin C, anthocyanins, and carotenoids. It has been shown to moderately improve the antioxidant defense mechanism in healthy females (Riso et al. 2005). As vitamin C markedly improves endothelium-dependent responses in chronic smokers (Heitzer and Mu 1996), blood orange juice, being a bioavailable

source of antioxidants, especially vitamin C, can help in repairing oxidative damage in smokers.

- *n-3 Polyunsaturated fatty acids*: n-3 Polyunsaturated fatty acids, especially eicosapentaenoic acid and docosahexaenoic acid, are found in fish. They have been shown to reduce the risk of chronic bronchitis, emphysema, and chronic obstructive pulmonary disease (COPD) in smokers in a quantity-dependent fashion—that is, the higher the intake of n-3 polyunsaturated fatty acids, the lower the chances of chronic respiratory disease (Shahar et al. 2008).
- *Olive oil*: Olive oil, the main source of fat in the Mediterranean diet, has been shown to be effective against oxidative stress–associated diseases (Fito et al. 2007). Olive mill waste water, a byproduct of olive oil, has been shown to be effective in protecting against oxidative stress caused by passive smoking in rats (Visioli et al. 2000).
- *Mediterranean diet*: The Mediterranean diet is characterized by high intakes of vitamins, antioxidants, and fiber through the increased consumption of olive oil, wild greens, fruits, legumes, whole wheat bread, walnuts, and almonds and the moderate consumption of fish, meat, and dairy products. This dietary pattern has been linked to the prevention of cardiovascular diseases, cancers, and respiratory illness by protecting against biochemical processes leading to these diseases. Studies have shown that diseases such as lung cancer, asthma, and cardiovascular disease related to smoking are inversely related to certain antioxidants. As the Mediterranean diet is rich in antioxidants, it may protect against oxidative damage and hence the diseases attributed to smoking (Vardavas et al. 2011). The Mediterranean diet has also been linked to weight loss (Esposito et al. 2011). The Diet, Spirometry and Tobacco (DIET) study, a 2-year randomized controlled trial to increase the adherence of smokers to the Mediterranean diet, is underway to explore the association of adherence to the Mediterranean diet and lung functions in smokers (Sorli-Aguilar et al. 2015).

12.8 NUTRITIONAL HOME REMEDIES FOR SMOKING CESSATION AND REPAIRING DAMAGE CAUSED BY SMOKING

Many remedies have been suggested that may help to quit smoking and repair the damage caused by smoking, though evidence regarding these is limited. Some of these are

- *Water*: Drinking water is recommended to reduce cigarette cravings. It is one of the Ds in the "4Ds" remedy (delay, deep breathing, drink water, do something else), as suggested by Quit Victoria, Australia (Quit Victoria 2016).
- *Spices*: Spices are widely used in Asia and the Middle East to enhance flavor and aroma while cooking and also in preserving foods (e.g., pickles). Spices possess antioxidant, anti-inflammatory, antitumor, and immunomodulatory activities. Ginger, caraway, cumin, and fennel significantly inhibit DNA

damage and ginger, pepper, and long pepper are the most effective in inhibiting nicotine-induced cancer cell migration (Jayakumar and Kanthimathi
2012). Some people might have allergies to spices and caution should be
taken in these cases.

- *Apple, pear, and orange juice*: The juice of an apple, a pear, and 200 mL of
  orange juice per day administered for 26 days reduces the levels of cholesterol
  and LDL and the LDL/HDL ratio in smokers (Alvarez-Parrilla et al. 2010).
- *Grape juice*: Purple grape juice, 480 mL/day for 8 weeks, has been shown
  to protect against DNA damage and improves the antioxidant defense system in Korean smokers (Park et al. 2004). In the same cohort, grape juice
  reduced diastolic blood pressure by 6.5% and inhibited free radical generation, while it led to an increase in total plasma cholesterol, HDL, and LDL
  in smokers (Kim et al. 2004).
- *Medicinal herb tea*: A study in Korea found that the consumption of 11
  species of medicinal herb tea (*Eugenia aromaticum* and *Astragalus mem-
  branaceus* having the highest antioxidant and nicotine degradation activity)
  for 4 weeks led to smoking cessation in 38% of the smokers compared with
  17% in those not consuming medicinal herb tea. Moreover, the intervention
  group had less smoking withdrawal symptoms compared with the control
  group (Lee and Lee 2005).
- *Green tea*: Intake of 8 g/day of green tea for 2 weeks improves endothelial
  function in chronic smokers, and thus might be effective in the prevention
  of cardiovascular diseases (Kim et al. 2006). Ingestion of 600 mL of green
  tea for 4 weeks can significantly reduce plasma-soluble P-selectin level and
  oxidized LDL concentration in smokers (Lee et al. 2005).

12.9 NUTRITIONAL COUNSELING FOR SMOKING CESSATION

Primary health care, which is the first point of contact for the community, plays an
important role in counseling for smoking cessation. According to the Behavioral
Risk Factor Surveillance System (BRFSS) in the United States, 55% of 10,582 smokers who had one or more clinical encounters in the year 2000 reported receiving
advice on quitting smoking (Lucan and Katz 2006). Delivery of the 5As (ask, advise,
assess, assist [talk about quitting, recommend stop smoking medications, or recommend counseling], and arrange follow-up) ranged from 10.4% for "arrange follow-
up" to 77.2% for "ask" 1 year after the national lung-screening trial in the United
States. "Assist" was associated with 40% odds of quitting, while "arrange follow-up"
was associated with 46% odds of quitting (Park et al. 2012). The prevalence of anti-
smoking counseling is 62.3% in primary care settings in Spain, as reported by the
patients (Lumbreras et al. 2002). Advice to quit was provided to 42% of the patients
in hospital settings according to a meta-analysis of published studies from 1994–
2005 (Freund et al. 2008). Nutrition counseling occurs in 24% of all patients attend-
ing family physician practices in the United States (Eaton et al. 2002). Smoking
cessation counseling should be increased at primary health-care facilities and nutrition counseling should be embedded to improve quit rates. Figure 12.2 shows nutrition counseling in smokers.

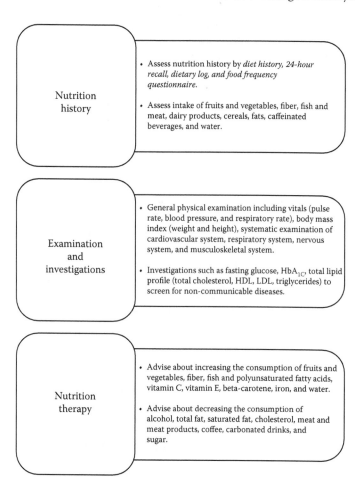

FIGURE 12.2 Nutritional counseling for smokers.

12.10 CASE STUDIES

12.10.1 CASE STUDY 1

A middle-aged woman, 54 years old, has been a smoker for 26 years and smokes 20 cigarettes a day. She tried to quit smoking 5 years ago, remaining abstinent for 4 months. The reason she resumed smoking was that giving up increased her weight. In the previous year, she developed type 2 diabetes and wants to quit smoking. She has concerns about weight gain after quitting smoking. As a dietician/nutritionist/health counselor, give responses to the following:

- What methods will you use to assess her dietary intake? (*Hint*: Refer to Figure 12.2).
- What food will you suggest to make the taste of cigarettes nonpalatable? (*Hint*: Refer to Section 12.6).

- Which diet will you suggest for weight loss and weight maintenance? (*Hint*: Refer to Sections 12.6 and 12.7).

12.10.2 CASE STUDY 2

A 40-year-old male quit smoking 5 months ago. He wants to consume foods and use dietary patterns to repair the damage caused by smoking. As a dietician/nutritionist/ health counselor, give responses to the following:

- What foods would you suggest he consume? (*Hint*: Refer to Section 12.7.)
- What home remedies would you like to consider in this case? (*Hint*: Refer to Section 12.8.)

REFERENCES

Alvarez-Parrilla, Emilio, Laura A. De La Rosa, Patricia Legarreta, Laura Saenz, Joaquan Rodrigo-Garcia, and Gustavo A. Gonzalez-Aguilar. 2010. Daily consumption of apple, pear and orange juice differently affects plasma lipids and antioxidant capacity of smoking and non-smoking adults. *Int J Food Sci Nutr* 61 (4):369–380.

Ambrose, John A., and Rajat S. Barua. 2004. The pathophysiology of cigarette smoking and cardiovascular disease: An update. *J Am Colle Cardiol* 43 (10):1731–1737.

Aubin, Henri-Jean, Amanda Farley, Deborah Lycett, Pierre Lahmek, and Paul Aveyard. 2012. Weight gain in smokers after quitting cigarettes: Meta-analysis. *BMJ* 345:e4439.

Aveyard, Paul, Rachna Begh, Amanda Parsons, and Robert West. 2012. Brief opportunistic smoking cessation interventions: A systematic review and meta-analysis to compare advice to quit and offer of assistance. *Addiction* 107 (6):1066–1073.

Aycicek, Ali, Ozcan Erel, and Abdurrahim Kocyigit. 2005. Decreased total antioxidant capacity and increased oxidative stress in passive smoker infants and their mothers. *Pediatr Int* 47 (6):635–639.

Barnoya, Joaquin, and Stanton A. Glantz. 2005. Cardiovascular effects of secondhand smoke nearly as large as smoking. *Circulation* 111 (20):2684–2698.

Bhowmik, Debjit, K. P. Sampath Kumar, Shravan Paswan, and Shweta Srivastava. 2012. Tomato: A natural medicine and its health benefits. *J Pharmacogn Phytochem* 1 (1):33–43.

BinDhim, Nasser F., Kevin McGeechan, and Lyndal Trevena. 2014. Who uses smoking cessation apps? A feasibility study across three countries via smartphones. *JMIR Mhealth Uhealth* 2 (1):e4.

Bonita, Ruth, John Duncan, Thomas Truelsen, Rodney T. Jackson, and Robert Beaglehole. 1999. Passive smoking as well as active smoking increases the risk of acute stroke. *Tob Control* 8 (2):156–160.

Bricker, Jonathan B., Kristin E. Mull, Julie A. Kientz, Roger Vilardaga, Laina D. Mercer, Katrina J. Akioka, and Jaimee L. Heffner. 2014. Randomized, controlled pilot trial of a smartphone app for smoking cessation using acceptance and commitment therapy. *Drug Alcohol Depend* 143:87–94.

Burns, David M. 2003. Epidemiology of smoking-induced cardiovascular disease. *Prog Cardiovasc Dis* 46 (1):11–29.

Chen, Zhengming, and Jillian Boreham. 2002. Smoking and cardiovascular disease. *Semin Vasc Med* 2:243–252.

Coogan, Patricia F., Nelsy Castro-Webb, Jeffrey Yu, George T. O'Connor, Julie R. Palmer, and Lynn Rosenberg. 2015. Active and passive smoking and the incidence of asthma in the Black Women's Health Study. *Am J Respir Crit Care Med* 191 (2):168–176.

Dallongeville, Jean, Nadine Marecaux, Jean-Charles Fruchart, and Philippe Amouyel. 1998. Cigarette smoking is associated with unhealthy patterns of nutrient intake: A meta-analysis. *J Nutr* 128 (9):1450–1457.

Danielsson, Tobias, Kevin Jones, Stephan Rossner, and Åke Westin. 1999. Open randomised trial of intermittent very low energy diet together with nicotine gum for stopping smoking in women who gained weight in previous attempts to quit: Commentary; Results are unlikely to be as good in routine practice. *BMJ* 319 (7208):490–493.

Eaton, Charles B., Meredith A. Goodwin, and Kurt C. Stange. 2002. Direct observation of nutrition counseling in community family practice. *Am J Prev Med* 23 (3):174–179.

Esposito, Katherine, Christina-Maria Kastorini, Demosthenes B. Panagiotakos, and Dario Giugliano. 2011. Mediterranean diet and weight loss: Meta-analysis of randomized controlled trials. *Metab Syndr Relat Disord* 9 (1):1–12.

Etter, Jean-Francois, and John A. Stapleton. 2006. Nicotine replacement therapy for long-term smoking cessation: A meta-analysis. *Tob Control* 15 (4):280–285.

Ezzati, Majid, and Alan D. Lopez. 2004. Regional, disease specific patterns of smoking-attributable mortality in 2000. *Tob Control* 13 (4):388–395.

Fiore, Michael C., Carlos Roberto Jaen, Timothy B. Baker, William C. Bailey, N. Benowitz, and Susan J. Curry. 2008. Treating tobacco use and dependence: 2008 update. U.S. Public Health Service Clinical Practice Guideline executive summary. *Respir Care* 53 (9):1217–1222.

Fito, Montserrat, Rafael de la Torre, and Maria-Isabel Covas. 2007. Olive oil and oxidative stress. *Mol Nutr Food Res* 51 (10):1215–1224.

Forey, Barbara A., Alison J. Thornton, and Peter N. Lee. 2011. Systematic review with meta-analysis of the epidemiological evidence relating smoking to COPD, chronic bronchitis and emphysema. *BMC Pulm Med.* 11:36.

Freedman, Neal D., Christian C. Abnet, Neil E. Caporaso, Joseph F. Fraumeni, Gwen Murphy, Patricia Hartge, Albert R. Hollenbeck, Yikyung Park, Meredith S. Shiels, and Debra T. Silverman. 2015. Impact of changing U.S. cigarette smoking patterns on incident cancer: Risks of 20 smoking-related cancers among the women and men of the NIH-AARP cohort. *Int J Epidemiol* pii: dyv175. (Epub ahead of print.)

Freund, Megan, Elizabeth Campbell, Christine Paul, Patrick McElduff, Raoul A. Walsh, Rebecca Sakrouge, John Wiggers, and Jenny Knight. 2008. Smoking care provision in hospitals: A review of prevalence. *Nicotene Tob Res* 10 (5):757–774.

Fujii, Fumitaka, Toshitsugu Hashimoto, Naoko Suzuki, Ryoko Suzuki, and Kiminori Mohr. 2008. Pilot study of the standardized oats herb extract for smoking reduction. *Pharmacometrics* 75 (3/4):47–53.

Gao, Chang-Ming, Jian-Hua Ding, Su-Ping Li, Yan-Ting Liu, Yun Qian, Jun Chang, Jin-Hai Tang, and Kazuo Tajima. 2013. Active and passive smoking, and alcohol drinking and breast cancer risk in Chinese women. *Asian Pac J Cancer Prev* 14 (2):993–996.

Glantz, Stanton, and Mariaelena Gonzalez. 2012. Effective tobacco control is key to rapid progress in reduction of non-communicable diseases. *Lancet* 379 (9822):1269–1271.

Hagstad, Stig, Anders Bjerg, Linda Ekerljung, Helena Backman, Anne Lindberg, Eva Ronmark, and Bo Lundback. 2014. Passive smoking exposure is associated with increased risk of COPD in never smokers. *Chest* 145 (6):1298–1304.

Haibach, Jeffrey P., Gregory G. Homish, R. Lorraine Collins, Christine B. Ambrosone, and Gary A. Giovino. 2015. An evaluation of fruit and vegetable consumption and cigarette smoking among youth. *Nicotene Tob Res* 17 (6):719–726.

Haibach, Jeffrey P., Gregory G. Homish, and Gary A. Giovino. 2013. A longitudinal evaluation of fruit and vegetable consumption and cigarette smoking. *Nicotine Tob Res* 15 (2):355–363.

Hawkins, Brian T., Rachel C. Brown, and Thomas P. Davis. 2002. Smoking and ischemic stroke: A role for nicotine? *Trends Pharmacol Sci* 23 (2):78–82.

He, Jiang, Suma Vupputuri, Krista Allen, Monica R. Prerost, Janet Hughes, and Paul K. Whelton. 1999. Passive smoking and the risk of coronary heart disease: A meta-analysis of epidemiologic studies. *N Engl J Med* 340 (12):920–926.

Heitzer, Thomas, and Thomas Mu. 1996. Antioxidant vitamin C improves endothelial dysfunction in chronic smokers. *Circulation* 94 (1):6–9.

Herman, Patricia M., and Michele E. Walsh. 2011. Hospital admissions for acute myocardial infarction, angina, stroke, and asthma after implementation of Arizona's comprehensive statewide smoking ban. *Am J Public Health* 101 (3):491–496.

Hirayama, Takeshi. 2000. Non-smoking wives of heavy smokes have a higher risk of lung cancer: A study from Japan. *Bull World Health Organ* 78 (7):940–942.

Hoeppner, Bettina B., Susanne S. Hoeppner, Lourah Seaboyer, Melissa R. Schick, Gwyneth W. Y. Wu, Brandon G. Bergman, and John F. Kelly. 2015. How smart are smartphone apps for smoking cessation? A content analysis. *Nicotene Tob Res* pii:ntv117.

Holay, M. P., N. P. Paunikar, P. P. Joshi, V. S. Sahasrabhojney, and S. R. Tankhiwale. 2004. Effect of passive smoking on endothelial function in healthy adults. *J Assoc Physicians India* 52:114–117.

Hu, W., T. Zhang, J. Shi, W. Qin, L. Tong, and Y. Shen. 2014. Association between cigarette smoking and hypertension in men: A dose response relationship analysis. *Zhonghua Xin Xue Guan Bing Za Zhi* 42 (9):773–777.

Hymowitz, Norman, K. Michael Cummings, Andrew Hyland, William R. Lynn, Terry F. Pechacek, and Tyler D. Hartwell. 1997. Predictors of smoking cessation in a cohort of adult smokers followed for five years. *Tob Control* 6 (Suppl 2):S57–S62.

Jayakumar, R., and M. S. Kanthimathi. 2012. Dietary spices protect against hydrogen peroxide-induced DNA damage and inhibit nicotine-induced cancer cell migration. *Food Chem* 134 (3):1580–1584.

Kalkhoran, Sara, and Stanton A. Glantz. 2016. E-cigarettes and smoking cessation in real-world and clinical settings: A systematic review and meta-analysis. *Lancet Respir Med* 4 (2):116–128.

Kim, Jung Shin, Hae Young Kim, Yoo Kyoung Park, Eunju Park, and Myung Hee Kang. 2004. The effects of purple grape juice supplementation on blood pressure, plasma lipid profile and free radical levels in Korean smokers. *Korean J Nutr* 37 (6):455–463.

Kim, Soon Kyung, Bo Young Yeon, and Mi Kyeong Choi. 2003. Comparison of nutrient intakes and serum mineral levels between smokers and non-smokers. *Korean J Nutr* 36 (6):635–645.

Kim, Weon, Myung Ho Jeong, Suk Hee Cho, Ji Hye Yun, Hong Jae Chae, Young Keun Ahn, Min Cheol Lee, Xianwu Cheng, Takahisa Kondo, and Toyoaki Murohara. 2006. Effect of green tea consumption on endothelial function and circulating endothelial progenitor cells in chronic smokers. *Circ J* 70 (8):1052–1057.

Kosecik, Mustafa, Ozcan Erel, Eylem Sevinc, and Sahabettin Selek. 2005. Increased oxidative stress in children exposed to passive smoking. *Int J Cardiol* 100 (1):61–64.

Kruger, Judy, Lauren Shaw, Jennifer Kahende, and Erica Frank. 2012. Health care providers' advice to quit smoking: National Health Interview Survey, 2000, 2005, and 2010. *Prev Chronic Dis* 9:E130.

Kurth, Tobias, Carlos S. Kase, Klaus Berger, Elke S. Schaeffner, Julie E. Buring, and J. Michael Gaziano. 2003. Smoking and the risk of hemorrhagic stroke in men. *Stroke* 34 (5):1151–1155.

Larkin, F. A., P. P. Basiotis, H. A. Riddick, K. E. Sykes, and E. M. Pao. 1990. Dietary patterns of women smokers and non-smokers. *J Am Diet Assoc* 90 (2):230–237.

Lee, Ho-Jae, and Jae-Hwan Lee. 2005. Effects of medicinal herb tea on the smoking cessation and reducing smoking withdrawal symptoms. *Am J Chin Med* 33 (1):127–138.

Lee, Woochang, Won-Ki Min, Sail Chun, Yong-Wha Lee, Hyosoon Park, Do Hoon Lee, You Kyoung Lee, and Ji Eun Son. 2005. Long-term effects of green tea ingestion on atherosclerotic biological markers in smokers. *Clin Bioc hem* 38 (1):84–87.

Leeman, Robert F., Stephanie S. O'Malley, Marney A. White, and Sherry A. McKee. 2010. Nicotine and food deprivation decrease the ability to resist smoking. *Psychopharmacology (Berl)* 212 (1):25–32.

Leone, Aurelio. 2011. Smoking and hypertension: Independent or additive effects to determining vascular damage? *Curr Vasc Pharmacol* 9 (5):585–593.

Lightwood, James M., and Stanton A. Glantz. 2009. Declines in acute myocardial infarction after smoke-free laws and individual risk attributable to secondhand smoke. *Circulation* 120 (14):1373–1379.

Lucan, Sean C., and David L. Katz. 2006. Factors associated with smoking cessation counseling at clinical encounters: The Behavioral Risk Factor Surveillance System (BRFSS) 2000. *Am J Health Promot* 21 (1):16–23.

Luger, Tana M., Jerry Suls, and Mark W. Vander Weg. 2014. How robust is the association between smoking and depression in adults? A meta-analysis using linear mixed-effects models. *Addict Behav* 39 (10):1418–1429.

Lumbreras, Garcia G., Ruiz M. D. Mena, Alvarez I. Calvo, Cano I. Perez, Miro J. Sanchez, Paris J. Molina, and Cuesta T. Sanz. 2002. Prevalence of anti-smoking counseling in a primary care clinic: Comparison of patient charts with patient reports. *Arch Bronconeumol* 38 (7):317–321.

Ma, Jun, Nancy M. Betts, and Jeff S. Hampl. 2000. Clustering of lifestyle behaviors: The relationship between cigarette smoking, alcohol consumption, and dietary intake. *Am J Health Promot* 15 (2):107–117.

Marcus, Bess H., Anna E. Albrecht, Teresa K. King, Alfred F. Parisi, Bernardine M. Pinto, Mary Roberts, Raymond S. Niaura, and David B. Abrams. 1999. The efficacy of exercise as an aid for smoking cessation in women: A randomized controlled trial. *Arch Intern Med* 159 (11):1229–1234.

Marley, Julia V., David Atkinson, Carmel Nelson, Tracey Kitaura, Dennis Gray, Sue Metcalf, Richard Murray, and Graeme P. Maguire. 2014. The protocol for the Be Our Ally Beat Smoking (BOABS) study, a randomised controlled trial of an intensive smoking cessation intervention in a remote Aboriginal Australian health care setting. *BMC Public Health* 14:32.

McClernon, F. Joseph, Eric C. Westman, Jed E. Rose, and Avery M. Lutz. 2007. The effects of foods, beverages, and other factors on cigarette palatability. *Nicotene Tob Res* 9 (4):505–510.

McMillen, Robert, Jeomi Maduka, and Jonathan Winickoff. 2012. Use of emerging tobacco products in the United States. *J Environ Public Health* 2012. doi:10.1155/2012/989474.

Midgette, Andre S., John A. Baron, and Thomas E. Rohan. 1993. Do cigarette smokers have diets that increase their risks of coronary heart disease and cancer? *Am J Epidemiol* 137 (5):521–529.

Morabia, Alfredo, Francois Curtin, and Martine S. Bernstein. 1999. Effects of smoking and smoking cessation on dietary habits of a Swiss urban population. *Eur J Clin Nutr* 53 (3):239–243.

Morrow, Jason D., Balz Frei, Atkinson W. Longmire, J. Michael Gaziano, Sean M. Lynch, Yu Shyr, William E. Strauss, John A. Oates, and L. Jackson Roberts. 1995. Increase in circulating products of lipid peroxidation (F2-isoprostanes) in smokers: Smoking as a cause of oxidative damage. *N Engl J Med* 332 (18):1198–1203.

Naiman, Alisa, Richard H. Glazier, and Rahim Moineddin. 2010. Association of anti-smoking legislation with rates of hospital admission for cardiovascular and respiratory conditions. *CMAJ* 182 (8):761–767.

Nakamura, Koshi, Federica Barzi, Tai-Hing Lam, Rachel Huxley, Valery L. Feigin, Hirotsugu Ueshima, Jean Woo et al., and the Asia Pacific Cohort Studies Collaboration. 2008. Cigarette smoking, systolic blood pressure, and cardiovascular diseases in the Asia-Pacific region. *Stroke* 39 (6):1694–1702.

Nierkens, Vera, Marieke A. Hartman, Mary Nicolaou, Charlotte Vissenberg, Erik J. A. J. Beune, Karen Hosper, Irene G. van Valkengoed, and Karien Stronks. 2013. Effectiveness of cultural adaptations of interventions aimed at smoking cessation, diet, and/or physical activity in ethnic minorities. A systematic review. *PloS One* 8 (10):e73373.

O'Connor, Richard J. 2012. Non-cigarette tobacco products: What have we learnt and where are we headed? *Tob Control* 21 (2):181–190.

Park, Elyse R., Ilana F. Gareen, Sandra Japuntich, Inga Lennes, Kelly Hyland, Sarah DeMello, JoRean D. Sicks, and Nancy A. Rigotti. 2012. Primary care provider-delivered smoking cessation interventions and smoking cessation among participants in the National Lung Screening Trial. *JAMA Intern Med* 175 (9):1509–1516.

Park, Eun Ju, Jung Shin Kim, Eun Jae Jeon, Hae Young Kim, Yoo Kyoung Park, and Myung Hee Kang. 2004. The effects of purple grape juice supplementation on improvement of antioxidant status and lymphocyte DNA damage in Korean smokers. *Korean J Nutr* 37 (4):281–290.

Parry, Charles D., Jayadeep Patra, and Jargen Rehm. 2011. Alcohol consumption and non-communicable diseases: Epidemiology and policy implications. *Addiction* 106 (10):1718–1724.

Patel, Raja, Lucy Sulzberger, Grace Li, Jonny Mair, Hannah Morley, Merryn N. Shing, Charlotte O'Leary et al. 2015. Smartphone apps for weight loss and smoking cessation: Quality ranking of 120 apps. *N Z Med J* 128:1421.

Pistelli, F., F. Aquilini, and L. Carrozzi. 2009. Weight gain after smoking cessation. *Monaldi Arch Chest Dis* 71 (2):81–87.

Poisson, T., J. Dallongeville, A. Evans, P. Ducimetierre, P. Amouyel, J. Yarnell, A. Bingham, F. Kee, and L. Dauchet. 2012. Fruit and vegetable intake and smoking cessation. *Eur J Clin Nutr* 66 (11):1247–1253.

Prochaska, Judith J., Kevin Delucchi, and Sharon M. Hall. 2004. A meta-analysis of smoking cessation interventions with individuals in substance abuse treatment or recovery. *J Consult Clin Psychol* 72 (6):1144.

Quit Victoria. 2016. Craving a smoke right now? Accessed April 17, 2016. http://www.quit.org.au/staying-quit/craving-a-cigarette-right-now.

Reed, Mark B., Rong Wang, Audrey M. Shillington, John D. Clapp, and James E. Lange. 2007. The relationship between alcohol use and cigarette smoking in a sample of undergraduate college students. *Addict Behav* 32 (3):449–464.

Reynolds, Peggy, Susan Hurley, Debbie E. Goldberg, Hoda Anton-Culver, Leslie Bernstein, Dennis Deapen, Pamela L. Horn-Ross, David Peel, Richard Pinder, and Ronald K. Ross. 2004. Active smoking, household passive smoking, and breast cancer: Evidence from the California Teachers Study. *J Natl Cancer Inst* 96 (1):29–37.

Riso, Patrizia, Francesco Visioli, Claudio Gardana, Simona Grande, Antonella Brusamolino, Fabio Galvano, Giacomo Galvano, and Marisa Porrini. 2005. Effects of blood orange juice intake on antioxidant bioavailability and on different markers related to oxidative stress. *J Agric Food Chem* 53 (4):941–947.

Roura, Esther, Xavier Castellsagué, Michael Pawlita, Noémie Travier, Tim Waterboer, Núria Margall, F. Xavier Bosch et al. 2014. Smoking as a major risk factor for cervical cancer and pre-cancer: Results from the EPIC cohort. *Int J Cancer* 135 (2):453–466.

Seet, Raymond C. S., Chung-Yung J. Lee, Wai Mun Loke, Shan Hong Huang, Huiwen Huang, Woan Foon Looi, Eng Soh Chew, Amy M. L. Quek, Erle C. H. Lim, and Barry Halliwell. 2011. Biomarkers of oxidative damage in cigarette smokers: Which biomarkers might reflect acute versus chronic oxidative stress? *Free Radic Biol Med* 50 (12):1787–1793.

Shahar, Eyal, Aaron R. Folsom, Sandra L. Melnick, Melvyn S. Tockman, George W. Comstock, Valerio Gennaro, Millicent W. Higgins, Paul D. Sorlie, Wen-Jene Ko, and Moyses Szklo. 2008. Dietary n-3 polyunsaturated acids and smoking-related chronic obstructive pulmonary disease. *Am J Epidemiol* 168 (7):796–801.

Siddiqi, Kamran, Amir Khan, Maqsood Ahmad, Omara Dogar, Mona Kanaan, James N. Newell, and Heather Thomson. 2013. Action to stop smoking in suspected tuberculosis (ASSIST) in Pakistan: A cluster randomized, controlled trial. *Ann Intern Med* 158 (9):667–675.

Silagy, Christopher, David Mant, Godfrey Fowler, and Mark Lodge. 1994. Meta-analysis on efficacy of nicotine replacement therapies in smoking cessation. *Lancet* 343 (8890):139–142.

Siroux, Vimn, I. Pin, M. P. Oryszczyn, N. Le Moual, and F. Kauffmann. 2000. Relationships of active smoking to asthma and asthma severity in the EGEA study. Epidemiological study on the Genetics and Environment of Asthma. *Eur Respir J* 15 (3):470–477.

Sorli-Aguilar, Mar, Francisco Martin-Lujan, Antoni Santigosa-Ayala, Josep Lluas Pinol-Moreso, Gemma Flores-Mateo, Josep Basora-Gallisa, Victoria Arija-Val, and Rosa Sola-Alberich. 2015. Effects of Mediterranean diet on lung function in smokers: A randomised, parallel and controlled protocol. *BMC Public Health* 15:74.

Taylor, Gemma, Ann McNeill, Alan Girling, Amanda Farley, Nicola Lindson-Hawley, and Paul Aveyard. 2014. Change in mental health after smoking cessation: Systematic review and meta-analysis. *BMJ* 348:g1151.

Teo, Koon K., Stephanie Ounpuu, Steven Hawken, M. R. Pandey, Vicent Valentin, David Hunt, Rafael Diaz, Wafa Rashed, Rosario Freeman, and Lixin Jiang. 2006. Tobacco use and risk of myocardial infarction in 52 countries in the INTERHEART study: A case-control study. *Lancet* 368 (9536):647–658.

Touvier, M., M. Niravong, J. L. Volatier, L. Lafay, S. Lioret, F. Clavel-Chapelon, and M. C. Boutron-Ruault. 2009. Dietary patterns associated with vitamin/mineral supplement use and smoking among women of the E3N-EPIC cohort. *Eur J Clin Nutr* 63 (1):39–47.

Uddin, Md Jalal, Badrul Alam Mondol, Shahrukh Ahmed, A. K. M. Anwar Ullah, M. A. Jabbar, and Quazi Deen Mohammad. 2008. Smoking and ischemic stroke. *Bangladesh J Neurosci* 24 (1):50–54.

Ussher, Michael, Paola Nunziata, Mark Cropley, and Robert West. 2001. Effect of a short bout of exercise on tobacco withdrawal symptoms and desire to smoke. *Psychopharmacology (Berl)* 158 (1):66–72.

Vardavas, Constantine, Andreas Flouris, Aristides Tsatsakis, Anthony G. Kafatos, and Wim H.M. Saris. 2011. Does adherence to the Mediterranean diet have a protective effect against active and passive smoking? *Public Health* 125 (3):121–128.

Veenstra, J., J. A. Schenkel, A. M. van Erp-Baart, H. A. Brants, K. F. Hulshof, C. Kistemaker, G. Schaafsma, and Th Ockhuizen. 1993. Alcohol consumption in relation to food intake and smoking habits in the Dutch National Food Consumption Survey. *Eur J Clin Nutr* 47 (7):482–489.

Virdis, A., C. Giannarelli, M. Fritsch Neves, S. Taddei, and L. Ghiadoni. 2010. Cigarette smoking and hypertension. *Curr Pharm Des* 16 (23):2518–2525.

Visioli, Francesco, Claudio Galli, Elena Plasmati, Serena Viappiani, Alicia Hernandez, Claudio Colombo, and Angelo Sala. 2000. Olive phenol hydroxytyrosol prevents passive smoking-induced oxidative stress. *Circulation* 102 (18):2169–2171.

Wan Ghazali, Wan S., and Mahaneem Mohamed. 2015. An open-label pilot study to assess honey supplementation in improving lipid profiles among chronic smokers. *J Integr Med Ther* 2 (1):5.

Wan Ghazali, Wan Syaheedah, Mahaneem Mohamed, Siti Amrah Sulaiman, Aniza Abdul Aziz, and Harmy Mohamed Yusoff. 2015. Tualang honey supplementation improves oxidative stress status among chronic smokers. *Toxicol Environ Chem* 97 (8):1017–1024.

Wannamethee, Goya, A. G. Shaper, P. W. Macfarlane, and Mary Walker. 1995. Risk factors for sudden cardiac death in middle-aged British men. *Circulation* 91 (6):1749–1756.

Whittaker, Robyn, Hayden McRobbie, Chris Bullen, Ron Borland, Anthony Rodgers, and Yulong Gu. 2012. Mobile phone–based interventions for smoking cessation. *Cochrane Database Syst Rev* 11:CD006611.

Willi, Carole, Patrick Bodenmann, William A. Ghali, Peter D. Faris, and Jacques Cornuz. 2007. Active smoking and the risk of type 2 diabetes: A systematic review and meta-analysis. *JAMA* 298 (22):2654–2664.

World Health Organization. 2015. Tobacco. Accessed February 25, 2016. http://www.who.int/mediacentre/factsheets/fs339/en.

WHO. 2016a. Cancer prevention. Accessed March 14, 2016. http://www.who.int/cancer/prevention/en.

WHO. 2016b. Prevalence of tobacco smoking. Accessed February 20, 2016. http://www.who.int/gho/tobacco/use/en.

Ybarra, Michele L., Jodi Summers Holtrop, Tonya L. Prescott, Mohammad H. Rahbar, and David Strong. 2013. Pilot RCT results of stop my smoking USA: A text messaging–based smoking cessation program for young adults. *Nicotine Tob Res* 15 (8):1388–1399.

Zimmerman, Rick S., George J. Warheit, Patricia M. Ulbrich, and Joanne Buhl Auth. 1990. The relationship between alcohol use and attempts and success at smoking cessation. *Addict Behav* 15 (3):197–207.

Index